The Coherence of Personality

THE COHERENCE OF PERSONALITY

Social-Cognitive Bases of Consistency, Variability, and Organization

Editors

DANIEL CERVONE
YUICHI SHODA

THE GUILFORD PRESS
New York   London

© 1999 The Guilford Press
A Division of Guilford Publications, Inc.
72 Spring Street, New York, NY 10012
http://www.guilford.com

Printed in the United States of America

This book is printed on acid-free paper.

Last digit is print number: 9   8   7   6   5   4   3   2   1

Library of Congress Cataloging-in-Publication Data

The coherence of personality: social-cognitive bases of consistency,
   variability, and organization / edited by Daniel Cervone, Yuichi
Shoda.
       p.   cm.
   Includes bibliographical references and index.
   ISBN 1-57230-436-7 (hard)
   1. Personality and cognition.   2. Personality and emotions.
3. personality—Social aspects.   I. Cervone, Daniel.   II. Shoda,
Yuichi.
   [DNLM: 1. Personality.   2. Cognition.   3. Social Environment.   BF
698.9.C63 C678 1999]
BF698.9.C63C67   1999
155.2—dc21
DNLM/DLC
for Library of Congress   98-52114
                                                                 CIP

About the Editors

DANIEL CERVONE, PhD, an associate professor of psychology at the University of Illinois at Chicago, earned his doctorate in psychology from Stanford University in 1985. He is a former Fellow at the Center for Advanced Study in the Behavioral Sciences, Stanford, CA.

YUICHI SHODA, PhD, an assistant professor of psychology at the University of Washington, Seattle, was born in Japan and studied geophysics at Hokkaido University. He then studied psychology at the University of California at Santa Cruz, Stanford University, and Columbia University, and he received his doctorate at Columbia in 1990.

Contributors

Mark W. Baldwin, PhD, Department of Psychology, McGill University, Montreal, Quebec, Canada

Albert Bandura, PhD, Department of Psychology, Stanford University, Stanford, California

Nancy Cantor, PhD, Department of Psychology, University of Michigan, Ann Arbor, Michigan

Kenneth A. Dodge, PhD, Department of Public Policy Studies, Duke University, Durham, North Carolina

Carol S. Dweck, PhD, Department of Psychology, Columbia University, New York, New York

Heidi Grant, MA, Department of Psychology, Columbia University, New York, New York

E. Tory Higgins, PhD, Department of Psychology, Columbia University, New York, New York

Shinobu Kitayama, PhD, Faculty of Integrated Human Studies, Kyoto University, Kyoto, Japan

Hazel Rose Markus, PhD, Department of Psychology, Stanford University, Stanford, California

Walter Mischel, PhD, Department of Psychology, Columbia University, New York, New York

Catherine A. Sanderson, PhD, Department of Psychology, Amherst College, Amherst, Massachusetts

Arnaldo Zelli, PhD, Department of Public Policy Studies, Duke University, Durham, North Carolina

Preface

This volume is about a phenomenon, a theoretical perspective, and how the two go together.

The phenomenon is personality coherence. Modern lives require multiple roles and impose disruptive life transitions. People must adapt to social demands that vary across contexts and across the life course. Despite all this, the individual's life is rarely chaotic, disorganized, or fragmented. People somehow manage to achieve an integrated sense of self. They plan courses of action that organize their lives over extended periods. They display stable patterns of behavior that distinguish them from one another. Understanding this coherence in psychological functioning is a central goal of the field of personality psychology.

The theoretical perspective is social-cognitive theory. Social-cognitive theories explain personality functioning by reference to basic cognitive and affective processes. They explore the dynamic interactions between cognitive mechanisms and social contexts. Personality thus is contextualized. Individuals are understood, in part, by an exploring of the personal and social tasks they confront and the cultural contexts that give meaning to their actions.

Social-cognitive approaches view personality coherence as a natural product of the interactions among psychological mechanisms and between persons and social environments. Social-cognitive and affective processes are interconnected, and thus function as coherent systems. These personality systems enable people to select and shape their environments, to adapt to social demands, and thus to attain coherence in their experience and behavior. The contributions to this volume reveal how interactions among basic psychological mechanisms give rise to the coherent, distinctive patterns of experience and action that are the hallmark of "personality."

More generally, this volume addresses the question of how to build a theory of personality. Personality theories have, in the past, been disconnected from the mainstream of psychological research. This reflects two factors. Some of the field's most prominent theories were not developed by research psychologists, but rather by individuals trained as physicians or as counselors. Although research psychologists hold no monopoly on understanding persons, they are far better positioned than others to bring a broad array of psychological knowledge to bear on questions of personality functioning. Second, many psychologists have chosen to organize personality theories around dispositional constructs, that is, variables that capture people's average tendency to perform a particular class of behavior. Whatever the potential merits of this approach, a primary drawback is that the psychological mechanisms underlying the hypothesized dispositional tendencies generally have not been well understood. This has served further to divorce developments in personality psychology from advances in the study of basic psychological processes.

When addressing questions of personality functioning and differences among individuals, psychologists need not exchange well-understood psychological mechanisms for poorly understood dispositional tendencies. Each of our contributors reveals how questions of personality psychology can be answered by examining basic social-cognitive processes that are well understood thanks to extensive research efforts both in the field and the laboratory. The contributors, then, show how a personality theory can be built on psychology's broader base of knowledge about cognitive and affective systems. This approach to theory building does not yield a reductionistic view of persons. Instead, it reveals how personality coherence arises from transactions between the sociocultural environment and a dynamic, complex, self-regulating personality system.

*   *   *

We note here that the task of organizing the chapters of this volume was a particularly difficult one. The phenomenon of personality coherence can be understood to encompass a set of subissues, including coherence among psychological mechanisms, the expression of stable patterns of behavior, and the experience of an integrated sense of self (see our introductory chapter). Personality coherence also can be understood to arise from interactions among a set of social-cognitive personality variables, including social and self-knowledge, personal goals and standards, expectations about the world, reflections upon oneself, and affective experiences that interact dynamically with these cognitive mechanisms. Yet, we found that subdivisions of the book according to phenomena or to social-cognitive variables were not satisfactory. The reason for this is a tribute to the breadth of the individual chapters. Each of our contributors examines how multiple psychological mechanisms contribute to multiple aspects of personality coherence. Thus, arranging the chapters according to "subissues" would have misrepresented their scholarly breadth.

We have chosen instead to arrange the volume according to three broad themes. Personality coherence arises from the ways in which people assign meaning to, or encode, social information; from self-knowledge and self-reflective processes that give people causal agency over their lives; and from goals and life tasks through which people organize multiple life events. These three themes define the subsections of the text. Readers should bear in mind that these themes are themselves related and that individual contributions to this volume commonly address more than one theme. We hope this lends a sense of coherence to the volume as a whole.

*   *   *

On a more personal note, this project has been an extremely exciting one for us, because of both the content of its ideas and the individuals who contributed them. The chapters are authored by people without whom "we wouldn't even be here." The authors, in other words, are people whose ideas and research findings inspired us to pursue these topics in the first place. We thus are far more indebted than the usual volume editors to our contributors.

This project originated while DC was a residential fellow at the Center for Advanced Study in the Behavioral Sciences, Stanford, California. The Center is a remarkably fertile breeding ground for ideas and the sense of efficacy required to act on them. DC is deeply grateful not only to the Center's staff, but to the fellows during his year in residence, a number of whom have contributed chapters to this volume and others of whom have contributed ideas that are felt throughout the text. A more specific moment of origin for this volume was a visit by YS to the Center one spring weekend (the only weekend in our collective memory that it snowed in Palo Alto). YS concurs with DC about the Center's contribution in encouraging intellectual adventures, which this project certainly has been. YS would also like to note the role of his coeditor, whose effect on others, in his encouragement and nurturance of interesting ideas, has an uncanny resemblance to that of the Center.

The development of the volume benefited from the efforts of students in a seminar at the University of Illinois at Chicago who provided valuable feedback on initial drafts of a number of chapters. These individuals include Amy Blickenstaff, Thomas Griffin, Eshkol Rafaeli-Mor, Nilly Rafaeli-Mor, Karen Rausch, and Julie Weitlauf. It has also benefited from National Institute of Mental Health Grant No. MH39349 and the University of Washington Royalty Research Fund. We also wish to thank Seymour Weingarten, Editor-in-Chief at The Guilford Press, for his encouragement and invaluable assistance.

Finally, we thank our friends and colleagues at Stanford, Columbia, the University of Illinois at Chicago, and the University of Washington, for sharing their ideas and thereby shaping ours over many years.

Daniel Cervone
Yuichi Shoda

Contents

The Coherence of Personality

I

Introduction

1

Social-Cognitive Theories
and the Coherence of Personality

DANIEL CERVONE
YUICHI SHODA

Were it not for the coherence of personality functioning, there might be little need for a psychology of personality. Most of the other concerns of the personality psychologist (motivation, emotion, self-concept, etc.) are addressed in psychology's other subdisciplines. The study of individual differences distinguishes the field for some investigators, yet others contend that individual-difference analyses are not germane to the development of personality theory (Lamiell, 1997; Rorer, 1990). On the question of personality coherence, however, all can agree. Understanding the coherent functioning of the individual is the central, unique charge of the field (Allport, 1937).

Almost all the major theories in the history of the field have accepted this charge. Writers as different as Jung and Rogers have explored people's striving toward a coherent sense of self. The disparate "grand theories" of the mid-20th century (e.g., Allport, 1937; Cattell, 1950; Lewin, 1935; Murray, 1938; Murphy, 1947) all "emphasize the consistency and coherence of normal personality and view the individual organism as an organized and complexly structured whole" (McAdams, 1997, p. 12). The variety of contemporary trait theories adopt, as their basic units of analysis, personality variables that correspond to coherent patterns of social behavior. The present volume shares this historic commitment to the study of personality coherence.

Although this volume continues an historic tradition, in another respect it breaks with the past. The contributors to this volume address the question of personality coherence through methodologies and theory that are novel to this area—indeed, so novel that their nontraditional nature has sometimes resulted in their being misconstrued as an attack on the phenomenon of personality coherence rather than a novel way of explaining it.

The contributors to this volume advance what have come to be known as "social-cognitive" theories of personality. Since they themselves define the approach, we provide only a cursory overview here. Social-cognitive theories are most clearly defined by the units of analysis through which they conceptualize personality functioning and differences among individuals. Personality is understood by reference to basic cognitive and affective processes (e.g., Higgins & Kruglanski, 1996). These psychological mechanisms have social foundations (Bandura, 1986; Levine, Resnick, & Higgins, 1993; also see Baltes & Staudinger, 1996). They develop in social and cultural contexts and are activated by social settings. They thus are "social-cognitive" mechanisms. The social-cognitivist strives to understand how multiple mechanisms operate, in concert, as coherent psychological systems. Coherence in personality functioning is viewed as an emergent property of interactions among multiple psychological mechanisms (Cervone, 1997; Mischel & Shoda, 1995).

In this analysis of social-cognitive and affective mechanisms in personality functioning, persons and social settings are viewed as reciprocally interacting systems (Bandura, 1978). People select and shape their environments (e.g., Caspi, 1998) and give meaning to events by interpreting them according to their personal beliefs (Higgins, 1990). The sociocultural environment, in turn, shapes self-views, knowledge mechanisms, and psychological tendencies. People construct a coherent sense of identify through psychological processes that are "attuned to" (Kitayama, Markus, Matsumoto, & Norasakkunit, 1997, p. 1246) their surrounding social and cultural contexts.

A second defining feature of social-cognitive theories is the goal of developing a common language for understanding both consistency and variability in social behavior (e.g., Grant & Dweck, Chapter 10, this volume; Higgins, Chapter 3, this volume). People's defining attributes include not only average response tendencies that are evident across contexts, but distinctive variations in action from one context to another (Shoda, Mischel, & Wright, 1994). The social-cognitivist does not write off this variability as statistical "error" that lies beyond the grasp of the personality psychologist. Instead, one works toward models of personality that can account for both stability and variability in action across time and place. Doing so requires that one attend not only to persons but to the social tasks they confront and construct (Sanderson & Cantor, Chapter 11, this volume).

Social-cognitive theories also are marked by their methodological strategies. Social-cognitivists commonly bring both correlational and experimental methods to bear on questions of personality functioning. This volume presents numerous research programs in which a given personality mechanism is studied correlationally, to relate an individual's typical level of the variable to a target outcome, as well as experimentally, to clarify causal relations among personality processes and outcomes of interest.

Finally, social-cognitive theories are notable for being "social" in a broad sense of the word. Personality theories must be judged in part on their ability to deliver useful solutions to social and personal problems. Social-cognitivists historically have attended to this need, devoting much attention to the analysis of social problems and the development of psychosocial interventions (e.g., Bandura, 1969, 1973; Dodge, 1993, in press; Wilson, 1989). The area's continuing efforts in this regard are evident throughout this volume, as well as in numerous other applications to problems of health (O'Leary & Brown, 1995; Miller, Shoda, & Hurley, 1996), education (Berry, 1989; Schunk & Zimmerman, 1994), societal aggression (Huesmann, 1998; Huesmann & Guerra, 1997), and therapeutic behavior change (Williams, 1995).

Of these four defining features of social-cognitive theories, the latter three follow from the first. The ability to address both consistency and variability in action, to marshall converging correlational and experimental evidence, and to develop theory-guided psychosocial interventions all stem from the initial decision to ground a personality theory in the study of basic psychological mechanisms of cognition, affect, and action. The advantages of this decision seem obvious in retrospect. Yet this approach contrasts with the field's popular attempts to build a psychology of personality on the study of dispositional constructs whose relation to underlying psychological mechanisms is unknown (Goldberg, 1993; John, 1990).

In this introductory chapter, we briefly outline the history of social-cognitive theories, comment on their contemporary status in the field, and relate the perspective to others in the field. We then delineate the various aspects of "coherence" in personality functioning and, as a way of previewing the contributions to this volume, overview the ways in which social-cognitive mechanisms contribute to each of these aspects of personality coherence.

A BRIEF HISTORY OF SOCIAL-COGNITIVE THEORIES OF PERSONALITY

Ideas emerge from previous ideas. Any intellectual tradition thus can be traced arbitrarily far into the past. A more complete history of social-cognitive theories than that presented here might trace their 20th-century roots in Hullian and Tolmanian learning theory, gestalt psychology, and Lewinian field theory (see Loevinger, 1987; Woodward, 1982). Turning to the post-World War II era, it would outline the influence of Dollard and Miller (1950), Sears and colleagues (Sears, Maccoby, & Levin, 1957; Sears, Rau, & Alpert, 1965), Kelly (1955), and Rotter (1954; see Cantor & Kihlstrom, 1987). It would detail the impact of Skinnerian behaviorism (1953)—an approach that was thoroughly rejected as an explanatory paradigm but that left its mark in the social-cognitivist's care in tying theoretical constructs to well-specified research methods (Mahoney, 1974). However, since our coverage is brief, we merely mention this longer history and turn, instead, to two developments in the 1960s.

In his research on social learning processes with Richard Walters, Albert Bandura (Bandura & Walters, 1963) laid critical foundations for contemporary social-cognitive theories. Bandura's modeling research showed how basic principles of social learning uncovered in the laboratory could illuminate complex social problems. Of equal importance, it shifted psychology's focus from peripheral learning mechanisms to central ones. The finding that people can acquire new skills and adapt to environmental contingencies through observation (Bandura, 1965), rather than exclusively through firsthand experience, forced the development of detailed accounts of high-level cognitive processes in observational learning (e.g., Rosenthal & Zimmerman, 1978). Bandura's work ushered in further change. The therapeutic power of observational and other cognitive techniques contributed to a revolution in the conceptualization of behavior-change processes (Bandura, 1969) that set the intellectual tone for a generation of cognitive-behavioral therapists (Meichenbaum, 1990) and that is felt throughout clinical psychology to the present day. Advances in the study of self-regulatory capabilities (Bandura, 1977) changed psychology's conception of human nature. People no longer were viewed as responders to environmental stimuli (Skinner, 1971) but as causal agents whose personal agendas and capabilities shaped the conditions of their lives and the course of their development (Bandura, 1974). Bandura's contributions helped to fuel psychology's ever-greater recognition of proactive, agentic functions in personality development (Baltes, Linderberger, & Staudinger, 1998; Lerner & Busch-Rossnagel, 1981).

Walter Mischel provided a second cornerstone for social-cognitive theories. In what originally was intended as a simple review of personality theory, Mischel (1968) provided the field's most penetrating critique. He questioned whether traditional individual-difference conceptions of personality structure were adequate to capture the complexity of personality functioning, particularly as revealed in individuals' attempts to meet the shifting demands of their lives. His answer of "No" resounded through the field. As with any complex critique, there was more than one way to read its conclusion. Some viewed Mischel's work as an attack on the very concept of personality. They rallied to defend the concept by showing that, in the signal-and-noise of traditional personality research, there at least is "enough signal . . . to make it worthwhile to turn on the radio" (Kenrick & Funder, 1988, p. 31). An alternative reading recognized that Mischel was not questioning the existence of personality but the existence of adequate personality theory (Shadel & Cervone, 1993). Read this way, Mischel's work inspired novel attempts to account for consistency, variability, and uniqueness in personality structure and functioning (e.g., Cantor & Kihlstrom, 1981). Mischel himself provided a map for this enterprise in his 1973 *Psychological Review* article, an enduring manifesto for the social-cognitive perspective presented in this volume. His empirical research showed how analyses of basic cognitive processes could illuminate classic problems that had bedeviled personality psychologists for decades (e.g., Mischel, 1974, 1979).

Bandura and Mischel are both historical figures and contemporary ones. Their work moves the field ahead to the present day, as is evident in their contributions to this volume.

A third development in our understanding of the social-cognitive bases of personality coherence derived from experimental social psychology. Researchers in social cognition identified not only general psychological processes in social thinking but enduring individual differences in the cognitive structures that underlie judgment, affect, and action. People were found to differ in the personal domains in which they develop elaborate self-knowledge (Markus, 1977), the constructs through which they chronically interpret social events (Higgins, King, & Mavin, 1982), and, more generally, the repertoire of declarative and procedural knowledge that they bring to bear on life's problems (Cantor & Kihlstrom, 1987). These cognitively based individual differences proved central to phenomena ranging from motivation (Dweck & Leggett, 1988) to aggression (Dodge, 1993) to interpersonal relations (Baldwin, 1992). Thus, although deriving from a field known for the study of situational influences, these social-psychological analyses revealed enduring person-based sources of variance in experience and action.

Finally, we note that brief histories cannot be comprehensive ones. The development of social-cognitive theories of personality has benefited enormously from the contributions of both our present authors and many other investigators whose writing does not happen to appear in this volume.

The Evolution of Social-Cognitive Theories

Personality theories commonly change over the years in light of new findings and conceptualizations. Psychodynamically oriented investigators no longer view the mind as a hydraulic energy system, and trait theorists no longer debate whether 3 versus 16 dimensions characterize the phenotypic structure of individual differences. Similarly, social-cognitive theories have evolved significantly in the past decades.

Changes in social-cognitive theories reflect a movement away from two paradigms popular in the 1960s. The first is behaviorism. By the early 1970s, social-cognitivists had fully rejected behaviorism's situationist account of human action. This was due, in part, to research findings that showed that people are capable of overcoming situational constraints and thereby exerting control over their own behavior (Bandura, 1974; Mischel, 1974). Self-regulatory functions are a central feature of the contemporary social-cognitive approach. Although some undergraduate textbooks persist in grouping social-cognitive theory with the behavioristic "learning theories," such characterizations seriously misrepresent a quarter-century of theoretical and research developments.

The second paradigm is the linear, serial information-processing approach to cognition. This paradigm was not so much rejected as modified. Symbolic information-processing functions still are critical to social-cognitive theories. However, contemporary investigators recognize that information systems are not linear. Elements reciprocally interact with one another, and the individual's information-processing system itself develops in reciprocal interaction with biological factors and social conditions (Crick & Dodge, 1994; Dodge, in press; Shoda & Mischel, 1998). Further, serial information-processing models tended to depict the cognitive system as a passive one that merely reacts to a given input. In contrast, contemporary dynamic models recognize that cognitive systems process and reprocess information in the absence of input, and therefore cannot be characterized as simple input–output devices. These two paradigm shifts underlie many of the theoretical and research contributions presented in this volume.

One other change is of note. Social-cognitivists have devoted ever greater attention to affective processes in personality functioning. Indeed, a number of writers have come to recognize personality as a "cognitive-affective system" (Mischel, Chapter 2, this volume; Mischel & Shoda, 1995; Shoda, Chapter 6, this volume). A key feature of this system is that cognitive and affective mechanisms, while distinct, are also reciprocally linked. Cognitive structures and processes influence emotional response (Higgins, 1987; Lazarus, 1991), and affective states, in turn, shape cognition (Forgas, 1995; Schwarz, 1990). Interconnected cognitive-affective elements constitute enduring personality structures that foster stable patterns of experience and action (Mischel & Shoda, 1995).

THE CONTEMPORARY STATUS OF SOCIAL-COGNITIVE THEORIES IN THE FIELD OF PERSONALITY PSYCHOLOGY

Tracing a history of social-cognitive theories of personality is easier than characterizing their current status in the field. On the one hand, the contributions that we have just outlined did not go unappreciated. Social-cognitive theories have achieved a unique stature. Impartial observers characterize the approach as "the current favorite among academic personality psychologists" (Pervin & John, 1997, p. 444). Edited volumes on personality theory commonly feature a social-cognitivist as the only contemporary writer represented (e.g., Frick, 1995). Proponents of the social-cognitive approach number among the most impactful psychologists in the discipline (Mayer & Carlsmith, 1997). Proponents of alternative approaches acknowledge the need to reconcile their work with the social-cognitive tradition (McCrae & Costa, 1996).

But as anyone familiar with the field of personality psychology realizes, there is a second side to this story (Cervone, 1991). The social-cognitive approach, so visible in some quarters, is nearly invisible in others. Commentators judge that social-cognitive contributions are irrelevant to the core concerns of the discipline (Hogan, 1982). Reviewers portray social-cognitive theories as disregarding personal factors that contribute to personality coherence (Revelle, 1995), as questioning whether personality exists (Goldberg, 1993), and as harboring the "villian[s]" of the field (Wiggins & Pincus, 1992, p. 474).

These characterizations of social-cognitive theories reflect, we believe, a confusion of two issues: the phenomena to be addressed by the personality psychologist and the units of analysis through which these phenomena are understood. Some writers equate the field of personality psychology with the study of traits (e.g., Buss, 1989). Since social-cognitive theories lack traditional trait variables, they appear irrelevant to the discipline. But, as most commentators recognize, "trait" has multiple meanings. If "trait" refers merely to a phenomenon—the existence of enduring, coherent patterns of action that distinguish individuals from one another—then traits indeed are central to the field, and social-cognitive approaches represent a strategy for explaining people's "traits." But "trait" commonly takes on an additional meaning. It refers to an internal psychological structure or system that is responsible for consistencies in action across sets of behaviors and situations (Allport, 1937; Tellegen, 1991). Used in this second sense, traits and trait theory are simply one possible way of understanding the phenomenon of personality coherence. Social-cognitive theories are another. No matter what one's assessment of these and other theoretical paradigms, one should not equate a field of study with one possible way of explaining its core phenomena.

SOCIAL-COGNITIVE THEORIES
AND CONCEPTUAL ALTERNATIVES

What one stands for is, as the saying goes, more important than what one stands against. Most of the pages of this volume are devoted to exploring how an analysis of social-cognitive mechanisms can contribute to our understanding of personality coherence.

Despite this generally positive tone, the present volume also is critical. Social-cognitive theories are not the only perspective in the discipline, as we have just noted. Many of our contributors recognize the need to differentiate their work from alternative viewpoints. In particular, many contributors contrast their approach to an interrelated set of viewpoints known as the "Big Five" (Goldberg, 1993; John, 1990) and the "five-factor" (McCrac & Costa, 1996) models of personality structure. These approaches describe people by locating them along a set of five psychometrically derived linear dimensions.

Each dimension describes an average tendency to display a particular class of affect and action. To five-factor theorists, the dimensions also correspond to inferred structures that are causally responsible for the individual's dispositional tendencies (McCrae & Costa, 1995, 1996). McCrae and Costa (1996) contend that the core of human nature is a set of five dispositional structures that are possessed by all people in varying amounts. A corollary is that the five dispositional structures purportedly shape the content of social-cognitive variables (McCrae & Costa, 1996). In this view, then, social-cognitive variables are mediators of the effect of core personality factors on social behavior.

This merger of trait and social-cognitive theories is appealing at first. However, if "traits" are construed as universal psychological structures that correspond to, and cause, broad patterns of response, then this merger is generally not accepted by social-cognitive theorists. Indeed, a number of contributors to this volume explicitly reject the contention that "trait" approaches, defined in this manner, provide an adequate foundation for understanding social-cognitive processes or for building a personality theory. It is important to note that they reject trait approaches on at least three distinct grounds.

The first point is a familiar one, having formed the basis of the "person–situation debate" of the 1970s and 1980s: Personality functioning is sensitive to variations in social context. Context-free trait variables thus account for only a small fraction of the variance in social behavior. The empirical evidence, then, does not compel one to adopt a trait model of personality structure. Although one may tire of hearing this well-known argument, it remains that deconditionalized trait variables predict behavior no better now than they did decades ago (Pervin, 1994).

The other two points are less familiar. In this regard, it would be a complete misreading of this volume to view it as a simple restatement of arguments made a quarter century ago about the "personality-and-prediction" data. Indeed, the second reason for rejecting dispositional models is, in a sense, the opposite of the first: There exist important forms of personality coherence that trait models fail to capture. By implicitly equating "coherence" with consistency in behavior across a fixed set of trait indicators (Jackson & Paunonen, 1985), nomothetic trait approaches truncate the phenomenon of personality coherence and thereby overlook significant patterns of coherence that one observes empirically. Much of the research reported in this volume reveals patterns of coherence in personality functioning that go beyond simple consistency or stability in response. Coherence across time is revealed not only in stability of action, but in meaningful patterns of change when people face changing environmental demands (Sanderson & Cantor, Chapter 11). Coherence across contexts is revealed not only in stable mean levels of response, but in variations in cognition and action from one context to another (Baldwin, Chapter 5; Shoda, Chapter 6; Zelli & Dodge, Chapter 4). Further, when consistency in response is observed, it is found across sets of situations that vary idiosyncratically from person to person and that often bear little relation to nomothetic trait categories (Cervone, Chapter 9). Trait approaches, then, do not fail because personality lacks coherence. They fail because individuals exhibit complex patterns of coherence that would be missed if personality functioning were viewed solely through the filter of nomothetic trait categories.

The third reason for rejecting trait models of personality structure is not empirical, but conceptual: Trait constructs do not provide an adequate explanatory foundation for a science of personality. Nomothetic dispositional constructs, in other words, fail to provide a scientifically adequate causal account of an individual's experiences and actions. In this volume, some contributors completely reject the contention that trait constructs have explanatory power (Bandura, Chapter 7; Zelli & Dodge, Chapter 4) whereas others judge that their explanatory power is so weak, especially in light of criteria articulated in the philosophy of science, that a strong trait position is untenable (Cervone, Chapter 9). A number of writers note that, unlike trait models, social-cognitive approaches seek "bottom-up" causal explanations (Salmon, 1989) in which personality coherence is understood as a product of interactions among multiple psychological structures and processes, none of which directly corresponds to the phenotypic psychological disposition that is to be explained (see Cervone, 1997 and Chapter 9, this volume; Shadel, Niaura, & Abrams, in press; Zelli & Dodge, Chapter 4, this volume).

Surprising patterns of personality coherence often are revealed through careful analysis of the individual case. Idiographic analyses reported in this volume reveal patterns of organization among social-cognitive processes and resulting coherence in social behavior that might never have been found if individuals had been forced into a nomothetic system of dispositional tendencies. These findings are part of a larger body of recent idiographic findings that severely question the adequacy of nomothetic analyses. Feldman (1995) finds that the structure of affect revealed at the level of the individual may differ markedly from the population-level structure. Although dispositional tendencies toward positive and negative affectivity may be orthogonal in the population (Watson & Clark, 1997), they are highly related for many individuals (Feldman, 1995). In the study of smoking cessation and relapse, Shadel and colleagues find that relations among personality structures and the social situations that trigger relapse are so highly idiosyncratic that they would be obscured in any nomothetic scheme (Shadel et al., in press). Such findings are particularly noteworthy in clinical domains, where the practicing psychologist must manage the individual case. Finally, in work that speaks directly to the logic of the five-factor model, Fleeson (1998) recently has analyzed dispositional tendencies via within-subject factor analyses. Findings suggest that the dispositional structures found at the level of the individual commonly differ from the five-factor structure found at the level of the population (Fleeson, 1998). Some years ago, Tellegen (1991) noted that, "if encountered," idiosyncratic variations in personality structure would "undoubtedly force us to rethink certain nomothetic trait constructs and current personality assessment practices" (p. 29). The findings that have become available in the intervening years suggest that the time for rethinking may have arrived.[1]

A rejection of nomothetic dispositional models such as five-factor theory (McCrae & Costa, 1996) is in no sense a rejection of the fact inherited neuro-anatomical and neurochemical factors contribute to coherence in personality functioning (also see Mischel, Chapter 2, this volume). The question here is not whether biological factors are important but how to conceptualize their role in personality structure and functioning. Acknowledging the importance of biological temperament is not at all equivalent to adopting a trait model of personality structure. This point is underscored by the fact that scholars who study biological temperament are among the five-factor model's severest critics (Kagan, 1994). As Zuckerman (1995) reminds us, "We do not inherit personality traits" (1995, p. 331). Molecular genetic findings (Lesch et al., 1996) reinforce this important, yet often ignored, fact. We inherit genes that code for proteins that are structural components of the nervous system. Genetic factors only partly determine the overall structure of neural systems, which are influenced by experiential factors in the course of ontogenesis (Gottlieb, 1991, 1998; Edelman, 1992; Kandel, Schwartz, & Jessell, 1991). Further, temperament mechanisms may not give rise to broad, trait-like dispositions, but to contextualized reactions to particular classes of stimuli (Kagan, 1994). Genetic factors may contribute not only to consistencies in action but to variations in behavior across contexts (Saudino, 1997). Recent work by Dodge (1996) indicates how biological factors can be incorporated into a dynamic social-cognitive model.

The fact that social-cognitivists study personality coherence while rejecting personality trait constructs can be further understood by analogy to the field of intelligence. Many investigators study human intelligence without reference to constructs such as "generalized intelligence" or similar individual-difference factors (see Neisser et al., 1996). Instead, they examine the multiple information-processing mechanisms that underlie the individual's capacity for intelligent action (e.g., Gardner, 1983; Sternberg, 1985). These mechanisms are generally found to be more contextualized, or domain-specific, than a global IQ perspective suggests. However, a cognitive analysis is not mute to questions of generality in intelligence. Generality can, for example, be understood by reference to abstract cognitive schemas that individuals apply to problems in multiple domains (Ohlsson, 1993, 1998). Efforts to explain both specificity and generality in human intelligence without reference to psychometric individual-difference factors parallel the social-cognitivists' efforts to explain specificity and generality in personality functioning without reference to personality traits (also see Cantor & Kihlstrom, 1987).

Investigators who pursue information-processing analyses of intelligence share with many investigators in personality (e.g., Epstein, 1994; Mischel & Shoda, 1994) the recognition that the statistical analysis of individual differences is not a reliable route to discovering underlying causal structure. This point is made obvious by considering well-understood domains; a factor analysis of automobiles, for example, may yield factors such as maximum speed and reliability that shed little light on the causal components under the hood (Epstein, 1994). In any domain, the causal components of a system are not necessarily revealed by factor analyses of individual differences among multiple instances of the system.

Although the social-cognitive perspective differs fundamentally from contemporary trait theories, it does share an affinity with other viewpoints in personality psychology that do not happen to employ a "social-cognitive" label. Many analyses of goal systems in personality functioning (e.g., Emmons, 1997; Little, 1989; see Pervin, 1989) share the social-cognitivist's focus on purposive mechanisms that organize coherent patterns of action. Work on autobiographical memory, narrative processes, and personal identity (Greenwald, 1980; McAdams, 1996; Ross, 1989; Singer & Salovey, 1996) contributes greatly to the social-cognitivist's attempt to identify memory-based processes that contribute to a coherent sense of self (Cantor & Kihlstrom, 1987). Cognitive appraisal models of emotion (e.g., Lazarus, 1991; Smith & Lazarus, 1990, 1993) share with social-cognitive theories a concern with both self-appraisal mechanisms that are proximal determinants of psychological experience and knowledge structures that foster coherence in appraisals of oneself and the environment. Coherence that results from the dynamic interplay between persons and situations is a concern of interactionist approaches in personality psychology (Magnusson & Torestad, 1993), especially those that stress agentic, goal-directed processes in personality functioning (Hettema, 1979). Finally, contemporary psychodynamically oriented investigators share the social-cognitivist's goal of identifying coherent cognitive-affective structures that characterize the individual (Horowitz, 1991; Westen, 1991). Indeed, the development of social-cognitive models of psychodynamic processes (Chen & Andersen, in press; Baldwin, Chapter 5, this volume; Newman, Duff, & Baumeister, 1997) is a particularly exciting recent advance in the field.

Trends in social-cognitive theories also are congruent with developments outside of personality psychology. In cognitive psychology, research findings bolster two long-standing tenets of social-cognitive theories, namely, that cognition involves contextualized mental processes and that cognitive mechanisms develop in reciprocal interaction with social systems. Much work shows cognitive processes to be domain-linked, with rates of learning and cognitive skills often showing little transfer from one domain or context to another (Detterman & Sternberg, 1993; Gelman & Williams, 1998). The importance of reciprocal influence processes is highlighted by the "situative perspective" (Greeno et al., 1998) on cognition, which posits that cognitive processes function in reciprocal interaction with environmental constraints and affordances, as well as by work in cultural psychology, which uncovers significant cross-cultural variations in social-cognitive mechanisms (Lillard, 1998).

Work in the social-cognitive theories also is complemented by advances in developmental psychology. For example, the comprehensive analysis of life-span development by Baltes and colleagues (Baltes, 1997; Baltes et al., 1998; Maciel, Heckhausen, & Baltes, 1994) reaches conclusions about personality functioning that are fully congruent with the social-cognitive emphasis on self-referent processes, personal agency, and person–situation interactions: "A central feature of personality development is the emergence of . . . self-regulatory mechanisms that mediate successful transactional adaptation (Baltes et al., 1998, pp. 1111). From this perspective, "Structural organization and coherence of personality, self, and self-regulatory mechanisms are a necessary precondition (constraint) for adaptive fitness and . . . growth" (p. 121). It is noteworthy that life-span research reveals greater perceived change in personality attributes across the life course than dispositional models would predict (Fleeson & Heckhausen, 1997). Finally, the social-cognitivist's guiding causal principle of reciprocal determinism (Bandura, 1978, Chapter 7, this volume) is congruent with theory and research in community psychology. For example, the ecological perspective of Kelly and associates has long highlighted "the impact of social settings on individuals and, reciprocally, how persons respond to varied environments" (Kelly, 1979, p. 4). In this work, "the principle of interdependence is superordinate to the premises of psychological or sociological causation" (Kelly, 1979, p. 4).

In the decade past, much inquiry in personality psychology has been guided by the view that human nature consists of a small set of dispositional tendencies that are universal, unaffected by social experiences, and unchanging across the life course (McCrae & Costa, 1996, 1997). A guiding metaphor for understanding persons was not energy (Freud, 1923) or information (Simon, 1983), but "plaster" (Costa & McCrae, 1994; cf. Roberts, 1997). Many extolled the benefits of this view. Others were concerned about its costs. The belief that personality consists primarily of static, genetically-determined trait structures (McCrae & Costa, 1996) may deflect attention from the dynamic psychological processes and person–environment transactions through which people's distinctive characteristics develop (Block, 1995). Recent advances in the study of individuals, cognition, cultures, communities, and human development suggest that we may be entering a period that more fully appreciates and illuminates the unique ways in which individuals construct a coherent sense of self and maintain stable patterns of social behavior as they negotiate the varied tasks and developmentally shifting demands of their lives (Cervone & Shoda, in press).

The Evolutionary Alternative

Finally, one other theoretical alternative deserves careful consideration. Recent years have seen greater awareness of the possibility that the mind consists of a large number of "modules" (Fodor, 1983) or "mental organs" (Pinker, 1997), each of which evolved through natural selection to solve a distinct adaptive problem (Barkow, Cosmides, & Tooby, 1992). These adaptive mechanisms are seen to perform computations on only a particular class of inputs and to generate solutions that have been evolutionarily effective in solving the problem presented by the given input. Inputs such as problems of social exchange or mate attraction, for example, trigger mechanisms that generate strategies such as detecting cheaters (Cosmides, 1989) or displaying resources to attract females (Buss, 1988).

Although both evolutionary psychology and social-cognitive theories analyze personality functioning through contextualized personality variables, "contextualized" has a different meaning in these two very different approaches. The adaptive mechanisms posited by evolutionary psychology are contextualized in that each mechanism processes only a very limited class of inputs. In contrast, each of the mechanisms posited by social-cognitive theory (e.g., the "fundamental capabilities" of Bandura, Chapter 7, this volume, or the cognitive-affective person variables of Mischel & Shoda, 1995) processes a spectrum of potential inputs. These variables are contextualized by social-learning processes that cause certain inputs to become particularly salient to the individual or to become grouped into an equivalence class with other inputs. In Fodor's (1983) language, then, evolutionary psychology posits "modules," whereas social-cognitive theory is concerned with "central" mechanisms.

Evolutionary psychologists promote their view as an overarching theoretical framework for the fields of personality and social psychology (Buss, 1991, 1996; Buss & Kenrick, 1998). In so doing, they commonly suggest that nonadherents ignore the principles of natural selection or maintain the outmoded view that the brain consists of an undifferentiated mass of neurons. Social-cognitivists generally do not ground their work in evolutionary psychology. Yet we suspect that they are aware of the basic tenets of evolutionary theory and do not view the brain as an undifferentiated neural lump. The question here is not whether the mind evolved or whether it consists, at least in part, of input-specific modules. The work of Darwin and the existence of input-specific perceptual systems, for example, should convince anyone of these facts. The question is whether current evolutionary psychology can serve as a viable theoretical foundation for explaining the coherence of personality functioning and individual differences in social behavior. To this end, evolutionary psychology would appear to face obstacles of such severity that even the informed personality psychologist might not embrace the approach. Some of these obstacles, as discussed below, are underscored by social-cognitive research.

Evolutionary psychology proposes that a given adaptive mechanism (e.g., a cheating detector) explains an individual's actions as she or he acts on a problem of adaptive significance (e.g., social exchange). The approach thus solves the problem of identifying causal mechanisms. But it leaves another problem unsolved, namely, the problem of identifying acts. In the complex flow of social events, how do we know when the person is engaged in social exchange? This seemingly simple problem of act identification is actually vexing (Vallacher & Wegner, 1987). Suppose I am playing cards. Am I engaged in social exchange? Or, as a novice player, am I engaged exclusively in esteem-protecting impression management as I struggle to avoid violating a rule and disrupting the game? Suppose I am playing cards against an attractive opponent. Am I engaged in social exchange or mate attraction? Different people performing the same act may be attempting to solve different problems. Without resolving the problem of act identification, there is no way of knowing what adaptive problem people are working on and, therefore, what module to invoke to explain their behavior (Cervone, in press). This concern is not mere speculation. Social science research has long documented that even single acts that seemingly serve a unitary biological purpose can, in fact, serve diverse purposes for different people, and therefore cannot be traced to a common causal mechanism. For example, anthropological research has examined causes underlying the seemingly simply act of act of boiling water prior to its consumption (Wellin, 1955). In deciding whether to boil their water, all people might be seen to be doing the same thing. One might search for a singular mechanism underlying the seemingly common act. But ethnographic research revealed that different people performing the same act were doing very different things. Some were solving a problem of hygiene. Others were rebelling against social norms, one of which dictated that only ill persons should boil their drinking water. Yet others were adhering to social norms; they chose *not* to boil water, even if they understood the hygienic advantages (Wellin, 1955). Resolving the problem of act identification requires that one attend to the processes through which people encode social situations and to the goal structures that lend meaning to action. These psychological mechanisms are a central focus of the research presented in this volume.

A second limitation derives from the fact that any given social task may activate multiple adaptive mechanisms. As proponents of the evolutionary viewpoint recognize, "behavior is the result of an internal struggle among many mental modules" (Pinker, 1997, p. 42). This fact raises serious practical problems. Predicting and explaining complex social behavior requires not only that one identify an adaptive mechanism, but that one identify the multiple modules that might come into play and provide a method for determining which of the modules have relatively greater strength in a given circumstance. Evolutionary psychology currently provides no tools for doing this.

Finally, as noted, evolutionary psychologists posit psychological mechanisms that process only a selected class of inputs. Indeed, they chide other social scientists for assuming that psychological mechanisms function in a similar manner across problems of diverse content (e.g., Cosmides & Tooby, 1987; Pinker, 1997). Much evidence, however, suggests that important personality mechanisms do indeed function in a similar manner across diverse content domains. In this volume, for example, Grant and Dweck (Chapter 10) report that goal mechanisms shape motivation and affect in a similar manner across interpersonal and achievement domains. The wealth of research on perceived self-efficacy (Bandura, 1997) suggests that this social-cognitive mechanism regulates affect and action in a similar manner across a spectrum of activities. Much can be learned about personality coherence by studying such contextualized, central cognitive processes.

SOCIAL-COGNITIVE BASES OF PERSONALITY COHERENCE

The central argument of this book is that social-cognitive processes account for much of the coherence of personality functioning. To advance this argument, we delineate the various phenomena that constitute personality "coherence" and outline how social-cognitive mechanisms give rise to these phenomena. In doing so, we primarily draw upon theory and research presented in this volume.

The Phenomena of Personality Coherence

It is useful to distinguish among three interrelated phenomena that each comprise an important component of coherence in personality functioning. The first is organization among multiple personality processes. Personality variables do not function as independent mechanisms but as coherent, integrated systems. The within-person organization among personality processes has been of central importance to the field since its outset (Allport, 1937).

A second element of personality coherence is coherence among social behaviors and experiences. Experiences and actions across different situations and time periods often are interconnected. People respond in a consistent manner across some contexts and display meaningful patterns of variation in response across others. They create stable patterns of personal experience by selecting and shaping the circumstances that make up their day-to-day lives. This phenotypic coherence is key to both psychologists' and layperson's inferences about personality.

The third aspect of coherence is phenomenological. People generally achieve a coherent sense of self. They have a stable sense of their preferences, values, and tendencies, their strengths and weaknesses, and the attributes they wish to develop. They develop and update a coherent life story that reflects both their past experiences and their current aspirations (Greenwald, 1980; McAdams, 1994; Ross, 1989). People strive to achieve a sense of meaning in their lives. The development of meaning enables people to see the events of their lives as meaningfully interconnected (Baumeister, 1991). A comprehensive theory of personality must address each of these three aspects of personality coherence.

Social-Cognitive Bases of Personality Coherence

A basic premise of the social-cognitive approach is that these various aspects of personality coherence cannot be fully understood without a model of the individual's social information-processing system. Although personality coherence can be explained at various levels, a key level of explanation is one that addresses the organization of knowledge and the dynamic interplay among cognition, affect, and behavior as a person interacts with the social world. This model must be capable of capturing not only typical patterns of social thinking but the social information-processing system of particular, potentially idiosyncratic, individuals.

In constructing such a model, the social-cognitive approach to personality draws on an over-arching theory, or "meta-theory," of social information processing that has emerged from work in various domains of research (e.g., Higgins & Kruglanski, 1996). This meta-theory provides the "common language" for analyzing individual differences *and* intraindividual dynamics (Higgins, Chapter 3, this volume). A key principle of this approach is that the activation of mental representations plays a central role in the processing of social information (Higgins, 1996; Higgins & Bargh, 1987). Personal and situational factors determine the activation level of alternative knowledge structures. Active knowledge structures, in turn, shape the meaning people assign to new social inputs. Key mental representations include knowledge of social situations; representations of self, others, and prospective events; personal goals, beliefs, and expectations; and knowledge of behavioral alternatives and task strategies.

As noted earlier, this model of social information processing recognizes reciprocal links between cognitive and affective processes. Cognitive elements trigger affective responses. Affect, in turn, influences cognitive processing and the activation level of cognitive content.

The question of personality coherence can now be stated more specifically in light of this general model: How does one go from a general model of information processes to the construction of a specific model of a given individual? And how does this model speak to the three aspects of coherence in personality functioning outlined above? If we use a page of text, or an entire volume of a book, as an analogy for an individual, then the general model of human social information processing provides the vocabulary and the grammatical rules. But can any combination of words and sentences be chosen arbitrarily? Or do some combinations make more sense, have more coherence, and form poetry, while other combinations don't?

Organization among Cognitive-Affective Elements

In emerging general models of social information processing, then, individuals are seen as an organized system of multiple processes mutually influencing one another (Shoda, Chapter 6, this volume). The parameters of that system, such as the accessibility of a given knowledge representation, are not entirely free to vary independently, because one part of the system imposes constraints on other parts, forming a system of mutual constraints. Such a system is self-organizing, in that not all configurations of the parameters are likely or stable, and the system tends to "snap in" to a configuration that makes a coherent pattern that satisfies the constraints (e.g., Thagard, 1989). This process can be illustrated by the famous black and white design that is often used to show the gestalt principle of figure and ground. It has two mutually exclusive interpretations, of an old or young woman. After a moment of initial confusion, a viewer is likely to see one or another interpretation of the figure as the various parts of the design become consistent with each other and form a coherent whole. Similarly, a complex system of social-cognitive mediating processes does not result in an infinite number of configurations or freely variable parameters. Rather, they tend to self-organize into a coherent configuration. The system generally has multiple possible stable configurations into which it can "settle." In short, then, the individual's social-cognitive information-processing system is not just an arbitrary listing of independent variable parameters. It tends, instead, to take on a good, meaningful configuration that "coheres."

How might such distinctive configurations form? The contributions to this volume highlight a range of social-cognitive processes that contribute to coherent information processing. Much personality coherence derives from the impact of personal goals. People's goals, life tasks, and self-regulatory standards influence the situations they seek and the cognitive, affective, and behavioral reactions to situations that they experience (Bandura, Chapter 7, this volume; Sanderson & Cantor, Chapter 11, this volume). Goals that people bring to situations partly determine which aspects of a situation are most closely attended (Grant & Dweck, Chapter 10, this volume; Higgins, Chapter 3, this volume), which, in turn, influences the situation's psychological meaning and the information and competencies people acquire from encounters. Stable goal systems, then, foster stable organizations among beliefs, competencies, and affective experiences. Expectancies are another source of coherence. Expectancies about other people's intentions, feelings, and behaviors affect the interpretations of ambiguous events. In so doing, they foster distinctive, contextualized patterns of response (Baldwin, Chapter 4, this volume; Zelli & Dodge, Chapter 5, this volume). Expectancies, goals, and beliefs about the self are themselves coherently interconnected by virtue of their influences upon one other (Dweck, 1996). People partly base their goals on self-assessments of their efficacy for performance (Bandura, Chapter 7, this volume). Mastery beliefs differentially relate to affect and motivation depending upon the nature of people's goals (Dweck & Leggett, 1988; Grant & Dweck, Chapter 10, this volume).

Recurring social experiences also foster stable configurations in the cognitive-affective system. Exposure to violent behavior creates salient beliefs about hostility that guide social inferences (Zelli & Dodge, Chapter 4, this volume). Interpersonal experiences cause distinct beliefs about the self, others, and social interactions to form into coherent cognitive structures (Baldwin, Chapter 5, this volume).

These cognitive mechanisms do not leave people "lost in thought." Instead, they form the basis for human agency. People draw upon interconnected personal and situational beliefs when gauging their efficacy for performance (Cervone, Chapter 9, this volume). Coherent systems of efficacy beliefs, goals, and self-regulatory skills enable people to organize meaningful courses of action and to maintain a coherent sense of self, even when their personal lives feature conflicting roles and disruptive transitions (Bandura, Chapter 7, this volume).

Functional interrelations among social-cognitive and affective processes provide constraints that help to explain why some configurations are relatively more common than others. It is these common configurations that may be intuitively recognized, at a molar level, as personality "types." We may consider, as but one example, the interrelation between two person variables: standards for self-evaluation and affective experiences. Although these are distinct personality mechanisms, they do not vary in a free, unconstrained manner. Higher standards foster negative mood by making normatively acceptable outcomes appear disappointingly inadequate (Rehm, 1982). Conversely, lower mood fosters higher standards by coloring people's subjective evaluations of prospective outcomes (Cervone, Kopp, Schaumann, & Scott, 1994; Scott & Cervone, 1998; also see Wright & Mischel, 1982). These functional interrelations among cognition and affect may make certain configurations (e.g., the constellation of negative mood and stringent, "perfectionistic" standards) far more likely than others (e.g., the combination of dysphoric mood and lenient personal standards). Indeed, depression is found to be associated with perfectionistic attitudes (Frost, Marten, Lahart, & Rosenblate, 1990; Hewitt & Dyck, 1986; Hewitt & Flett, 1991). Intuitively, we easily recognize a person "type" that combines depressed mood with perfectionistic, self-critical thinking.

Interrelations among different aspects of the social-cognitive personality system, then, yield cognitive-affective configurations that "make sense," cohere, and thus are more stable. These stable configurations form the basis of an individual's unique personality. They contribute to the individual's recurrent style of planning, interpreting, and responding to events. Other configurations, in contrast, do not cohere and thus are not likely to become the basis of an individual's stable information-processing system.

The forms that such stable organizations do and do not take reflect not only intrapsychic, interpersonal, and social factors, but also broad "cultural narratives." Cultural narratives, for example, enable Japanese people who are characterized by the "balance view" of personality coherence (Kitayama & Markus, Chapter 8, this volume) to entertain a set of beliefs that might appear to be contradictory in the minds of those who are characterized by the more Western "consistency view" of personality coherence.

Behavioral Expressions of the Social-Cognitive Personality System

In social-cognitive theories, the structure of the personality system, that is, the configuration of social-cognitive variables that form a system of social information-processing, is assumed to remain relatively stable and invariant across situations. But as a person moves across situations that contain different psychological features, different cognitions and affects become activated in the system, resulting in wide variations in behaviors across situations. However, contrary to the field's long-standing tendency to view such cross-situational variation as antithetical to the role of personality, social-cognitive theories views patterns of behavior variation as a key expression, or "behavioral signature," of the personality of the individual (Shoda et al., 1994; Mischel & Shoda, 1995). This is because the individual's unique characteristic organization of cognitions and affects, which channels the activation of the mediating units, fosters stable patterns of behavior variation and consistency across situations. The stability in the individual's personality structure is thus reflected in the stable *if...then...* contingencies between the psychological conditions and the cognitions and affects that become activated (Shoda, Chapter 6, this volume).

Many examples of such stable cross-situational behavior patterns can be found in the work of the contributors. For example, an individual's relational schemas, representations of self, others, and their relationships, are manifested in *if...then...* contingencies (e.g., "if in an achievement situation, then dominant; if with a romantic partner, then submissive"; Baldwin, Chapter 5, this volume). Because any given situation contains a myriad of features, situations can form different idiographic equivalence classes (Cervone, Chapter 9, this volume) depending on the situation features that are attended to. For example, for one individual, the presence or absence of the opportunity to learn may be a salient situation feature, whereas the possibility of being evaluated may function as the salient feature for a second individual. These different situational construals would give rise to different cross-situational organization in the behaviors and experiences of these two individuals. Their goals would affect the features of situations to which they attend. Individuals with different goals are expected to differ in the units of situations that serve as the basic "ifs" in their characteristic organization of behaviors across situations (Grant & Dweck, Chapter 10, this volume). Thus for the first individual in the example above, the key "if" is the perceived opportunity to learn; for the second individual, it is the perceived evaluation by others. Different phases of one's life may also constitute different "situations"; hence the individual for whom the life task of establishing independence is salient may, upon entering college, seek friends in order to separate from parents, but after graduation, the same person may focus on career at the expense of social life, in order to maintain independence (Sanderson & Cantor, Chapter 11, this volume).

An analysis of social-cognitive processes also can speak to the behavioral expressions described by traditional dispositional constructs. Interactions among a stable set of social-cognitive mechanisms may, in other words, explain behavioral expressions that are captured by well-known personality variables. Such explanations do not merely "translate" trait terms into a social-cognitive language; they often force a reconceptualization of the original personality variable. Higgins (Chapter 3, this volume) provides a lucid example. Dispositional tendencies to achieve success and to fear failure (McClelland, Atkinson, Clark, & Lowell, 1953) need not be explained by reference to corresponding hypothetical constructs (e.g., a motive to achieve). Instead, they can be understood by reference to an interacting set of social-cognitive mechanisms including expectations, standards, and strategies (Higgins, Chapter 3, this volume). This explanation reconceptualizes the original variable in that tendencies to achieve success and to avoid failure are understood as but two of a possible eight combinations of the underlying self-regulatory dynamics (Higgins, Chapter 3, this volume). The social-cognitive analysis, then, both explains the original dispositional tendency and provides a richer, more differentiated understanding of how individuals differ one from another.

Toward a Coherent, Integrated Sense of Self

The third type of personality coherence that must be addressed in a comprehensive theory is the individual's subjective sense of personal coherence. Rooted in its phenomenological tradition (e.g., Kelly, 1955; Rotter, 1954), social-cognitive theories approach this question from the standpoint of people trying to make sense of the vast array of experiences they encounter. That is, people create explanations for their experiences and try to tie them together into a coherent theory that encompasses many aspects of their lives. Ideally, such a theory not only accounts for the present experiences but also integrates the individual's memory of his or her past and future aspirations (McAdams, 1994). Although efforts to address this question have only begun relatively recently (e.g., Ross, 1989), there is already an emerging theme in the social cognitive approaches to this question.

Specifically, research and theorizing on "explanatory coherence" has yielded basic principles (Thagard, 1989) as well as specific models of social explanation (e.g., Miller & Read, 1991). These models integrate not only work on explanatory coherence but also the knowledge structure approach to understanding (e.g., Galambos, Abelson, & Black, 1986; Schank & Abelson, 1977; Wilensky, 1983) and models of discourse comprehension (e.g., Kintsch, 1988). Whereas these models have so far focused on explanatory coherence in the construction of mental models of others, the same principle can readily be applied to understanding how people construct a mental model of themselves and their lives.

The work in this area so far has shown that, in their efforts to make sense of self and others, people sometimes do act like social-cognitive theorists, particularly when they care about achieving a deeper understanding (e.g., Shoda & Mischel, 1993). Specifically, when people try to explain other people's behavior, upon observing them, they activate in their minds such constructs as the goals, plans, resources, beliefs, and scripts (Miller & Read, 1991). The constructs are activated initially rather "promiscuously" (Kintsch, 1988), without regard to the consistency and coherence among them. But as soon as these constructs are activated, they become a part of the "shakedown" process, which occurs mostly without conscious effort, so that the constructs that are mutually consistent support each other, while those that are inconsistent lose their activation. The result is an emergence of a set of constructs—goals, beliefs, and so forth—that are consistent to form a coherent picture of one's life, similar to the process of generating a coherent perception of a gestalt figure, as mentioned earlier. Only here the "picture" that emerges is that of one's life: past, present, and future. Furthermore, in this process, the perception and impact of new experiences are influenced by the current set of explanations about one's life, which ultimately determine how new experiences are incorporated into an evolving set of coherent explanations about personal history and the future.

Thus, in the social-cognitive theories, the same constructs and processes that have been used to understand the behavior-generation process, such as the activation of knowledge representations (e.g., Higgins, Chapter 3, this volume), also can be applied to understand the process of phenomenological aspects of personal coherence. The work on actor–observer differences suggests that social-cognitive constructs probably play a more prominent role in understanding self. People are less likely to use static traits in explaining their own behavior and are more likely to pay attention to situations (e.g., McGuire & McGuire, 1986). When they pay attention to situational variations in an individual's behavior, and when they try to explain, rather than merely describe, such situational variations, they resort to social-cognitive constructs (Shoda, Chapter 6, this volume).

The work presented in this volume provides ample evidence for the unique organization of social-cognitive variables that forms a coherent whole within each individual (Cervone, Chapter 9). The contributions highlight the importance of goals as a theme that connect one's past to the future (Bandura, Chapter 7; Grant & Dweck, Chapter 10; Sanderson & Cantor, Chapter 11) and illustrate how beliefs about self and others contribute to stable patterns of interpersonal interaction (Baldwin, Chapter 5; Zelli & Dodge, Chapter 4) that, in turn, are integral to one's sense of self. Finally, just as social-cognitive theories strive to form a meta-theory about forms of personal coherence and relations between behaviors and social contexts, each individual's sense of being "fully human" is rooted in a theory of personal coherence that is inherent in his or her given culture (Kitayama & Markus, Chapter 8).

SOCIAL-COGNITIVE THEORY AS A THEORY OF PERSONALITY

The postmodern trend sensitizes us to the pitfalls of "grand theory." We don't call our work "The Behavior of Organisms" (Skinner, 1938) anymore, and for good reason. As Kelly (1955) instructed, even the grandest theories are temporary constructions of limited scope. At best, they are not "true" but useful. Modesty is the order of the day.

Despite this trend, theory remains critical. Personality psychology contains no theory-free research. Personality theories dictate the questions one asks, the theoretical constructs one adopts, and the evidence one accepts as valid. This paramount role of theory has sustained personality psychology's historic concern with theoretical and meta-theoretical issues and its continued search for a viable, unifying grand theory.

In the past, the grand theories of personality generally were products of individual writers working in relative isolation. Their theories contained idiosyncratic constructs that could not easily be integrated with the larger body of psychological knowledge. Personality theory lived outside of the psychological mainstream (Hall & Lindzey, 1957; also see Higgins, Chapter 3, this volume). In these respects, social-cognitive theory does not fit the "grand theory" mold. It is the product of multiple investigators (although some individuals have made extraordinarily seminal contributions). These investigators directly draw upon, and contribute to, general knowledge in the psychological sciences. Social-cognitive theory is very much a part of psychology's mainstream. But this makes social-cognitive theory no less a theory of personality than the grand systems of the past. A personality theory is a systematic, testable framework for explaining the coherent patterns of psychological experience and behavior that distinguish individuals from one another. Such a theory can be grounded in psychology's detailed understanding of the social-cognitive and affective processes that underlie coherence in personality functioning. The advantages of this approach are compellingly illustrated by the contributions to this volume.

NOTE

1. Although they do not employ idiographic methods, the work of Kaiser and Ozer (1998) is relevant to the present discussion of the relation between trait and social-cognitive models. These investigators study a psychological mechanism that is central to social-cognitive theory, namely, personal goal systems. In contrast to the expectations of five-factor theory (McCrae & Costa, 1996), they find "no evidence here that the structure of goals reduces to the five-factor model" (Kaiser & Ozer, 1998, p. 7).

REFERENCES

Allport, G. (1937). *Personality: A psychological interpretation.* New York: Holt, Rinehart & Winston.

Baldwin, M. W. (1992). Relational schemas and the processing of social information. *Psychological Bulletin, 112,* 461–484.

Baltes, P. B. (1997). On the incomplete architecture of human ontogeny. *American Psychologist, 52,* 366–380.

Baltes, P. B., Linderberger, U., & Staudinger, U. M. (1998). Life-span theory in developmental psychology. In W. Damon (Series Ed.) & R. M. Lerner (Vol. Ed.), *Handbook of child psychology: Vol. 1. Theoretical models of human development* (5th ed., pp. 1029–1143). New York: Wiley.

Baltes, P. B., & Staudinger, U. M. (Eds.). (1996). *Interactive minds: Life-span perspectives on the social foundation of cognition.* New York: Cambridge University Press.

Bandura, A. (1965). Vicarious processes: A case of no-trial learning. In L. Berkowitz (Ed.), *Advances in experimental social psychology* (Vol. 2, pp. 1–55). New York: Academic Press.

Bandura, A. (1969). *Principles of behavior modification.* New York: Holt, Rinehart, & Winston.

Bandura, A. (1973). *Aggression: A social learning analysis.* Englewood Cliffs, NJ: Prentice-Hall.

Bandura, A. (1974). Behavior theory and the models of man. *American Psychologist, 29,* 859–869.

Bandura, A. (1977). *Social learning theory.* Englewood Cliffs, NJ: Prentice-Hall.

Bandura, A. (1978). The self-system in reciprocal determinism. *American Psychologist, 33,* 344–358.

Bandura, A. (1986). *Social foundations of thought and action: A social cognitive theory.* Englewood Cliffs, NJ: Prentice-Hall.

Bandura, A. (1997). *Self-efficacy: The exercise of control.* New York: Freeman.

Bandura, A., & Walters, R. H. (1963). *Social learning and personality development.* New York: Holt, Rinehart & Winston.

Barkow, J. H., Cosmides, L., & Tooby, J. (Eds.). (1992). *The adapted mind: Evolutionary psychology and the generation of culture.* New York: Oxford University Press.

Baumeister, R. F. (1991). *Meanings of life.* New York: Guilford Press.

Berry, J. M. (1989). Cognitive efficacy across the life span: Introduction to the special series. *Developmental Psychology, 25,* 683–686.

Block, J. (1995). A contrarian view of the five-factor approach to personality description. *Psychological Bulletin, 117,* 187–215.

Buss, A. H. (1989). Personality as traits. *American Psychologist, 44,* 1378–1388.

Buss, D. M. (1988). The evolution of human intrasexual competition: Tactics of mate attraction. *Journal of Personality and Social Psychology, 54,* 616–628.

Buss, D. M. (1991). Evolutionary personality psychology. *Annual Review of Psychology, 42,* 459–491.

Buss, D. M. (1996). The evolutionary psychology of human social strategies. In E. T. Higgins & A. W. Kruglanski (Eds.), *Social psychology: Handbook of basic principles* (pp. 3–38). New York: Guilford Press.

Buss, D. M., & Kenrick, D. T. (1998). Evolutionary social psychology. In D. T. Gilbert, S. T. Fiske, & G. Lindzey (Eds.), *The handbook of social psychology* (4th ed., Vol. 1, pp. 982–1026). Boston: McGraw-Hill.

Cantor, N., & Kihlstrom, J. F. (Eds.). (1981). *Personality, cognition, and social interaction.* Hillsdale, NJ: Erlbaum.

Cantor, N., & Kihlstrom, J. F. (1987). *Personality and social intelligence.* Englewood Cliffs, NJ: Prentice-Hall.

Caspi, A. (1998). Personality development across the life course. In W. Damon (Series Ed.) & N. Eisenberg (Vol. Ed.), *Handbook of child psychology: Vol. 3. Social, emotional, and personality development* (5th ed., pp. 311–388). New York: Wiley.

Cattell, R. B. (1950). *Personality: A systematic, theoretical, and factual study.* New York: McGraw-Hill.

Cervone, D. (1991). The two disciplines of personality psychology. *Psychological Science, 2,* 371–377.

Cervone, D. (1997). Social-cognitive mechanisms and personality coherence: Self-knowledge, situational beliefs, and cross-situational coherence in perceived self-efficacy. *Psychological Science, 8,* 43–50.

Cervone, D. (in press). Evolutionary psychology and explanation in personality psychology: How do we know which module to invoke? *American Behavioral Scientist.*

Cervone, D., Kopp, D. A., Schaumann, L., & Scott, W. D. (1994). Mood, self-efficacy, and performance standards: Lower moods induce higher standards for performance. *Journal of Personality and Social Psychology, 67,* 499–512.

Cervone, D., & Shoda, Y. (in press). Beyond traits in the study of personality coherence. *Current Directions in Psychological Science.*

Chen, S., & Andersen, S. M. (in press). Relationships in the past in the present: Significant-other representations and transference in everyday interpersonal life. In M. P. Zanna (Ed.), *Advances in experimental social psychology* (Vol. 31). Mahwah, NJ: Erlbaum.

Cosmides, L. (1989). The logic of social exchange: Has natural selection shaped how humans reasons? Studies with the Wason selection task. *Cognition, 31,* 187–276.

Cosmides, L., & Tooby, J. (1987). From evolution to behavior: Evolutionary psychology as the missing link. In J. Dupre (Ed.), *The latest on the best: Essays on evolution and optimality* (pp. 277–306). Cambridge, MA: MIT Press.

Costa, P. T., & McCrae, R. R. (1994). Set like plaster? Evidence for the stability of the adult personality. In T. F. Heatheron & J. L. Weinberger (Eds.), *Can personality change?* (pp. 21–40). Washington, DC: American Psychological Association.

Crick, N. R., & Dodge, K. A. (1994). A review and reformulation of social information-processing mechanisms in children's social adjustment. *Psychological Bulletin, 115,* 74–101.

Detterman, D. K., & Sternberg, R. J. (Eds.). (1993). *Transfer on trial.* Norwood, NJ: Ablex.

Dodge, K. A. (1993). Social-cognitive mechanisms in the development of conduct disorder and depression. *Annual Review of Psychology, 44,* 559–584.

Dodge, K. A. (1996). Biopsychosocial perspectives on the development of conduct disorder. In J. A. Linney (Ed.), *Proceedings of the Fifth National Prevention Research Conference.* Washington, DC: National Institute of Mental Health.

Dodge, K. A. (in press). Conduct disorder. In M. Lewis & A. J. Sameroff (Eds.), *Handbook of developmental psychopathology* (2nd ed.). New York: Plenum Press.

Dollard, J., & Miller, N. E. (1950). *Personality and psychotherapy: An analysis in terms of learning, thinking, and culture.* New York: McGraw-Hill.

Dweck, C. S. (1996). Implicit theories as organizers of goals and behavior. In P. M. Gollwitzer & J. A. Bargh (Eds.), *The psychology of action: Linking cognition and motivation to behavior* (pp. 69–90). New York: Guilford Press.

Dweck, C. S., & Leggett, E. L. (1988). A social-cognitive approach to motivation and personality. *Psychological Review, 95,* 256–273.

Edelman, G. M. (1992). *Bright air, brilliant fire: On the matter of the mind.* New York: Basic Books.

Emmons, R. A. (1997). Motives and goals. In R. Hogan, J. Johnson, & S. Briggs (Eds.), *Handbook of personality psychology* (pp. 485–512). San Diego, CA: Academic Press.

Epstein, S. (1994). Trait theory as personality theory: Can a part be as great as the whole? *Psychological Inquiry, 5,* 120–122.

Feldman, L. A. (1995). Valence focus and arousal focus: Individual differences in the structure of affective experience. *Journal of Personality and Social Psychology, 69*(1), 153–166.

Fleeson, W. (1998). Across-time within-person structures of personality: Common and individual traits. In G. V. Caprara & D. Cervone (Chairs), *Personality and social cognition.* Symposium conducted at the 9th European Conference on Personality, Guildford, UK.

Fleeson, W., & Heckhausen, J. (1997). More or less "me" in past, present, and future: Perceived lifetime personality during adulthood. *Psychology and Aging, 12,* 125–136.

Fodor, J. A. (1983). *The modularity of mind.* Cambridge, MA: MIT Press.

Forgas, J. P. (1995). Mood and judgment: The affect infusion model (AIM). *Psychological Bulletin, 117,* 39–66.

Freud, S. (1923). *The ego and the id.* New York: Norton.

Frick, W. B. (1995). *Personality: Selected readings in theory.* Itasca, IL: Peacock.

Frost, R., Marten, P., Lahart, C., & Rosenblate, R. (1990). The dimensions of perfectionism. *Cognitive Therapy and Research, 14,* 449–468.

Galambos, J. A., Abelson, R. P., & Black, J. B. (1986). *Knowledge structures.* Hillsdale, NJ: Erlbaum.

Gardner, H. (1983). *Frames of mind: The theory of multiple intelligences.* New York: Basic Books.

Gelman, R., & Williams, E. M. (1998). Enabling constraints for cognitive development and learning: Domain specificity and epigenesis. In W. Damon (Series Ed.) & D.

Kuhn & R. S. Siegler (Vol. Eds.), *Handbook of child psychology: Vol. 2. Cognition, perception, and language* (5th ed., pp. 575–630). New York: Wiley.

Goldberg, L. R. (1993). The structure of phenotypic personality traits. *American Psychologist, 48,* 26–34.

Gottlieb, G. (1991). Experiential canalization of behavioral development: Theory. *Developmental Psychology, 27,* 4–13.

Gottlieb, G. (1998). Normally occurring environmental and behavioral influences on gene activity: From central dogma to probabilistic epigenesis. *Psychological Review, 105,* 792–802.

Greeno, J. G., & The Middle School Mathematics through Applications Project Group. (1998). The situativity of knowing, learning, and research. *American Psychologist, 53,* 5–26.

Greenwald, A. G. (1980). The totalitarian ego: Fabrication and revision of personal history. *American Psychologist, 35,* 603–618.

Hall, C. S., & Lindzey, G. (1957). *Theories of personality.* New York: Wiley.

Hettema, P. J. (1979). *Personality and adaptation.* Amsterdam: North-Holland.

Hewitt, P. L., & Dyck, D. G. (1986). Perfectionism, stress, and vulnerability to depression. *Cognitive Therapy and Research, 10,* 137–142.

Hewitt, P. L., & Flett, G. L. (1991). Dimensions of perfectionism in unipolar depression. *Journal of Abnormal Psychology, 100,* 98–101.

Higgins, E. T. (1987). Self-discrepancy: A theory relating self and affect. *Psychological Review, 94,* 319–340.

Higgins, E. T. (1990). Personality, social psychology, and person–situation relations: Standards and knowledge activation as a common language. In L. A. Pervin (Ed.), *Handbook of personality: Theory and research* (pp. 301–338). New York: Guilford Press.

Higgins, E. T. (1996). Knowledge activation: Accessibility, applicability, and salience. In E. T. Higgins & A. E. Kruglanski (Eds.), *Social psychology: Handbook of basic principles* (pp. 133–168). New York: Guilford Press.

Higgins, E. T., & Bargh, J. A. (1987). Social cognition and social perception. *Annual Review of Psychology, 38,* 369–425.

Higgins, E. T., King, G. A., & Mavin, G. H. (1982). Individual construct accessibility and subjective impressions and recall. *Journal of Personality and Social Psychology, 43,* 35–47.

Higgins, E. T., & Kruglanski, A. W. (1996). *Social psychology: Handbook of basic principles.* New York: Guilford Press.

Hogan, R. (1982). On adding apples and oranges in personality psychology. *Contemporary Psychology, 27,* 851–852.

Horowitz, M. J. (Ed.). (1991). *Person schemas and maladaptive interpersonal patterns.* Chicago: University of Chicago Press.

Huesmann, L. R. (1998). The role of social information processing and cognitive schema in the acquisition and maintenance of habitual aggressive behavior. In R. G. Geen & E. Donnerstein (Eds.), *Human aggression: Theories, research, and implications for policy* (pp. 73–109). New York: Academic Press.

Huesmann, L. R., & Guerra, N. G. (1997). Children's normative beliefs about aggression and aggressive behavior. *Journal of Personality and Social Psychology, 72,* 408–419.

Jackson, D. N., & Paunonen, S. V. (1985). Construct validity and the predictability of behavior. *Journal of Personality and Social Psychology, 49,* 554–570.

John, O. P. (1990). The "Big Five" factor taxonomy: Dimensions of personality in the natural language and in questionnaires. In L. A. Pervin (Ed.), *Handbook of personality: Theory and research* (pp. 66–100). New York: Guilford Press.

Kagan, J. (1994). *Galen's prophecy.* New York: Basic Books.

Kaiser, R. T., & Ozer, D. J. (1998). *The structure of personal goals and their relation to personality traits.* Unpublished manuscript, Department of Psychology, University of California, Riverside.

Kelly, G. A. (1955). *The psychology of personal constructs.* New York: Norton.

Kelly, J. G. (1979). The high school: Students and social contexts—An ecological perspective. In J. G. Kelly (Ed.), *Adolescent boys in high school: A psychological study of coping and adaptation* (pp. 3–14). Hillsdale, NJ: Erlbaum.

Kandel, E. R., Schwartz, J. H., & Jessell, T. M. (1991).*Principles of neural science* (3rd ed.). New York: Elsevier.

Kenrick, D. T., & Funder, D. C. (1988). Profiting from controversy: Lessons from the person-situation debate. *American Psychologist, 43*, 23–34.

Kintsch, W. (1988). The role of knowledge in discourse comprehension: A construction-integration model. *Psychological Review, 95*, 163–182.

Kitayama, S., Markus, H. R., Matsumoto, H., & Norasakkunit, V. (1997). Individual and collective processes in the construction of the self: Self-enhancement in the United States and self-criticism in Japan. *Journal of Personality and Social Psychology, 72*, 1245–1267.

Lamiell, J. T. (1997). Individuals and the differences between them. In R. Hogan, J. Johnson, & S. Briggs (Eds.), *Handbook of personality psychology* (pp. 117–141). San Diego, CA: Academic Press.

Lazarus, R. S. (1991). *Emotion and adaptation.* New York: Oxford University Press.

Lerner, R. M., & Busch-Rossnagel, N. (Eds.). (1981). *Individuals as producers of their development: A life-span perspective.* New York: Academic Press.

Lesch, K.-P., Bengel, D., Heils, A., Sabol, S. Z., Greenberg, B. D., Petri, S., Benjamin, J., Muller, C. R., Hamer, D. H., & Murphy, D. L. (1996). Association of anxiety-related traits with a polymorphism in the serotonin transporter gene regulatory region. *Science, 274*, 1527–1531.

Levine, J. M., Resnick, L. B., & Higgins, E. T. (1993). Social foundations of cognition. *Annual Review of Psychology, 44*, 585–612.

Lewin, K. (1935). *A dynamic theory of personality: Selected papers.* New York: McGraw-Hill.

Lillard, A. (1998). Ethnopsychologies: Cultural variations in theories of mind. *Psychological Bulletin, 123*, 3–32.

Little, B. (1989). Personal projects analysis: Trivial pursuits, magnificent obsessions and the search for coherence. In D. M. Buss & N. Cantor (Eds.), *Personality psychology: Recent trends and emerging directions* (pp. 15–31). New York: Springer-Verlag.

Loevinger, J. (1987). *Paradigms of personality.* New York: Freeman.

Maciel, A. G., Heckhausen, J., & Baltes, P. B. (1994). A life-span perspective on the interface between personality and intelligence. In R. J. Sternberg & P. Ruzgis (Eds.), *Personality and intelligence.* New York: Cambridge University Press.

Magnusson, D., & Torestad, B. (1993). A holistic view of personality: A model revisited. *Annual Review of Psychology, 44*, 427–452.

Mahoney, M. J. (1974). *Cognition and behavior modification.* Cambridge, MA: Ballinger.

Markus, H. (1977). Self-schemata and processing information about the self. *Journal of Personality and Social Psychology, 35*, 63–78.

Mayer, J. D., & Carlsmith, K. M. (1997). Eminence rankings of personality psychologists as a reflection of the field. *Personality and Social Psychology Bulletin, 23*, 707–716.

McAdams, D. P. (1994). Personality, modernity, and the storied self: A contemporary framework for studying persons. *Psychological Inquiry, 7*, 295–321.

McAdams, D. P. (1996). Narrating the self in adulthood. In J. E. Birren & G. M. Kenyon (Eds.), *Aging and biography: Explorations in adult development.* (pp. 131–148). New York: Springer.

McAdams, D. P. (1997). A conceptual history of personality psychology. In R. Hogan, J. Johnson, & S. Briggs (Eds.), *Handbook of personality psychology* (pp. 3–39). San Diego, CA: Academic Press.

McClelland, D. C., Atkinson, J. W., Clark, R. A., & Lowell, E. L. (1953). *The achievement motive.* New York: Appleton-Century-Crofts.

McCrae, R. R., & Costa, P. T., Jr. (1995). Trait explanations in personality psychology. *European Journal of Personality, 9*, 231–252.

McCrae, R. R., & Costa, P. T., Jr. (1996). Toward a new generation of personality theories: Theoretical contexts for the five-factor model. In J. S. Wiggins (Ed.), *The five-factor model of personality: Theoretical perspectives* (pp. 51-87). New York: Guilford Press.

McCrae, R. R., & Costa, P. T., Jr. (1997). Personality trait structure as a human universal. *American Psychologist, 52*, 509–516.

McGuire, W. J., & McGuire, C. V. (1986). Differences in conceptualizing self versus conceptualizing other people as manifested in contrasting verb types used in natural speech. *Journal of Personality and Social Psychology, 51*, 1135–1143.

Meichenbaum, D. (1990). Paying homage: Providing challenges [Review of the book *Social foundations of thought and action*]. *Psychological Inquiry, 1*, 96–100.

Miller, L. C., & Read, S. J. (1991). On the coherence of mental models of persons and relationships: A knowledge structure approach. In G. J. O. Fletcher & F. Fincham (Eds.), *Cognition in close relationships* (pp. 69–99). Hillsdale, NJ: Erlbaum.

Miller, S. M., Shoda, Y., & Hurley, K. (1996). Applying cognitive-social theory to health-protective behavior: Breast self-examination in cancer screening. *Psychological Bulletin, 119*, 70–94.

Mischel, W. (1968). *Personality and assessment.* New York: Wiley.

Mischel, W. (1973). Toward a cognitive social learning reconceptualization of personality. *Psychological Review, 80*, 252–283.

Mischel, W. (1974). Processes in delay of gratification. In L. Berkowitz (Ed.), *Advances in experimental social psychology* (Vol. 7, pp. 249–292). San Diego, CA: Academic Press.

Mischel, W. (1979). On the interface of cognition and personality: Beyond the person–situation debate. *American Psychologist, 34*, 740–754.

Mischel, W., & Shoda, Y. (1994). Personality psychology has two goals: Must it be two fields? *Psychological Inquiry, 5*, 156–158.

Mischel, W., & Shoda, Y. (1995). A cognitive-affective system theory of personality: Reconceptualizing situations, dispositions, dynamics, and invariance in personality structure. *Psychological Review, 102*, 246–286.

Murphy, G. (1947). *Personality: A biosocial approach to origins and structure.* New York: Harper.

Murray, H. A., and collaborators. (1938). *Explorations in personality.* New York: Oxford University Press.

Neisser, U., Boodoo, G., Bouchard, T. J., Boykin, A. W., Ceci, S. J., Halpern, D. F., Loehlin, J. C., Perloff, R., Sternberg, R. J., & Urbina, S. (1996). Intelligence: Knowns and unknowns. *American Psychologist, 51,* 77–101.

Newman, L. S., Duff, K. J., & Baumeister, R. F. (1997). A new look at defensive projection: Thought suppression, accessibility, and biased person perception. *Journal of Personality and Social Psychology, 72,* 980–1001.

Ohlsson, S. (1993). Abstract schemas. *Educational Psychologist, 28,* 51–66.

Ohlsson, S. (1998). Spearman's *g* = Anderson's ACT?: Reflections on the locus of generality in human cognition. *Journal of the Learning Sciences, 7,* 135–145.

O'Leary, A., & Brown, S. (1995). Self-efficacy and the physiological stress response. In J. E. Maddux (Ed.), *Self-efficacy, adaptation, and adjustment: Theory, research, and application* (pp. 227–246). New York: Plenum Press.

Pervin, L. A. (Ed.). (1989). *Goal concepts in personality and social psychology.* Hillsdale, NJ: Erlbaum.

Pervin, L. A. (1994). A critical analysis of current trait theory. *Psychological Inquiry, 5,* 103–113.

Pervin, L. A., & John, O. P. (1997). *Personality: Theory and research* (7th ed.). New York: Wiley.

Pinker, S. (1997). *How the mind works.* New York: Norton.

Rehm, L. P. (1982). Self-management in depression. In P. Karoly & F. H. Kanfer (Eds.), *Self-management and behavior change: From theory to practice.* New York: Pergamon Press.

Revelle, W. (1995). Personality processes. *Annual Review of Psychology, 46,* 295–328.

Roberts, B. W. (1997). Plaster or plasticity: Are work experiences associated with personality change in women? *Journal of Personality, 65,* 205–232.

Rorer, L. G. (1990). Personality assessment: A conceptual survey. In L. A. Pervin (Ed.), *Handbook of personality: Theory and research* (pp. 693–720). New York: Guilford Press.

Rosenthal, T. L., & Zimmerman, B. J. (1978). *Social learning and cognition.* New York: Academic Press.

Ross, M. (1989). Relation of implicit theories to the construction of personal histories. *Psychological Review, 96,* 341–357.

Rotter, J. B. (1954). *Social learning and clinical psychology.* Englewood Cliffs, NJ: Prentice-Hall.

Salmon, W. C. (1989). Four decades of scientific explanation. In P. Kitcher & W. C. Salmon (Eds.), *Minnesota studies in the philosophy of science: Vol. XIII. Scientific explanation.* Minneapolis: University of Minnesota Press.

Saudino, K. J. (1997). Moving beyond the heritability question: New directions in behavioral genetic studies of personality. *Current Directions in Psychological Science, 6,* 86–90.

Schank, R. C., & Abelson, R. P. (1977). *Scripts, plans, goals, and understanding.* Hillsdale, NJ: Erlbaum.

Schunk, D. H., & Zimmerman, B. J. (1994). *Self-regulation of learning and performance: Issues and educational applications.* Hillsdale, NJ: Erlbaum.

Schwarz, N. (1990). Feelings as information: Information and motivational functions of affective states. In E. T. Higgins & R. M. Sorrentino (Eds.), *Motivation and cognition: Foundations of social behavior* (Vol. 2, pp. 527–561). New York: Guilford Press.

Scott, W. D., & Cervone, D. (1998). *The influence of negative affect on self-regulatory cognition.* Unpublished manuscript, University of Miami.

Sears, R. R., Rau, L., & Alpert, R. (1965). *Identification and child rearing.* Stanford, CA: Stanford University Press.

Sears, R. R., Maccoby, E., E., & Levin, H. (1957). *Patterns of child rearing.* Evanston, IL: Row, Peterson.

Shadel, W. G., & Cervone, D. (1993). The big five versus nobody? *American Psychologist, 48,* 1300–1302.

Shadel, W. G., Niaura, R., & Abrams, D. (in press). An idiographic approach to understanding personality structure and individual differences among smokers. *Cognitive Therapy and Research.*

Shoda, Y., & Mischel, W. (1993). Cognitive social approach to dispositional inferences: What if the perceiver is a cognitive-social theorist? *Personality and Social Psychology Bulletin, 19,* 574–585.

Shoda, Y., & Mischel, W. (1998). Personality as a stable cognitive-affective activation network: Characteristic patterns of behavior variation emerge from a stable personality structure. In S. J. Read & L. C. Miller (Ed.), *Connectionist and PDP models of social reasoning and social behavior* (pp. 175–208). Mahwah, NJ: Erlbaum.

Shoda, Y., Mischel, W., & Wright, J. C. (1994). Intra-individual stability in the organization and patterning of behavior: Incorporating psychological situations into the idiographic analysis of personality. *Journal of Personality and Social Psychology, 67,* 674–687.

Singer, J. A., & Salovey, P. (1996). Motivated memory: Self-defining memories, goals, and affect regulation. In L. L. Martin & A. Tesser (Eds.), *Striving and feeling: Inter actions among goals, affect, and self-regulation* (pp. 229–250). Hillsdale, NJ: Erlbaum.

Simon, H. A. (1983). *Reason in human affairs.* Stanford, CA: Stanford University Press.

Skinner, B. F. (1938). *The behavior of organisms.* New York: Appleton-Century-Crofts.

Skinner, B. F. (1953). *Science and human behavior.* New York: Macmillan.

Skinner, B. F. (1971). *Beyond freedom and dignity.* New York: Knopf.

Smith, C. A., & Lazarus, R. S. (1990). Emotion and adaptation. In L. A. Pervin (Ed.), *Handbook of personality: Theory and research* (pp. 609–637). New York: Guilford Press.

Smith, C. A., & Lazarus, R. S. (1993). Appraisal components, core relational themes, and the emotions. *Cognition and Emotion, 7,* 233–269.

Sternberg, R. J. (1985). *Beyond I.Q.: A triarchic theory of human intelligence.* New York: Cambridge University Press.

Tellegen, A. (1991). Personality traits: Issues of definition, evidence, and assessment. In W. M. Grove & D. Cicchetti (Eds.), *Thinking clearly about psychology: Vol. 2. Personality and psychopathology* (pp. 1–35). Minneapolis: University of Minnesota Press.

Thagard, P. (1989). Explanatory coherence. *Behavioral and Brain Sciences, 12,* 435–467.

Vallacher, R. R., & Wegner, D. M. (1986). What do people think they're doing? Action identification in human behavior. *Psychological Review, 94,* 3–15.

Watson, D., & Clark, L. A. (1997). Extraversion and its positive emotional core. In R. Hogan, J. Johnson, & S. Briggs (Eds.), *Handbook of personality psychology* (pp. 767–793). San Diego, CA: Academic Press.

Wellin, E. (1955). Water boiling in a Peruvian town. In B. D. Paul (Ed.), *Health, culture, and community: Case studies of public reactions to health programs* (pp. 71–103). New York: Russell Sage Foundation.

Westen, D. (1991). Social cognition and object relations. *Psychological Bulletin, 109,* 429–455.

Wiggins, J. S., & Pincus, A. L. (1992). Personality: Structure and assessment. *Annual Review of Psychology, 43,* 473–504.

Wilensky, R. (1983). *Planning and understanding: A computational approach to human reasoning.* New York: Addison-Wesley.

Williams, S. L. (1995). Self-efficacy, anxiety, and phobic disorders. In J. Maddux (Ed.), *Self-efficacy, adaptation, and adjustment: Theory, research, and application* (pp. 69–107). New York: Plenum Press.

Wilson, G. T. (1989). The treatment of bulimia nervosa: A cognitive-social learning analysis. In A. J. Stunkard & A. Baum (Eds.), *Eating, sleep and sexual disorders* (pp. 73–98). Hillsdale, NJ: Erlbaum.

Woodward, W. R. (1982). The "discovery" of social behaviorism and social learning theory, 1870–1980. *American Psychologist, 37,* 396–410.

Wright, J., & Mischel, W. (1982). Influence of affect on cognitive social learning person variables. *Journal of Personality and Social Psychology, 43,* 901–914.

Zuckerman, M. (1995). Good and bad humors: Biochemical bases of personality and its disorders. *Psychological Science, 6,* 325–332.

II

Knowledge Structures and Encoding Processes as a Source of Coherence

2

Personality Coherence and Dispositions in a Cognitive-Affective Personality System (CAPS) Approach

WALTER MISCHEL

In the last decade, fundamental controversies and debates in the search for personality coherence have been replaced by discoveries and reconceptualizations that identify and explain its nature and structure. These efforts promise to resolve paradoxes that have long split the area of personality and to advance personality theory in line with exciting progress in other areas of social and cognitive science. In this chapter, I consider personality coherence, dispositions, dynamics, and structure from the perspective of a social-cognitive-affective processing approach (e.g., Mischel & Shoda, 1995, 1998). After quickly sketching some of the history that impacts on the present scene, I turn to the current agenda, focusing on aspects of personality coherence and personality theory that merit attention but that risk being neglected within the contemporary social-cognitive framework. Cervone (Chapter 9, this volume) points to that neglect, noting on his opening page the common critique (by traditional personality psychologists) of social-cognitive approaches as "containing lists of seemingly disconnected personality processes that fail to explain the coherent functioning of the whole person."

On one hand, these principles, both singly and collectively, advance our understanding of basic social-cognitive-motivational processes and are among the most important gains emerging from a century of personality psychology. On the other hand, if the field is to retain its most basic goal, these principles must be applied in concert to understand the individual as an organized coherent functioning system—the fundamental unit of analysis to which personality psychology has been committed since its inception (Allport, 1937). That seems a challenge that needs to be taken seriously if the perspectives represented in this volume are to have the impact on personality psychology that they merit. This chapter addresses that challenge and considers the framework required to encompass both the dispositions that characterize the person and the processes that underlie them.

My particular emphasis will be on the construct of personality dispositions and its role and potential value within a processing approach to personality in a broadly social-cognitive framework. I try to show that dispositions can readily be incorporated within such a framework at several different levels of analysis that are easily confused and need to be distinguished. A unitary approach in the study of personality that encompasses both dispositions and the processes that underlie them seems to me sorely needed given the depth of the unconstructive splits that have occurred within the area of personality, as also discussed in this chapter. But first, I consider the history that has led us here and that needs to be understood in an effort to resolve the issues that remain.

THE PAST: CONSISTENCY LOST?

Paradigm Perturbations

This volume goes to press in the 70th anniversary year of the discoveries by Hartshorne and May (1928), and concurrently by Newcomb (1929), that the cross-situational consistency of behavior—which they assessed empirically in school and camp settings with such laborious care and at high cost—seemed to be grossly discrepant from the assumptions of the classical personality trait conceptions that guided their search: Namely, it was assumed that individuals are characterized by behavioral dispositions (like the tendency to be conscientious or honest or sociable) that are manifested relatively stably and consistently across many different types of situations. Their failure to find strong support for this belief only briefly perturbed the then-young field (although it did lead Newcomb to switch his career from personality to social psychology). But their studies did not challenge the traditional trait paradigm: Mainstream work within it continued and accelerated—as it still does.

The assessment needs of World War II demanded quick personality trait measurements and further stimulated work within the traditional paradigm with little time or opportunity to evaluate the utility or the theoretical implications of the results. It was not until 40 years after the discoveries of Hartshorne, May, and Newcomb, that the paradigm itself was challenged (Mischel, 1968; Peterson, 1968). That confrontation, now having its 30th anniversary, grew out of the embarrassing discrepancy between the numbers found in the extensive data that had accumulated and the still-regnant and unruffled classic trait theoretical assumptions of the field. It became apparent to quite a few personality researchers that we were ending our discussion sections with more apologies and self-criticisms than conclusions.

Paradigm Crisis

The upsets that spiraled into a paradigm crisis converged from several directions: A core assumption of trait psychology concerning the cross-situational consistency of behavior was contradicted by the small albeit nonzero (but not by much) cross-situational consistency coefficients found when researchers actually assessed people's behavior across even seemingly similar situations. Simultaneously, analyses of the utility of the approach for the prediction of behavior in particular situations, as well as its explanatory power, cast deep doubts on both.

Classic psychodynamic theory was the major alternative available at that time and hence the tempting option. It made no assumption of cross-situational consistency in behavior (nor claimed any predictive utility) but relied crucially on clinical judgments. The theory's Achilles heel was that the accuracy and utility of those inferences and judgments were undermined by evidence documenting the limitations of clinicians and their proneness to self-deceptive illusions of confidence (Chapman & Chapman, 1969; Mischel, 1968; Peterson, 1968). Consequently both routes to personality coherence and to personality itself—behavioral dispositions and underlying dynamics—were vulnerable.

Although *Personality and Assessment* (Mischel, 1968) was started with the intention of reviewing the state of the field, it was seen as a glove hurled to the ground. The first reactions in the early 1970s seemed devoted to arguing against the legitimacy of the critique and tried to deny its validity. (When first published, it was reviewed briefly on a back page of *Contemporary Psychology* and dismissed under the header "Personality Unvanquished.") In the next decade, the controversies and paradoxes of the field concerning the nature, locus, and even existence of personality coherence were articulated and debated and in time researched. Various routes both for continuing business as usual or for finding constructive alternatives and solutions were outlined and pursued.

The heated disputes that then raged sharpened and often exaggerated the differences between approaches. One fallout was the warfare between social and personality psychologists. In those battles, for at least a decade, the former were seen as the champions of the situation and its power (Nisbett & Ross, 1980), and the latter felt themselves the beleaguered defenders of the person and the construct of personality (e.g., Carlson, 1971). Although that may by now seem like ancient history, it remains relevant for the current agenda as background for understanding the almost reflexive hostility that developed between two subdisciplines that previously had been unified in a constructive collaboration.

The early consequences of these confrontations included dividing the flagship *Journal of Personality and Social Psychology* into three separate unconnected sections, one for social cognition and attitudes, one for interpersonal processes, one for personality—a move virtually guaranteed to obstruct efforts to understand persons (including their minds, feelings, and relationships) in their contexts. For more than a decade in this new structure, the third part, Personality, defined its mission as welcoming articles devoted to personality "as traditionally defined," that is, in terms of broad traits, suggesting a perspective that seems more defensive than scientific. Overcoming that unfortunate way of parsing the variance and the enterprise has been perhaps the largest barrier in the search for personality coherence, in my view, and fortunately, there now are creative routes for doing so (e.g., Zelli & Dodge, Chapter 4, this volume; Grant & Dweck, Chapter 10, this volume; Higgins, Chapter 3, this volume; Shoda, Chapter 6, this volume).

Search for Solutions

The Classic Personality Paradox

There also were constructive proposals to identify the conditions under which cross-situational consistency could be demonstrated. Most notably, Bem and Allen (1974) hypothesized that while, on the one hand, our intuitions convince us that people have broad behavioral dispositions that we believe are seen in the individual's extensive behavioral consistency across situations, the research results persistently contradict those intuitions. Naming this the "personality paradox," Bem and Allen tried try to prove that our intuitions are better than our research. They reasoned that the inconsistency of those for whom the trait is irrelevant will obscure the real consistency of the subset of people for whom the trait is relevant. Consequently, researchers have to preselect those persons who perceive themselves as consistent in the given disposition (and for whom the trait is thus relevant): Then high cross-situational consistency will be visible in their behavior in that domain, but it will not be seen in the behavior of those who perceive themselves as inconsistent.

In Pursuit of Consistency: The Carleton College Study

To test this proposal comprehensively, the Carleton College field study extensively observed behavior relevant to conscientiousness (and friendliness) *in vivo* over multiple situations and occasions that had been preselected as relevant by the students themselves (Mischel & Peake, 1982). Conscientiousness was sampled in various situations such as in the classroom, in the dormitory, in the library, and the assessments occurred over repeated occasions in the course of the semester to enhance reliability. It was found that the actual consistency in the cross-situational behavior of students who perceived themselves as consistent in their conscientiousness was as low as it was for those who perceived themselves as variable. (Indeed, the same pattern was found in Bem-Allen's own results, as discussed in Mischel & Peake, 1982.)

The Carleton College results (Mischel & Peake, 1982) shocked and split the field further. They were generally viewed by trait-oriented personality psychologists as yet another hostile claim by the "situationists" that there is no personality consistency, except perhaps the sort that is an illusory construction (Bem, 1983; Epstein, 1983; Funder, 1983). Neglected was the possibility that those data also pointed the way to discovering a second type of personality coherence that could serve to resolve the personality paradox. Namely, a person's self-perceived consistency with regard to a behavior such as conscientiousness seemed to be rooted not in higher cross-situational consistency in behavior (as Bem and Allen and the traditional trait view assumed): Rather, it seemed to link to the temporal stability of some relevant prototypical behaviors—hardly an illusion, although not the locus of consistency expected by trait theory.

THE PRESENT: A SPLIT PERSONALITY PSYCHOLOGY

In retrospect, the Carleton College findings seem to have been a step, inadvertently, in leading to partitioning personality psychology into two distinct approaches—perhaps really splitting it into two different subdisciplines. After years of debate, at last there was consensus about the state of the data— the average cross-situational consistency coefficient is nonzero but not by much (Bem, 1983; Epstein, 1983; Funder, 1983). But there was and is deep disagreement about how to interpret the data and proceed in the field of personality psychology. Two main alternatives developed, often in seeming opposition and conflict.

The Mainstream Aggregation Solution: Remove the Situation to Find Broad Behavioral Dispositions

The most widely accepted strategy adopted within the mainstream behavioral disposition approach to personality acknowledges the low cross-situational consistency in behavior found from situation to situation: It then systematically removes the situation by aggregating the individual's behavior on a given dimension (e.g., "conscientiousness") over many different situations (or "items") to estimate an overall "true score" (as discussed in Epstein, 1979, 1980; Mischel & Peake, 1982). That approach can be extremely useful for many goals, but its limits—as well as its strengths—are seen by analogy to meteorology, as Mischel and Shoda (1995) discussed. Although overall climatic trends surely are worth knowing, if meteorologists were to focus only on the aggregate climatic trends, they would neglect the atmo-spheric processes that underlie the changing weather patterns, as well as give up the goal of more accurate specific weather predictions.

Thus bypassing the issues that had been raised in the "paradigm crisis," much of contemporary mainstream personality psychology proceeds in an atmosphere its advocates describe as "euphoria" within an unrevised and even more extreme global trait framework (e.g., Funder, 1991), particularly the optimistically named Big Five (e.g., Goldberg, 1993; McCrae & Costa, 1996, 1997). It focuses on identifying a few broad behavioral dispositions that will manifest themselves stably across many situations and that characterize the individual in trait terms with regard to their position on each of the five factors. It does so in coexistence with sharply critical reviews of the problems and data that continue to undermine this approach fundamentally (e.g., Block, 1995; McAdams, 1992; Pervin, 1994)—criticisms and data that seem unnervingly similar to those that stirred the crises three decades earlier—and that apparently still remain largely unheeded.

The Alternative Route: Search for Social-Cognitive-Motivational Processes Underlying Person × Situation Interactions

Social and personality psychologists who were unwilling to bypass the role of the situation and thus did not accept the field's mainstream solution—nor its sense of euphoria—have been pursuing their separate routes in a frame-work now called "social-cognitive" (or "cognitive-social"), as evident in this volume. Some of the main themes for this alternative route were outlined originally in the "cognitive social learning reconceptualization of personal-ity" (Mischel, 1973). Its goal was to make clear that the 1968 critique of the state of personality required not abandoning the construct of personality but rather *reconceptualizing* it to encompass within it the complex and often subtle interactions between person and situation that characterize individuals and types.

With that aim, the proposal identified the types of social-cognitive and motivational variables and principles required for a mediating process account of person–situation interactions and personality coherence. In this account, personality is conceptualized in terms of such constructs as how the individual encodes or appraises particular types of situations, the relevant expectancies and values that become activated, and the competencies and self-regulatory strategies available (Mischel, 1973, 1990). The behavior pat-terns that unfold depend on the interactions among these person variables in relation to the particular type of situation (e.g., Mischel & Shoda, 1995).

The last quarter-century has seen diverse creative efforts in this general framework (many illustrated in this volume) and in many novel directions to conceptualize and clarify personality-relevant processes and principles (e.g., Mischel, 1998). Although each has its distinctive features and focus, most share the goal of wanting to explain the nature of intraindividual coherence and the mechanisms and conditions that generate it. The contributions in this volume attest to the richness of the yield.

Reconceptualizing—and Finding—Coherence in Unexpected Places

Much of the research that Shoda and I and our colleagues pursued within this general framework in recent years was directed at clarifying the nature of personality consistency. Briefly, our reasoning (in accord with Mischel, 1973; Mischel & Shoda, 1995, 1998; Shoda, Chapter 6, this volume) was that if personality is a stable system that processes the information about the situations, external or internal, then it follows that, as individuals encounter different situations, their behaviors should vary across the situations. These variations should reflect important differences among the individuals in the psychologically active features for them and in the ways they process them. That is, they should reflect, in part, the structure and organization of their personality systems, for example, how they encoded the situations and the expectations, affects, and goals that became activated within them (Mischel & Shoda, 1995).

If... Then... Situation–Behavior Profiles

Over time this will generate distinctive and stable *if...then...* situation–behavior profiles of characteristic elevation and shape like those illustrated and discussed by Shoda (Chapter 6, this volume). So that even if two people are similar in their overall average "aggressiveness," for example, they will manifest distinctive, predictable patterns of behavioral variability in their *if...then...* signatures of when and with whom and where they do and do not aggress. As Shoda's chapter illustrates, these expectations have been extensively supported empirically (e.g., Shoda, Mischel, & Wright, 1993a, 1993b, 1994).

These profiles provide a glimpse of the pattern of behavior variation in relation to situations that is expressive of personality invariance but that is completely bypassed in the traditional search for cross-situational consistency. Instead of searching for the traditional cross-situational consistency coefficient that has been pursued for most of the century (e.g., Hartshorne & May, 1928; Mischel, 1968; Newcomb, 1929; Peterson, 1968; Vernon, 1964), personality coherence can be found—and should be expected—in the intraindividual stable pattern of variability.

The results also make it evident that a focus on the relationships between psychological features of situations and the individual's patterns of behavior, rather than undermining the existence of personality, has to become part of the assessment and conception of personality (e.g., Mischel, 1973, 1990; Wright & Mischel, 1987; Shoda & Mischel, 1993; Shoda et al., 1994). It is obvious of course that if situation units are defined in terms of features salient for the researcher but trivial for, or irrelevant to, the individuals studied, one cannot expect their behaviors to vary meaningfully across them. In that case, the resulting pattern of behavior variation may well be unstable and meaningless. To discover the potentially predictable patterns of behavior variability that characterize individuals, one first has to identify those features of situations that are meaningful to them and that engage their important psychological qualities (e.g., their ways of encoding or construing, their expectancies, and goals). Fortunately the methodology to make that possible is now becoming available (e.g., Shoda et al., 1994; Wright & Mischel, 1987).

Behavioral Signatures of Personality: The Locus of Self-Perceived Consistency and Dispositional Judgments

The profiles of situation–behavior relations that characterize a person constitute a sort of "behavioral signature of personality" that in turn is linked to the person's self-perceived consistency and sense of coherence (Mischel & Shoda, 1995; Shoda et al., 1993b). This was found in a reanalysis by Mischel and Shoda (1995) of the Carleton College field study (Mischel & Peake, 1982). In that study, college students were repeatedly observed on campus in various situations relevant to their conscientiousness in the college setting (such as in the classroom, in the dormitory, in the library, assessed over repeated occasions in the semester). Students who perceived themselves as consistent did not show greater overall cross-situational consistency than those who did not. But for individuals who perceived themselves as consistent, the average situation–behavior profile stability correlation was near .5, whereas it was trivial for those who viewed themselves as inconsistent. So it is the stability in the situation–behavior profiles (e.g., conscientious about homework but not about punctuality), not the cross-situational consistency of behavior that underlies the perception of consistency with regard to a type of behavior or disposition.

In sum, relatively stable situation–behavior profiles reflect characteristic intraindividual patterns in how the person relates to different psychological conditions or features of situations, forming a sort of behavioral signature of personality (Shoda et al., 1994). The stability of these situation–behavior profiles in turn predicts the self-perception of consistency as well. These profiles are also linked to the dispositional judgments made about the person by others (Shoda et al., 1994). The surprise is not simply that this type of behavioral signature of personality exists, but rather that it has so long been treated as error and deliberately removed by averaging behavior over diverse situations to remove their role. Ironically, although such aggregation was intended to capture personality, it actually can delete data that reflect the individual's most distinctive qualities and unique intraindividual patterning.

These expectations and findings are congruent with classic processing theories, most notably Freud's conception of psychodynamics. In that view, peoples' underlying processing dynamics and qualities—the construals and goals, the motives and passions, that drive them—may be reflected not only in how often they display particular types of behavior but also in when and where, and thus also, and most importantly, *why* that behavior occurs. In short, this type of model expects that the stable patterns of situation–behavior relationships that characterize persons provide potential keys to their dynamics. They are informative roads to the underlying system that produces them, not sources of error to be eliminated systematically by aggregating out the situation. Thus, in the present approach, the concept of the invariances in the expression of personality is broadened to encompass the profile of situation–behavior relations that might characterize the person, not just the overall average level of particular types of behavior aggregated across diverse situations (e.g., Shoda et al., 1993a, 1994).

PERSONALITY RECONSIDERED:
TOWARD A UNIFYING FRAMEWORK

The above findings—and the confirmation of the hypotheses that predicted them—directly violate the assumptions made if one conceptualizes personality in terms of traits as behavioral dispositions. In that classic view, the intraindividual variations in a type of behavior across situations, given that the main effects of situations are removed by standardization, should reflect only intrinsic unpredictability or measurement error. If that assumption were correct, then the stability of the intraindividual pattern of variation should on average be zero. The finding that the situation–behavior profiles reliably reflect a statistically significant, stable facet of individual differences in social behavior thus has major implications for how one thinks about personality coherence and the kind of personality model that is needed.

The data provide clear evidence at the level of *in vivo* behavior observed extensively as it unfolds across situations and over time in everyday life (Mischel & Shoda, 1995). They are consistent with parallel findings showing significant amounts of variance attributable to person × situation interaction in analysis of variance studies, based on questionnaire responses (e.g., Endler & Hunt, 1969; Endler & Magnusson, 1976; Endler, Hunt, & Rosenstein, 1962; Magnusson & Endler, 1977). Furthermore, as shown elsewhere (Shoda, 1990), the degree that an individual is characterized by stable patterns of situation–behavior relations is necessarily negatively related to the level of overall cross-situational consistency that can be expected, making it clear that the quest for higher cross-situational consistency coefficients is bound to be futile.

The need now is for a personality theory, or at least an approach to personality, designed to try to predict and explain these signatures of personality, rather than to eliminate or ignore them. Such an approach requires rethinking the nature of personality coherence, and of personality dispositions, structure, and dynamics, as discussed next.

Personality as an Organized Dynamic System

A first requirement is to develop a processing model of the personality system at the level of the individual (Mischel & Shoda, 1995). In such a model, person variables, no matter how important, function not just as single, isolated variables but as components that are interconnected within an organized system of relationships that in turn interacts with the social-psychological situations in which the system is activated (e.g., Shoda & Mischel, 1998). That also requires conceptualizing the "situation" not just as a setting but in psychological terms (Shoda et al., 1994).

In short, an urgent theoretical need is to conceptualize personality as an organized system that is interactive and dynamic—a system that accounts both for intraindividual coherence and stability, on the one hand, and for plasticity and discriminativeness in behavior, on the other hand. It needs to take account of the individual's characteristic dispositions as well as of the dynamic mediating processes that underlie them. It has to consider not only social-cognitive-motivational and affective determinants and processes but also biological and genetic antecedents and levels. And it must be able to deal with the complexity of human personality and the cognitive-affective dynamics, conscious and unconscious—both 'cool' and 'hot,' cognitive and emotional, rational and impulsive—that underlie the individual's distinctive, characteristic internal states and external behavioral expressions (see Metcalfe & Jacobs, 1998; Metcalfe & Mischel, 1999).

A number of recent processing models now focus not just on how much of a particular mental representation or unit (e.g., of self-efficacy expectations, of fear of failure) a person has, but rather on how the units are related to each other within the processing system. These interconnections form a unique network that functions as an organized whole—a dynamic interacting, processing system that can operate rapidly in parallel at multiple levels of accessibility, awareness, and automaticity. Rather than conceptualizing the individual as a bundle of mediating variables or as a flow chart of discrete procedures and decision rules, this provides a more parallel and distributed (rather than serial, centralized) processing system. Particularly promising developments come from recent work in cognitive neuroscience, such as the neural network theories and connectionist models (e.g., Anderson, 1996; Kandel & Hawkins, 1992; Rumelhart & McClelland, 1986). Within such a framework, one can begin to conceptualize social information processing in terms of a dynamic organized network of interconnected and interacting representations—cognitions and affects (e.g., Kunda & Thagard, 1996; Read &

Miller, 1998; Shultz & Lepper, 1996)—operating at various levels of aware-ness (e.g., Westen, 1990). Our own attempt to move personality theory in this direction is the recently proposed cognitive-affective personality system (CAPS) (Mischel & Shoda, 1995, 1998; Shoda & Mischel, 1998).

Cognitive-Affective Personality System (CAPS)

According to CAPS, individuals differ first of all in the "chronic accessibility," that is, the ease, with which particular cognitive-affective units become acti-vated. These units refer to the mental-emotional representations—the cognitions and affects or feelings—that are available to the person. Such mediating units were conceptualized initially in terms of five relatively stable person variables on which individuals differ in processing self-relevant infor-mation (Mischel, 1973). Over the years, these units have been modified by research (reviewed in Mischel & Shoda, 1995; Mischel, Cantor, & Feldman, 1996), and the units within the CAPS system now include affects and goals, as well as encodings, expectancies, beliefs, competencies, and self-regulatory plans and strategies.

Individual Differences in the Stable Organization of Relations among Units (Interconnections)

The CAPS model goes beyond the earlier focus on person variables (Mischel, 1973) in emphasizing that stable individual differences reflect not only the accessibility of particular cognitions and affects but also the distinctive *organi-zation of relationships* among them. This organization guides and constrains the activation of the particular cognitions, affects, and actions that are avail-able within the system. It is this organization that constitutes the basic stable structure of personality and that underlies the behavioral signatures of per-sonality described above.

CAPS is a system that interacts continuously and dynamically with the social world in which it is contextualized. It is activated in part by external situations and in part by its own internal cognitive and affective activities, including fantasy, daydreaming, and planning (Mischel et al., 1996; Shoda & Mischel, 1996). The interactions with the external word involve a two-way reciprocal interaction: behaviors that the personality system generates impact on the social world, partly shaping and selecting the interpersonal situations the person subsequently faces and that, in turn, influence the person (e.g., Bandura, 1986; Buss, 1987).

Dynamic, Transactional System: The Active–Proactive Person

Figure 2.1 shows a schematic, greatly simplified CAPS system that is character-ized by the available cognitive and affective units, organized in a distinctive

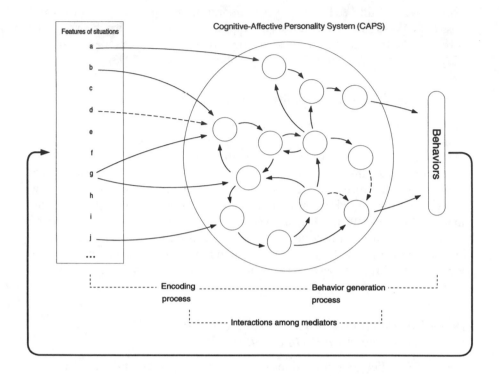

FIGURE 2.1. Simplified illustration of types of cognitive-affective mediating processes that generate an individual's distinctive behavior patterns. Situational features are encoded by a given mediating unit, which activates specific subsets of other mediating units, generating distinctive cognition, affect, and behavior in response to different situations. Mediating units become activated in relation to some situational features, deactivated (inhibited) in relation to others, and are unaffected by the rest. The activated mediating units affect other mediating units through a stable network of relations that characterize an individual. The relation may be positive (solid line), which increases the activation, or negative (dashed line), which decreases the activation. From Mischel and Shoda (1995). Copyright 1995 by the American Psychological Association, Inc. Reprinted by permission.

network of interrelations. When certain features of a situation are perceived by the individual, a characteristic pattern of cognitions and affects (shown schematically as circles) becomes activated through this distinctive network of connections. The personality structure refers to the person's stable system of interconnections among the cognitive and affective units, and it is this structure that guides and constrains further activation of other units throughout the network. Ultimately the result is the activation of plans, strategies, and potential behaviors in a characteristic pattern that is situationally contextualized.

In CAPS, mediating units become activated in relation to some situation features but are deactivated or inhibited in relation to others and not affected by the rest. That is, the connections among units within the stable network that characterizes the person may be positive, which increases the activation, or negative (shown as broken lines in Figure 2.1), which decreases the activation.

The personality system anticipates, interprets, rearranges, and changes situations as well as reacts to them. It thus is active and indeed proactive, not just reactive. It not only responds to the environment but also may generate, select, modify, and shape situations in reciprocal transactions (Figure 2.2).

Activation of Personality Dynamics and Dispositions in Context

People differ characteristically in the particular situational features (e.g., being teased, being approached socially, feeling lonely) that are the salient active ingredients for them and that thus activate their characteristic and relatively predictable patterns of cognitive, affective, and behavioral reactions to those situations, that is, their distinctive processing dynamics (Mischel & Shoda, 1995). For example, some individuals readily respond aggressively to

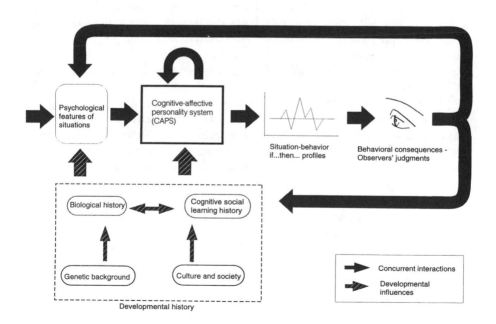

FIGURE 2.2. The cognitive-affective personality system (CAPS) in relation to concurrent interactions and developmental influences. From Mischel and Shoda (1995). Copyright 1995 by the American Psychological Association, Inc. Reprinted by permission.

such ambiguous stimuli as having milk spilled on them in the cafeteria line (Dodge, 1986). There also are internal feedback loops within the system through which self-generated stimuli (as in thinking, fantasizing, daydreaming) activate their distinctive pathways of connections, triggering characteristic cognitive-affective-behavioral reaction patterns (e.g., Shoda & Mischel, 1998). The behaviors the person constructs may in turn affect the interpersonal environment and social ecology, which changes the situational features that are encountered subsequently (e.g., Dodge 1986, 1993, 1997a, 1997b).

Variations across Situations: Stable Individual Differences in Situation–Behavior, If...Then... Relations

It follows from the assumptions of the CAPS model that the variation in the person's behavior in relation to changing situations in part constitutes a potentially meaningful reflection of the personality system itself. Different cognitions, affects, and behaviors become activated as the situation and its features change, even when the interconnections among them remain unchanged across situations. That is, the personality system determines the *relationships* among the types of situations encountered and the cognitive, affective, and behavioral responses: Thus, as the *ifs* change, so do the *thens*, but the *relationship* between them is stable as long as the personality system remains unchanged. This assumption leads the approach to predict characteristic, predictable patterns of variation in the individual's behavior across situations—that is, the sorts of stable situation–behavior, *if...then...* profiles that were in fact found in the empirical studies summarized above (Mischel & Shoda, 1995).

Further support that CAPS generates the theoretically expected *if... then...* profiles came from a computer simulation (Mischel & Shoda, 1995; Shoda & Mischel, 1998). It was shown that individual differences in the connections (patterns of activation pathways) among the internal representations determine the links between features of situations and the outcomes generated by the system. An individual's unique configuration of person variables is manifested in the uniqueness of the *if...then...* profiles that unfold. Thus, to recapitulate, the personality system is expressed in the pattern with which a type of behavior varies over a set of situations, as well as in the average level of the behavior: Predictable variability in relation to context becomes a key to the individual's stability and coherence, a sign of the underlying system that generates it.

The System in Action: Linking Processing Dynamics to Dispositions

To illustrate such a system in action, consider a person characterized by the disposition of "rejection sensitivity" (Downey & Feldman, 1996; Downey,

Freitas, Michaelis, & Khouri, 1997). When this person begins to discuss a relationship problem with a romantic partner, for example, his anxious expectations trigger the tendency to scan for evidence of imminent rejection and to focus on and encode those features of the situation most likely to provide such evidence (Downey & Feldman, 1996). These expectations, affects, and behaviors interact and combine to lead the person to readily perceive rejection even in ambiguous situations, which in turn tends to activate behavioral scripts for hostility (Ayduk, Downey, Testa, Yin, & Shoda, in press). The hostility that is enacted can then elicit the partner rejection that is most feared, eroding the relationship in a self-defeating pattern, thereby confirming and maintaining rejection expectations (Downey et al., 1997).

Rejection sensitivity also illustrates the conditional nature of dispositions insofar as the activation of the characteristic pattern depends both on the situational features and on the cognitive-affective organization of the system. For example, the rejection-sensitive person becomes hostile specifically in relation to perceived rejection from a romantic partner but can behave exceptionally caringly and supportively in other situations (e.g., early in the relationship). Thus a characteristic and defining situation–behavior profile for this disposition may include both a tendency to become very angry and coercive and a tendency to be exceptionally sensitive and caring, each in its own distinctive context (Downey & Feldman, 1996). So the same rejection-sensitive man who coerces and abuses his partner also can behave in exceedingly tender and loving ways (e.g., Walker, 1979). He is both hurtful and kind, caring and uncaring, abusive and gentle.

Traditional analyses of such "inconsistencies" in personality raise the question "which one of these two people is the real one? What is simply the effect of the situation?" In contrast, the CAPS approach allows the same person to have contradictory facets that are equally genuine. The surface contradictions become comprehensible when one analyzes the network of relations among cognitions and affects to identify their psychological organization. The research problem becomes to understand when and why different cognitions and affects become activated predictably in relation to different features of situations, external and internal. The theory views the individual's distinctive patterns of variability not necessarily as internal contradictions but as the potentially predictable expressions of an underlying system that itself may remain quite stable in its organization. To reiterate, the stability of the disposition, which reflects the stability of the underlying system, is seen in the predictability of the *if... then...* profile, not in the consistency of behavior across different types of situations. The challenge is to discriminate, understand, and predict when each aspect will be activated and the dynamics that underlie the pattern. For example, are the caring and uncaring behaviors two scripts in the service of the same goal? If so, how are they connected to, and guided by, the person's self-conceptions and belief system in relation to the psychological features of situations that activate them?

Refining and Redefining the Constructs of Dispositions, Dynamics, and Personality Structure

Although it is widely asserted that process-oriented approaches to personality ignore or deny stable personality dispositions (e.g., Funder, 1991; Goldberg, 1993), in fact, in the present approach they have a significant role. The issue that does have to be addressed is just how to conceptualize "personality traits" or "dispositions" within a processing approach.

Given the depths of the splits and disputes that have occurred between the two approaches—personality as trait dispositions and personality as mediating underlying processes—it will not be a trivial task to reconcile and construct a unified theory and approach to personality. As Block (1995) and Pervin (1994), as well as Cervone (Chapter 9, this volume) and the other contributors to this volume, make plain, the equation of the Big Five or any other set of global traits or factors with personality psychology is unacceptable and needs to be rejected. More generally, to understand intraindividual dynamics and the resultant behavioral signatures, one needs to reject making behavioral dispositions of any sort synonymous with personality (Shoda, Chapter 6, this volume). Nevertheless, it would be unwise to throw out with these false equations the concept of dispositions: That concept—a foundation stone in personality psychology—requires reanalysis and refinement rather than rejection.

Dispositional Levels

As a first step, it may be useful to distinguish some of the different levels of analysis in the study of dispositions, since at each level the definition and the relevant phenomena shift, and often the level is left unclear, easily leading to misunderstandings. Let us consider the following four levels.

Psychological Processing Level. At the "psychological processing level" of analysis, dispositions within the present perspective may be defined by a characteristic social cognitive-affective processing structure that underlies, and generates, distinctive processing dynamics within the personality system (Mischel & Shoda, 1995), depicted as CAPS in the solid rectangle of Figure 2.2. A characteristic set of cognitions, affects, and behavioral strategies in an organization of interrelations that guides and constrains their activation constitutes the processing structure of the disposition. The processing dynamics of the disposition refer to the patterns and sequences of activation among the mediating units—the mental representations—that are generated when these persons encounter or construct situations containing relevant features.

The processing dynamics are activated in relation to particular types of situational features (e.g., certain interpersonal encounters). Some of these stimuli are external, but others are internally generated in many ways, such as by thinking or ruminating about situations (e.g., Nolen-Hoeksema, Parker, & Larson, 1994), or through selective recall and reexperiences of past events and feelings, or by daydreaming, fantasies, and scenarios that are planned or imagined (e.g., Taylor & Schneider, 1989). Dynamics can also be self-activated by selective attention, such as to one's perceived strengths, resources, vulnerabilities, conflicts, ambivalences, and anticipated future (e.g., Bandura, 1986; Mischel, Ebbesen, & Zeiss, 1973, 1976; Norem & Cantor, 1986). The pattern of activation among cognitions and affects in the personality system at a given time may be defined as the *personality state*.

Behavioral Level. At the level of directly observable behavior, the manifestations of a disposition and its processing dynamics are seen in the distinctive elevations and shapes of the situation–behavior profiles—the dispositional signatures—that distinguish its exemplars (see Figure 2.2). Individuals who have similar organizations of relations among cognitions and affects that become activated in relation to a particular distinctive set of situational features may be said to have a particular "processing disposition." These dispositions generate distinctive processing dynamics that become activated and, over time and contexts, will generate the situation–behavior profiles that have the characteristic elevations and shapes that identify the dispositional exemplars. It should be clear that, in this approach, personality psychologists do not have to choose between the study of dispositions or processes but can simultaneously analyze both the distinctive *if...then...* profiles that characterize the disposition's exemplars and illuminate the processes underlying them.

Perceived Personality Level: The Observer's View. The behavioral manifestations of the personality system may be readily and consensually encoded by observers (the eye shown in Figure 2.2) as reflections of person prototypes or exemplars, (e.g., Cantor, Mischel, & Schwartz, 1982; Wright & Mischel, 1987, 1988) and of traits and types in everyday psycholexical terms, both by lay perceivers (e.g., Jones, 1990) and psychologists (e.g., John, 1990; Goldberg, 1993; McCrae & Costa, 1996).

These encodings are related not just to the mean levels of different types of behavior displayed by a person, but also to the shape of the *if...then...* profiles that express their pattern of variability across situations. This was illustrated in a study that obtained personality prototype judgments for the sample of participants in the summer camp described in the first part of this article. As predicted, judgments by observers of how well individuals fit particular dispositional prototypes (e.g., the "friendly" child, the "withdrawn" child, the "aggressive" child) were related clearly to the shape of the observed-behavior situation profiles as well as to their average level of prototype-relevant behaviors (Shoda et al., 1993b). When the pattern of variability is changed, so are the personality judgments (Shoda, Mischel, & Wright, 1989).

Exemplars of different personality prototypes thus are characterized by distinctive patterns of stable *if...then...* profiles, as well as by the average frequency in their prototype-relevant behaviors, with high agreement. A "friendly person," for example, is seen as such not just because of her average level of friendliness but also because of the stable pattern of *if...then...* relationships, as in "friendly with people she knows personally but not with casual acquaintances at work" (Shoda & Mischel, 1993). Moreover, while perceivers often encode other people and themselves in terms of traits, they also under some conditions infer the cognitions and affects—the motives, goals, plans, and other person variables—that may underlie the behavior, functioning more like social-cognitive theorists than like trait theorists (Shoda & Mischel, 1993).

However, as discussed by Shoda and Mischel (1993), most research on the perception of personality has been constrained by sharing the traditional trait assumption that equates personality with global behavioral dispositions (also see Shoda, Chapter 6, this volume). It thus construes personality and situations as mutually exclusive and opposite influences. Given that assumption, information about how the target's behavior varies across different situations is usually deliberately not given to the perceiver, leaving the role of situation–behavior relationships relatively unexamined in person-perception studies. Finally, as Figure 2.2 also indicates, the characteristic behavior patterns generated by the system impact not only on the perceptions of others and of oneself but also modify the types of situations that will be subsequently encountered, producing a continuous reciprocal interaction between the behaviors generated and the psychological situations experienced.

Biochemical–Genetic Level: Pre-Dispositions at the Biological Substrate. The long-term developmental influences on the system, and the personality structures and dispositions that emerge within it, depend importantly on biological and genetic history as well as on cognitive-social learning history, and cultural–social influences (lower-left rectangle in Figure 2.2). Individuals differ in diverse biochemical–genetic–somatic factors that may be conceptualized as *pre*-dispositions. These *pre*-dispositions ultimately influence such personality-relevant qualities as sensory and psychomotor sensitivities and vulnerabilities, skills and competencies, temperament (including activity level and emotionality), chronic mood, and affective states. These in turn impact on the psychological system—such as CAPS—that emerges and is seen at the psychological level of analysis.

There are great individual differences within virtually every aspect of the biological human repertoire and genetic heritage that can have profound predisposing implications for the personality and behavior that ultimately develop (e.g., Plomin, DeFries, McClearn, & Rutter, 1997). These differences occur, for example, in sensory, perceptual-cognitive, and affective systems, in metabolic clocks and hormones, in neurotransmitters—in short, in the person's total biochemical–genetic–somatic heritage. These *pre*-dispositions interact with conditions throughout development and play out in ways that influence what the person thinks, feels and does. Even small differences among individuals at the biochemical–somatic level (e.g., in sensory-perceptual sensitivity, in allergy and decease proneness, in energy levels) may manifest ultimately as considerable differences in their experiences and behavior and in what comes to be perceived as their personalities.

Consequently, an adequate approach to personality coherence requires addressing not only the structure and organization of the cognitive-affective-behavioral processing system at the psychological level but also its biochemical–genetic predisposing foundations (Plomin et al., 1997; Saudino & Plomin, 1996). These genetic individual differences presumably at least indirectly affect how people construe or encode—and shape—their environments, which in turn produce important person–context interactions throughout the life course (Plomin, 1994; Saudino & Plomin, 1996).

Both biochemical and social-cognitive influences, heritable and learned, impact on the personality system at the psychological level. They influence both the cognitive-affective units that become available in the system and their organization, although the effects often are indirect. Variables of temperament or reactivity, such as activity, irritability, tension, distress, and emotional lability, visible early in life (Bates & Wachs, 1994), for example, seem to have important, albeit complexly interactive links to emotional and attentional processing and self-regulation (Rothbart, Derryberry, & Posner, 1994). These processes, in turn, should influence the organization of relations among the mediating units in the system and are likely to have important effects, for example, on the types of self-regulatory strategies and competencies that develop and that enable (or hinder) effective impulse control. Because this system, in turn, generates the specific, *if...then...* situation–behavior relations manifested, the theory predicts that individual differences in genetic–biochemical *pre*-dispositions, in the present view, will be manifested not only in the mean level of various types of behaviors, but in the behavioral signatures of personality, that is, the stable configuration of *if...then...* situation–behavior relations. When the system changes, either due to modification in the biological substrates or due to developmental changes and significant life events, the effects will also be seen at the behavioral level as a change in the relationships between the "ifs" and the "thens" in the situation–behavior profiles that characterize the person.

Pursuing Dispositions and Dynamics in a Unitary Framework

Personality psychology has been committed since its beginnings to characterizing individuals in terms of their stable and distinctive qualities (e.g., Allport, 1937; Funder, 1991; Goldberg, 1993). Other personality theorists and researchers have focused instead on the processes that underlie these coherences and that influence how people function (e.g., Bandura, 1986; Cantor & Kihlstrom, 1987; Higgins (Chapter 3, this volume); Mischel, 1973; Pervin, 1990). These two goals —to identify and clarify personality dispositions or personality processes —have been pursued in two increasingly separated (and warring) subdisciplines with different agendas that seem to be in conflict with each other (Cervone, 1991; Cronbach, 1957, 1975; Mischel & Shoda, 1994).

The CAPS approach presented in this chapter suggests that both goals may be pursued in concert with no necessary conflict or incompatibility because, in this framework, dispositions and processing dynamics are two complementary facets of the same phenomena and of the same unitary personality system. The dispositional qualities of individuals are represented in the personality system in terms of particular enduring structures in the organization among cognitive-affective mediating units available to the person. This organization in the structure of the disposition guides and constrains the pattern of specific cognitions, affects, and potential behaviors and their interconnections that become activated by the relevant internal or external psychological features of situations. To illustrate, let us consider again the example of the disposition of rejection sensitivity. The expectations and anticipation of rejection, the readiness to encode even ambiguous experiences as rejecting, the tendency to overreact emotionally to such cues, the accessing of hostile and defensive scripts when these feelings arise—all these are characteristics of this disposition, and their activation in a distinct stable pattern defines its processing dynamics and enactment.

Misunderstandings in analyses of dispositions also can be avoided by realizing that they may be studied fruitfully at each of the four levels of analysis discussed above: at the psychological processing level of activated thoughts and feelings; at the behavioral level; at the level of the judgments of observers and of the self; and at the level of the predisposing biochemical–genetic and neural substrate. The basic caveat and crucial requirement for proceeding within a unitary framework, however, are that the construct of dispositions, and indeed of personality structure and dynamics, be revised and refined to take account of the data and theoretical developments on the nature of coherence—and thus of personality—that the last few decades have yielded. This chapter, and I suspect much in this volume, is intended as a step in that direction.

REFERENCES

Allport, G. W. (1937). *Personality: A psychological interpretation.* New York: Holt, Rinehart & Winston.

Anderson, J. R. (1996). ACT: A simple theory of complex cognition. *American Psychologist, 51,* 355–365.

Ayduk, O. N., Downey, G., Testa, S., Yin, Y., & Shoda, Y. (in press). Does rejection elicit hostility in rejection sensitive women? *Social Cognition.*

Bandura, A. (1986). *Social foundations of thought and action: A social cognitive theory.* Englewood Cliffs, NJ: Prentice-Hall.

Bates, J. E., & Wachs, T. D. (1994). *Temperament: Individual differences at the interface of biology and behavior.* Washington, DC: American Psychological Association.

Bem, D. J. (1983). Further déjà vu in the search for cross-situational consistency: A response to Mischel and Peake. *Psychological Review, 90,* 390–393.

Bem, D. J., & Allen, A. (1974). On predicting some of the people some of the time: The search for cross-situational consistencies in behavior. *Psychological Review, 81,* 506–520.

Block, J. (1995). A contrarian view of the five-factor approach to personality description. *Psychological Bulletin, 117,* 187–215.

Buss, D. M. (1987). Selection, evocation, and manipulation. *Journal of Personality and Social Psychology, 53,* 1214–1221.

Cantor, N., & Kihlstrom, J. F. (1987). *Personality and social intelligence.* Englewood Cliffs, NJ: Erlbaum.

Cantor, N., Mischel, W., & Schwartz, J. (1982). A prototype analysis of psychological situations. *Cognitive Psychology, 14,* 45–77.

Carlson, R. (1971). Where is the personality research? *Psychological Bulletin, 75,* 203–219.

Cervone, D. (1991). The two disciplines of personality psychology [Review of the *Handbook of personality: Theory and research*]. *Psychological Science, 2,* 371–376.

Chapman, L. J., & Chapman, J. P. (1969). Illusory correlations as an obstacle to the use of valid psychodiagnostic signs. *Journal of Abnormal Psychology, 74,* 271–280.

Cronbach, L. J. (1957). The two disciplines of scientific psychology. *American Psychologist, 12,* 671–684.

Cronbach, L. J. (1975). Beyond the two disciplines of scientific psychology. *American Psychologist, 30,* 116–127.

Dodge, K. A. (1986). A social information processing model of social competence in children. In M. Perlmutter (Ed.), *The Minnesota symposium on child psychology: Vol. 18. Cognitive perspectives on children's social behavioral development* (pp. 77–125). Hillsdale, NJ: Erlbaum.

Dodge, K. A. (1993). Social-cognitive mechanisms in the development of conduct disorder and depression. *Annual Review of Psychology, 44,* 559–584.

Dodge, K. A. (1997a, April). *Testing developmental theory through prevention trials.* Paper presented at the biennial meeting of the Society for Research in Child Development, Washington, DC.

Dodge, K. A. (1997b, April). *Early peer social rejection and acquired autonomic sensitivity to peer conflicts: Conduct problems in adolescence.* Paper presented at the biennial meeting of the Society for Research in Child Development, Washington, DC.

Downey, G., & Feldman, S. I. (1996). Implications of rejection sensitivity for intimate relationships. *Journal of Personality and Social Psychology, 70,* 1327–1343.

Downey, G., Freitas, A., Michaelis, B., & Khouri, H. (1997). The self-fulfilling prophecy in close relationships: Rejection sensitivity and rejection in romantic partners. *Journal of Personality and Social Psychology, 75,* 545–560.

Endler, N. S., & Hunt, J. (1969). Generalizability of contributions from sources of variance in the S-R inventories of anxiousness. *Journal of Personality, 37,* 1–24.

Endler, N.S., Hunt, J. M., & Rosenstein, A. J. (1962). An S-R inventory of anxiousness. *Psychological Monographs, 76*(536).

Endler, N. S., & Magnusson, D. (1976). Toward an interactional psychology of personality. *Psychological Bulletin, 83*, 956–974.

Epstein, S. (1979). The stability of behavior: I. On predicting most of the people much of the time. *Journal of Personality and Social Psychology, 37*, 1097–1126.

Epstein, S. (1980). The stability of behavior: II. Implications for psychological research. *American Psychologist, 35*, 790–806.

Epstein, S. (1983). The stability of confusion: A reply to Mischel and Peake. *Psychological Review, 90*, 179–184.

Funder, D. C. (1983). Three issues in predicting more of the people: A reply to Mischel and Peake. *Psychological Review, 90*, 283–289.

Funder, D. C. (1991). Global traits: a neo-Allportian approach to personality. *Psychological Science, 2*, 31–39.

Goldberg, L. R. (1993). The structure of phenotypic personality traits. *American Psychologist, 48*, 26–34.

Hartshorne, H., & May, A. (1928). *Studies in the nature of character: Vol. 1. Studies in deceit.* New York: Macmillan.

John, O. P. (1990). The big-five factor taxonomy: Dimensions of personality in the natural language and questionnaires. In L. A. Pervin (Ed.), *Handbook of personality: Theory and research* (pp. 66–100). New York: Guilford Press.

Jones, E. E. (1990). *Interpersonal perception.* New York: Macmillan.

Kandel, E. R., & Hawkins, R. D. (1992). The biological basis of learning and individuality. *Scientific American, 267*(3), 78–86.

Kunda, Z., & Thagard, P. (1996). Forming impressions from stereotypes, traits, and behaviors: A parallel-constraint-satisfaction theory. *Psychological Review, 103*, 284–308.

Magnusson, D., & Endler, N. S. (Eds.). (1977). *Personality at the crossroads: Current issues in interactional psychology.* Hillsdale, NJ: Erlbaum.

McAdams, D. P. (1992). The Five-Factor model in personality. *Journal of Personality, 60*, 329–361.

McCrae, R. R., & Costa, P. T., Jr. (1996). Toward a new generation of personality theories: Theoretical contexts for the five-factor model. In J. S. Wiggins (Ed.), *The five-factor model of personality: Theoretical perspectives* (pp. 51–87). New York: Guilford Press.

McCrae, R. R., & Costa, P. T. (1997). Conceptions and correlates of openness and to experience. In R. Hogan, J. Johnson, & S. Briggs (Eds.), *Handbook of personality psychology* (pp. 825–847). San Diego: Academic Press.

Metcalfe, J., & Jacobs W. J. (1998). Emotional memory: The effects of stress on "cool" and "hot" memory systems. In D. L. Medin (Ed.), *The psychology of learning and motivation: Vol. 38. Advances in research and theory* (pp. 187–222) . San Diego, CA: Academic Press.

Metcalfe, J., & Mischel, W. (1999). A hot/cool system analysis of delay of gratification: Dynamics of willpower. *Psychological Review, 6*.

Mischel, W. (1968). *Personality and assessment.* New York: Wiley.

Mischel, W. (1973). Toward a cognitive social learning reconceptualization of personality. *Psychological Review, 80*, 252–283.

Mischel, W. (1990). Personality dispositions revisited and revised: A view after three decades. In L. A. Pervin (Ed.), *Handbook of personality: Theory and research* (pp. 111–134). New York: Guilford Press.

Mischel, W. (1998). *Introduction to personality* (6th ed.). Fort Worth, TX: Harcourt Brace.

Mischel, W., Cantor, N., & Feldman, S. (1996). Principles of self-regulation: The nature of willpower and self-control. In E. T. Higgins & A. W. Kruglanski (Eds.), *Social psychology: Handbook of basic principles* (pp. 329–360). New York: Guilford Press.

Mischel, W., Ebbesen, E. B., & Zeiss, A. R. (1973). Selective attention to the self: Situational and dispositional determinants. *Journal of Personality and Social Psychology, 27*, 129–142.

Mischel, W., Ebbesen, E. B., & Zeiss, A. R. (1976). Determinants of selective memory about the self. *Journal of Consulting and Clinical Psychology, 44*, 92–103.

Mischel, W., & Peake, P. K. (1982). In search of consistency: Measure for measure. In M. P. Zanna, E. T. Higgins, & C. P. Herman (Eds.), *Consistency in social behavior: The Ontario symposium* (Vol. 2). Hillsdale, NJ: Erlbaum.

Mischel, W., & Shoda, Y. (1994). Personality psychology has two goals: Must it be two fields? *Psychological Inquiry, 5*, 156–158.

Mischel, W., & Shoda, Y. (1995). A cognitive-affective system theory of personality: Reconceptualizing situations, dispositions, dynamics, and invariance in personality structure. *Psychological Review, 102*(2), 246–268.

Mischel, W., & Shoda, Y. (1998). Reconciling processing dynamics and personality dispositions. *Annual Review of Psychology, 49*, 229–258.

Newcomb, T. M. (1929). *Consistency of certain extrovert–introvert behavior patterns in 51 problem boys.* New York: Columbia University, Teachers College, Bureau of Publications.

Nisbett, R. E., & Ross, L. D. (1980). *Human inference: Strategies and shortcomings of social judgment. Century Psychology Series.* Englewood Cliffs, NJ: Prentice-Hall.

Nolen-Hoeksema, S., Parker, L. E. & Larson, J. (1994). Ruminative coping with depressed mood following loss. *Journal of Personality and Social Psychology, 67*, 92–104.

Norem, J. K., & Cantor, N. (1986). Anticipatory and post hoc cushioning strategies: Optimism and defensive pessimism in "risky" situations. *Cognitive Therapy and Research, 10*, 347–362.

Pervin, L. A. (Ed.). (1990). *Handbook of personality: Theory and research.* New York: Guilford Press.

Pervin, L. A. (1994). A critical analysis of trait theory. *Psychological Inquiry, 5*, 103–113.

Peterson, D. R. (1968). *The clinical study of social behavior.* New York: Appleton.

Plomin, R. (1994). *Genetics and experience: The developmental interplay between nature and nurture.* Newbury Park, CA: Sage.

Plomin, R., DeFries, J. C., McClearn, G. E., & Rutter, M. (1997). *Behavioral genetics* (3rd ed.). New York: Freeman.

Read, S. J., & Miller, L. C. (Eds.). (1998). *Connectionist models of social reasoning and social behavior.* Mahwah, NJ: Erlbaum.

Rothbart, M. K., Derryberry, D., & Posner, M. I. (1994). A psychobiological approach to the development of temperament. In J. E. Bates & T. D. Wachs (Eds.), *Temperament: Individual differences at the interface of biology and behavior* (pp. 83–116). Washington, DC: American Psychological Association.

Rumelhart, D. E., & McClelland, J. L. (1986). *Parallel distributing processing: Explorations in the microstructure of cognition: Foundations* (Vol. 1). Cambridge, MA: MIT Press/Bradford Books.

Saudino, K. J., & Plomin, R. (1996). Personality and behavioral genetics: Where have we been and where are we going? *Journal of Research in Personality, 30*, 335–347.

Shoda, Y. (1990). *Conditional analyses of personality coherence and dispositions.* Unpublished doctoral dissertation, Columbia University, New York.

Shoda, Y., & Mischel, W. (1993). Cognitive social approach to dispositional inferences: What if the perceiver is a cognitive-social theorist? *Personality and Social Psychology Bulletin, 19,* 574–585.

Shoda, Y., & Mischel, W. (1996). Toward a unified, intraindividual dynamic conception of personality. *Journal of Research in Personality, 30,* 414–428.

Shoda, Y., & Mischel, W. (1998). Reconciling processing dynamics and personality dispositions. *Annual Review of Psychology, 49,* 229–258.

Shoda, Y., Mischel, W., & Wright, J. C. (1989). Intuitive interactionism in person perception: Effects of situation–behavior relations on dispositional judgments. *Journal of Personality and Social Psychology, 56,* 41–53.

Shoda, Y., Mischel, W., & Wright, J. C. (1993a). The role of situational demands and cognitive competencies in behavior organization and personality coherence. *Journal of Personality and Social Psychology, 56,* 41–53.

Shoda, Y., Mischel, W., & Wright, J. C. (1993b). Links between personality judgments and contextualized behavior patterns: Situation–behavior profiles of personality prototypes. *Social Cognition, 4,* 399–429.

Shoda, Y., Mischel, W., & Wright, J. C. (1994). intraindividual stability in the organization and patterning of behavior: Incorporating psychological situations into the idiographic analysis of personality. *Journal of Personality and Social Psychology, 65,* 1023–1035.

Shultz, T. R., & Lepper, M. R. (1996). Cognitive dissonance reduction as constraint satisfaction. *Psychological Review, 103,* 219–240.

Taylor, S. E., & Schneider, S. (1989). Coping and the simulation of events. *Social Cognition, 7,* 174–194.

Vernon, P. E. (1964). *Personality assessment: A critical survey.* New York: Wiley.

Walker, L. E. (1979). *The battered women.* New York: Harper & Row.

Westen, D. (1990). Psychoanalytic approaches to personality. In L. A. Pervin (Ed.), *Handbook of personality: Theory and research* (pp. 21–65). New York: Guilford Press.

Wright, J. C., & Mischel, W. (1987). A conditional approach to dispositional constructs: The local predictability of social behavior. *Journal of Personality and Social Psychology, 53,* 1159–1177.

Wright, J. C., & Mischel, W. (1988). Conditional hedges and the intuitive psychology of traits. *Journal of Personality and Social Psychology, 55,* 454–469.

3

Persons and Situations
Unique Explanatory Principles or Variability in General Principles?

E. TORY HIGGINS

What is personality? Most people, whether they are professional experts on personality or not, think of personality as an individual's predispositions to respond in specific ways to the world around him or her. The common view is that personality provides one kind of explanation for people's feelings, thoughts, strategies, and actions. Other areas of psychology, such as social psychology, are viewed as providing other kinds of explanations. It follows from this viewpoint that, if each area is to provide its own unique explanations, each area should develop its own unique principles to describe and account for psychological states.

Accordingly, the area of personality over time has developed its own set of psychological principles, such as personal constructs (Kelly, 1955) and achievement motives (Atkinson, 1964; McClelland, Atkinson, Clark, & Lowell, 1953). The implicit assumption is that these principles are personality principles of psychology that provide unique "person" explanations for people's psychological states. It is also assumed that there are social psychological principles of psychology, such as cognitive dissonance or obedience to authority, that provide unique "situation" explanations for people's psychological states.

Historically, then, personality as one area in psychology has had its own set of explanatory principles distinct from those in other areas of psychology, such as social psychology. In particular, "person" explanatory principles have been distinguished from "situation" explanatory principles. What has varied among different perspectives on personality is how variability across "situations" has been treated in conceptualizing personality.

The personality "traits" or "dimensions" perspective control for or remove the influence of situations on behavior in order to study cross-situational effects of "person" principles alone (see Epstein, 1979; John, 1990). The "psychoanalytic" perspective emphasizes the organization of interacting personality processes, such as characteristic conflicts and defenses, that reside within the person (see Westen, 1990). Situation principles, such as socialization styles, are transformed into personality principles, such as positive or negative fixations or strong or weak superego. Although these two classic perspectives on personality differ from one another in major respects, they use "person" principles to predict behavior.

Another classic approach to personality is the "interactionist" perspective (see Endler, 1982; Magnusson, 1990; Magnusson & Endler, 1977). This perspective neither removes nor internalizes situational variability such that only "person" principles remain. Instead, the interactions of "person" variability and "situation" variability are examined as combined influences on behavior. These "person" × "situation" interactive effects on behavior (e.g., Magnusson & Endler, 1977) are typically conceptualized as interactions between distinct sources of variability, each with its own underlying principle, comparable to the interactive effect of the nature of a material and situational stress on elasticity (see, e.g., Endler, 1982). A central concept in the classic "interactionist" perspective is "reciprocal determinism" (see Magnusson, 1990), which highlights both the assumption that "person" and "situation" forces influence each other *and* the assumption that "person" and "situation" explanatory principles are distinct.

Recent developments in the "interactionist" perspective treat the relation between "persons" and "situations" in a different way than the classic version. Mischel and Shoda (1995), for example, conceptualize personality dispositions in terms of stable profiles of "situation–behavior" relations in which each individual has a stable pattern of varying disposition-related behaviors across different situations. This approach includes situations as part of personality by describing dispositions in terms of situational variability. This is a powerful way of conceptualizing dispositions in which situational differences become part of personality rather than being separated from it. The question then becomes how to account for the variability in behavior across persons and situations.

To answer this question, Mischel and Shoda (1995) further develop the "social-cognitive learning" perspective (see Bandura, 1986; Cantor & Zirkel, 1990; Mischel, 1973) that has its roots in the work of Murray (1938), Kelly (1955), and Rotter (1954). This "social-cognitive learning" perspective attempts to link personality to individual differences in construals, expectancies, strategies, and so on. It differs from classic "interactionist" approaches in relating personality to individual differences in underlying psychological processes rather than to individual differences in needs or traits. The distinction between "person" principles and "situation" principles is retained, although "persons" and "situations" impact on one another and together influence behavior.

The emphasis of the "social-cognitive learning" perspective on underlying psychological processes is central to the approach I propose in this chapter as well. The approach I propose to identifying and selecting psychological processes differs in one respect, however. For the "social-cognitive learning" perspective on personality, psychological principles are identified that vary across persons, such as personal construals or encoding styles. Separate situational principles that vary across situations are also included as determinants of behavior that interact with the personality principles, such as positive versus negative interpersonal interactions with adults versus peers. As an alternative, I propose that *one* set of general principles be identified for which *both* persons and situations are sources of variability. In brief, I posit a *"general principles" perspective* on personality. From this perspective, "person" and "situation" variables can be understood in terms of the *same* general principles. Personality would be reconceptualized as simply one source of variability in the functioning of psychological principles that varies across situations as well (see also Higgins, 1990).

Let us first consider the issue of "source of variability." Imagine that one is interested in the psychological states of adults in the United States. From a personality perspective, one would investigate whether there are differences across individuals in people's psychological states. From a social-psychology perspective, one would investigate whether there are differences across situations in people's psychological states. From a cultural-psychology perspective, one would investigate whether there are differences across ethnic groups in people's psychological states.

Note that the investigation in each area involves comparing people's psychological states. Moreover, the exact same sample of psychological states of the same persons could be included in all of the investigations. The only difference is the choice of comparison. Thus, the difference between these areas of psychology is not in the psychological states as data but in which source of variability in this data is of interest to them. Interest in different sources of variability will lead to different descriptions of the data. But this does not mean the basic data itself, the psychological states, are different in these different areas. Moreover, given that these psychological states are just surface manifestations of underlying principles, the principles underlying the basic data also need not differ by area.

What does differ across areas is the source of variability that is chosen for investigation. Choosing a particular source of variability naturally influences how differences among the psychological states will be described. Because each description becomes the "phenomenon" of interest to an area, each area is then tempted to discover the unique psychological principles that underlie its own special phenomenon. But the fact that there are different sources of variability does not mean that different principles underlie each source. The same principle could underlie variability across individuals, situations, and groups. It is important to identify such common or general principles for a number of reasons (see Higgins, 1990). First, it would improve the economy of principles in psychology. Second, it would provide a common language of principles across areas in psychology that would facilitate examining interrelations and drawing general conclusions. Third, it would enrich our understanding of how each principle functioned across a broad range of conditions.

The goal of this chapter is to illustrate how a personality difference can be just one source of variability in the functioning of a general psychological principle that has situational sources of variability as well (see also Higgins, 1990). In it I show how personality can differ from other areas of psychology in its concern with variability across persons in the functioning of a principle without the principle itself being unique to personality. For this purpose of illustration, I have chosen a general "cognitive" principle of knowledge activation and a general "motivational" principle of self-regulation. The chapter begins by examining *accessibility* as a general principle of knowledge activation. "Persons" and "situations" as sources of variability in accessibility are described. Evidence is presented that a personality phenomenon such as the classic judgmental effects of "personal constructs" (e.g., Kelly, 1955) and a social-psychology phenomenon such as the well-known person perception effects of trait priming both reflect the *same* underlying principle of accessibility. The chapter next examines "regulatory focus" as a general principle of self-regulation. Regulatory focus distinguishes between self-regulation with a "promotion focus" on aspirations and accomplishments and self-regulation with a "prevention focus" on safety and responsibilities. Evidence is presented that the distinct motivations and emotions produced by a promotion focus versus a prevention focus occur both when "persons" are the source of variability in regulatory focus and when "situations" are the source of variability. The concluding section returns to the general question of whether personality can be conceptualized as just one source of variability in the functioning of general principles and the advantages of this conceptualization.

ACCESSIBILITY AS A GENERAL PRINCIPLE
OF KNOWLEDGE ACTIVATION

Psychologists have recognized for a long time that knowledge structures built up from past experiences are a major determinant of how people represent and categorize external stimuli (e.g., Wertheimer, 1923; Bartlett, 1932; Kelly, 1955; Bruner, 1957a, 1957b). The "new look" in perception that emerged in the 1940s proposed that needs, values, attitudes, and expectancies determine perception and result in people "going beyond the information given" (Bruner, 1957a). To capture the general role of expectancies and motivational states on perception, Bruner (1957b) introduced the notion of category "accessibility," which denoted "the ease or speed with which a given stimulus input is coded in terms of a given category under varying conditions."

Much of the research inspired by the "new look" was concerned with how people's long-term values, attitudes, and needs influenced the accessibility of stored constructs. In this sense, this early work treated accessibility as a personality variable. This personality emphasis became explicit in the work of Kelly (1955), who pointed out early on that "construct systems can be considered as a kind of scanning pattern which a person continually projects upon his world. As he sweeps back and forth across his perceptual field, he picks up blips of meaning" (p. 145). Mischel (1973) suggested that individual differences in the subjective meaning of social events may be especially evident in the personal constructs individuals employ and that these personal constructs may show the greatest resistance to situational presses. More generally, it has been proposed that there are individual differences in the "theories" or viewpoints that people have about human nature and personality (e.g., Kelly, 1955; Sarbin, Taft, & Bailey, 1960).

But is accessibility a personality variable? Is it *just* a personality variable? If it is not just a personality variable, does it function differently when it is a personality variable than when it is not? This section on accessibility will address each of these questions, but first, it is necessary to define accessibility more precisely and distinguish it from related concepts (see Higgins, 1996, for a fuller discussion of definitional issues).

Availability and Accessibility

Knowledge cannot be activated or brought to mind unless it is present in memory. "Availability" refers to whether or not some particular knowledge is actually stored in memory. Tulving and Pearlstone (1966) distinguished between accessibility and availability when considering the difference between free recall and cued recall. Information that is not retrieved in free recall may nevertheless be retrieved with cued recall. Thus, information can be stored in memory, that is, be "available," but not be easily retrieved or "accessible." Availability is a necessary condition for accessibility. If knowledge is available, it has at least some accessibility, but if it is not available, it has zero accessibility (Higgins & King, 1981). There can be variability across people both in which kinds of knowledge are available to them and in which kinds of available knowledge are most accessible to them. By distinguishing between availability and accessibility, "accessibility" can be defined as the activation potential of available knowledge (see Higgins, 1996).

Knowledge Activation and Knowledge Use

Bruner (1957b) conceptualized the "accessibility" of stored knowledge in terms of the readiness to use the stored knowledge to categorize stimulus information—"perceptual readiness." Similarly, Higgins and King (1981) proposed that accessible constructs are stored constructs that are readily used in information processing. Although these definitions reveal the general empirical relation between the accessibility of knowledge and the likelihood that the knowledge will be used in some way, they fail to distinguish conceptually between the activation and the use of knowledge. It is useful to distinguish between these concepts because there are variables that influence knowledge use beyond those involved in knowledge activation. It might be considered inappropriate to use activated knowledge, for example, when it was activated as part of an earlier task that is supposed to be kept separate from the current task (see Martin, 1986). It is preferable, therefore, to define "accessibility" in terms of potential for knowledge *activation* rather than potential for knowledge *use*.

Accessibility and Applicability

Two basic variables influence the likelihood that some stored knowledge will be activated—the accessibility of the stored knowledge prior to stimulus presentation and the "fit" between the stored knowledge and the presented stimulus (Bruner, 1957b). Like "fit," "applicability" refers to the relation between the features of some stored knowledge and the attended features of a stimulus (where the features are typically categorical in nature). The greater is the overlap between the features of some stored knowledge and the attended features of a stimulus, the greater is the applicability of the knowledge to the stimulus and the greater is the likelihood that the knowledge will be activated in the presence of the stimulus (see Higgins, 1996).

Applicability and Judged Usability

It is also important to distinguish between applicability and judged usability. "Judged usability" is the judged appropriateness or relevance of applying stored knowledge to a stimulus (see Higgins, 1996). There is substantial evidence that perceivers' judgment of the relevance or appropriateness of particular information for their response can determine their use of the information (for a review, see Higgins & Bargh, 1987). Even when stored information is activated because of its accessibility and applicability to a stimulus, it might not be consciously used if it is perceived as being irrelevant or inappropriate (see Martin & Achee, 1992). During a criminal trial, for example, jurists will attempt not to use evidence in their deliberations that has been ruled inadmissable by the trial judge. Nonprejudiced persons will attempt not to use stereotypic information in judging others when the momentary situation facilitates usability judgments. It has been suggested that information that is perceived as inappropriate is likely to be suppressed and that this can produce contrast effects of accessibility instead of the usual assimilation effects (see Martin, 1986). Rather than being an accessibility or applicability effect per se, such contrast would be an effect of judged usability.

Now that accessibility has been defined and distinguished from other variables involved in knowledge activation and knowledge use, we can return to the questions raised earlier.

Is Accessibility a Personality Variable?

It is clear from the work of Kelly (1955), Bruner (1957b), and others mentioned earlier that there are differences across persons in the relative accessibility of different kinds of stored constructs. The basic notion behind the Thematic Apperception Test, developed by Murray (1938) and used extensively to measure individual differences in need achievement (e.g., McClelland & Atkinson, 1948), was that thoughts that were related to a strong motive of a person should be chronically accessible (see Sorrentino & Higgins, 1986). One line of research inspired by the "new look" in perception examined how chronically accessible values influenced responses to stimulus information, such as how subjects with strong religious versus economic values perceive tachistoscopically presented pictures differently (Bruner, 1951). Even earlier, the defense mechanism of "projection" described in the psychodynamic literature includes the notion of heightened responding to others in terms of chronically accessible thoughts or feelings (see Cameron, 1963). More recent research has not only provided more direct evidence of individual differences in chronic accessibility, but it has also examined in more detail the nature and consequences of such individual differences.

How individual differences in the chronic accessibility of constructs influence the processing of behavioral information was directly examined by Higgins, King, and Mavin (1982). In one study, subjects' chronically accessible constructs were measured by asking them to list the traits of a type of person that they liked, disliked, sought out, avoided, and frequently encountered. Chronic accessibility was defined in terms of output primacy. For a given trait-related construct, individuals would be "chronic" on a construct if they listed that construct first in response to one or more questions, and they would be "nonchronic" on a construct if they did not list that construct in response to any question. About 1 week later, subjects participated in a supposedly unrelated study on "psycholinguistics" conducted by a different experimenter. Each subject read an individually tailored essay containing trait-related descriptions of a target person. Each subject was chronic for half of the traits and nonchronic for the other half of the traits. When a "quasi-yoking" design was used to control for the content of the trait-related descriptions, some subjects were chronics and some subjects were nonchronics for each of the traits described in the essays.

On both a measure of subjects' spontaneous impressions of the target person and a measure of their recall of the behavioral descriptions, the study found that subjects were significantly more likely to include information related to traits on which they were chronic than information related to traits on which they were nonchronic. These basic effects were also found in another study by Higgins et al. (1982) in which chronic accessibility was defined in terms of the frequency of output to different questions rather than the primacy of output. This study also found that the effects of chronic accessibility on impressions and memory can last for at least a couple of weeks. Moreover, using an alternative operationalization of chronic accessibility, Lau (1989) has found that chronically accessible constructs are relatively stable even over years and that they guide the processing of information about a wide variety of political objects.

Bargh and Pratto (1986) used the Stroop color-naming paradigm to test directly whether the activation potential of constructs on which individuals are chronic is higher than constructs on which individuals are nonchronics. Subjects were classified as chronic or nonchronic on different contructs according to the Higgins et al. (1982) criteria. Bargh and Pratto (1986) found that subjects' chronically accessible constructs were indeed at a higher level of activation readiness than their inaccessible constructs, as revealed by greater interference on the color-naming task from the chronically accessible constructs. Bargh and Thein (1985) tested whether chronic accessibility is associated with automatic processing. Again, subjects were classified as chronic or nonchronic on different contructs according to the Higgins et al. (1982) criteria. For constructs on which the subjects were chronic, Bargh and Thein (1985) found evidence of the processing efficiency expected with automatic processing for both subjects' impressions and recall of a target person's behaviors. No such evidence of processing efficiency was found for constructs on which the subjects were nonchronic.

Although not originally conceptualized in terms of individual differences in chronic accessibility, research comparing individuals for whom a construct is central ("schematics") or is not central ("aschematics") to their self-description can be interpreted as providing additional evidence for the role of chronic accessibility in social-information processing. Markus (1977) classified subjects as being independent schematics, for example, if they responded at the high end of both a self-descriptiveness and an importance scale for at least two of three independence-related traits and classified subjects as being independent aschematics if they responded in the middle of these scales. According to such criteria, schematics probably differ from aschematics in a number of ways (see Higgins & Bargh, 1987). Still, it is likely that independent schematics, for example, are chronic on the construct "independent," whereas aschematics are nonchronic.

Markus (1977) found that independent schematics (i.e., independent chronics) processed independent-related stimulus information faster and more consistently than did independent aschematics (i.e., independent nonchronics). Bargh (1982) also compared the processing of independent schematics and aschematics, classified according to Markus's (1977) criteria. Subjects were given a dichotic listening task in which independent-related words either appeared in the to-be-attended or the to-be-ignored channel. A probe reaction time was used to measure the amount of resources allocated to the listening task. Bargh (1982) found that compared to independent aschematics (i.e., independent nonchronics), independent schematics (i.e., independent chronics) used less resources when independent-related words appeared in the to-be-attended channel but used more resources when these words appeared in the to-be-ignored channel. These results support the notion that chronic accessibility is associated with automatic processing.

The initial studies on the effects of chronic accessibility on judging and remembering social behavior compared the effects of individuals who were chronic versus nonchronic on the target constructs. In a couple of recent studies, Higgins and Brendl (1995) have investigated the effects of chronic accessibility as a continuous variable with multiple levels of chronicity. Using the Higgins et al. (1982) measure of chronic accessibility, individuals were again classified as nonchronic on a construct if they did not list that construct in response to any question. An operationalization of individual differences in continuous levels of chronicity was introduced that involved a frequency of output score. This score was obtained by counting the total number of construct-related responses (in this case, "conceited" and its synonyms) to all five questions and dividing this number by the total number of all responses to these questions. Using the full range of subjects' chronicity scores for "conceited" that had been obtained weeks before the experiment, Higgins and Brendl (1995) found a strong positive relation between higher chronicity scores and stronger impressions that the vague or ambiguous behaviors of a target person reflected conceitedness.

Lau (1989) used a couple of similar measures of levels of chronicity to examine the relation between chronic accessibility for political constructs and evaluative responses to political candidates. One study investigated subjects' chronically accessible constructs for political candidates by measuring how frequently each subject mentioned person-related traits when answering open-ended questions about the good and bad points of the two major parties and their candidates. Lau (1989) found that subjects' preelection candidate opinions were more strongly related to their choice of candidate when the chronic accessibility of their candidate constructs was higher. Lau (1989) also provided evidence that the chronic accessibility of political constructs remains quite stable even over a period of 4 years.

Is Accessibility Just a Personality Variable?

The research findings of many studies make clear that there are differences across persons in how accessible different stored constructs are to them. Thus, accessibility is certainly a personality variable. But is it just a personality variable? There is equally substantial evidence from many studies that accessibility is also a situational variable. This evidence will be reviewed only briefly here because extensive and recent reviews are available in the literature (e.g., Higgins, 1996).

In an early study by Higgins, Rholes, and Jones (1977), subjects were initially exposed to one or another set of trait-related constructs as an incidental aspect of a supposed study on "perception." For example, half of the subjects were exposed to the word "stubborn" as an incidental part of a Stroop task, ostensibly functioning as a memory "load" to make the Stroop task more difficult, and the other half of the subjects were exposed to the word "persistent." The subjects later participated in a supposedly unrelated study on "reading comprehension" where they were asked to characterize the ambiguous behaviors of a target person, such as the following "stubborn/persistent" description: "Once Donald made up his mind to do something, it was as good as done no matter how long it might take or how difficult the going might be. Only rarely did he change his mind, even when it might well have been better if he had." The study found that the subjects were significantly more likely to use the trait-related constructs primed in the initial "perception" task to categorize the target person's behaviors in the second "reading comprehension" task than to use the equally applicable alternative constructs.

This basic phenomenon of situationally activating stored knowledge and thereby increasing the likelihood that this knowledge will influence subsequent responses to stimuli has been replicated many times using a wide variety of priming methods, types of responses, and types of stimuli (e.g., Bargh, Bond, Lombardi, & Tota, 1986; Smith & Branscombe, 1987; Srull & Wyer, 1979, 1980; for a fuller review, see Higgins, 1996). In the Higgins et al. (1977) study, as in many subsequent studies, the activated constructs were common trait-related concepts. It is likely that all subjects had each of the alternative constructs available to them. Given that these constructs were available, they had at least some activation potential. In addition, each behavior could be categorized by the alternative constructs. To reveal an accessibility effect, therefore, it is necessary that one construct be *more* accessible than an alternative construct that is equally applicable to the stimulus. These studies demonstrate that one way a construct can be made more accessible than alternatives is to prime that construct prior to stimulus exposure—"recent priming" as one situational condition for accessibility effects.

Recent priming increases the likelihood that the primed construct will be used to judge a subsequent stimulus. But how recent must the "recent" priming be? More generally, what is the effect of the delay from priming to stimulus exposure on the strength of accessibility effects? Several studies have found that the effect of recent priming tends to decrease as the delay from priming to stimulus exposure increases (e.g., Higgins, Bargh, & Lombardi, 1985; Higgins & Brendl, 1995; Srull & Wyer, 1979, 1980). When there is a competing accessible construct, the effect of recent priming on judgment can disappear in a couple of minutes or less. There are also cases, however, when situational priming effects can remain strong for a very long time. If the initial priming was frequent enough (e.g., over 30 primes), its effect on later judgments can be evident after even a 24-hour delay (see Srull & Wyer, 1979, 1980; see also Bargh & Pietromonaco, 1982). When a procedural knowledge unit is repeatedly activated and used in categorizing a specific behavior, then the effect of priming on later judgments of that same behavior can last several days (see, for example, Smith, Stewart, & Buttram, 1992). Whether it be minutes or days, the delay from priming to stimulus exposure is another situational condition for accessibility effects.

In sum, accessibility as a psychological principle is both a "person" and a "situation" variable. Does accessibility function differently when it is a "person" variable than when it is a "situation" variable? This question is addressed next.

Does Accessibility Function Differently as a "Person" Than a "Situation" Variable?

One way to address this question is to look at what happens when both "person" and "situation" sources of variability in accessibility are working together. Bargh et al. (1986), for example, selected subjects who were chronic or nonchronic on the construct "kind" weeks before the experiment and then primed or did not prime (subliminally) the construct "kind" a few minutes before the subjects' judged "ambiguously kind" behavioral descriptions. Bargh et al. (1986) found that subjects' construct-related impressions of the target person were stronger both when the subjects were chronic on the construct and when the construct was primed. Most important, there was a reliable effect of chronic accessibility even within the priming condition. Higgins and Brendl (1995) also found that the effect of higher levels of chronic accessibility on strengthening judgments did not interact with priming and was reliable even within the priming condition. These studies suggest that chronic accessibility as a "person" variable and increasing accessibility by priming as a "situation" variable have similar, independent effects on judgment. "Person" and "situation" sources of variability in accessibility can also work together when both are needed in order for the accessibility to be sufficiently high to compensate for extremely low applicability (see Higgins & Brendl, 1995).

What happens when "person" and "situation" sources of variability in accessibility are pitted against one another? Specifically, what happens when recent situational priming is pitted against chronic accessibility and subjects judge an ambiguous description where one competing alternative relates to the priming and the other relates to the chronicity? Bargh, Lombardi, and Higgins (1988) first selected subjects who were chronic on either "inconsiderate" or "outgoing." During the experiment weeks later, either the construct "inconsiderate" was primed or the construct "outgoing" was primed. The construct that was primed was always opposite to the subject's chronic construct (e.g., "inconsiderate" chronics were primed with "outgoing"). After either a 15-second, a 120-second, or a 180-second delay following the last priming trial, subjects judged what type of person was exemplified in a behavioral description ambiguous for "inconsiderate" and "outgoing." The subjects' judgments reflected the primed construct slightly more than the chronic construct after the 15-second delay, but the reverse was true after the 120-second delay. For this reversal to have occurred, there must have been some difference between the chronic "person" accessibility and the priming "situation" accessibility. Does this mean that accessibility functions differently as a "person" versus a "situation" variable? Before drawing this conclusion, let us consider what happens when two situational variables—recent versus frequent priming—are pitted against each other.

Most priming studies have primed only one construct per subject that could be used to judge the stimulus information. Higgins et al. (1985), however, primed two alternative constructs that were equally applicable to an ambiguous behavior. In this way, the effects of recent and frequent priming as two situational sources of accessibility could be pitted against each other. One of two alternative constructs was primed more frequently (four times), and the other was primed only once but most recently at the very end of the priming task. Following the final prime, there was either a 15-second or 120-second delay (filled by a "counting backwards" interference task) before subjects read the ambiguous target behaviors. After the shorter delay, the subjects tended to judge each behavior using the more recently primed construct. But after the longer delay, the subjects tended to judge each behavior using the more frequently primed construct (see also Lombardi, Higgins, & Bargh, 1987).

The results from the studies pitting recent versus frequent situational priming show the *same* reversal as was found in the studies pitting recent situational priming versus individual chronic accessibility. Thus, the latter reversal need not mean that accessibility functions differently as a "person" versus a "situation" variable. What might account for the reversal? In their "synapse" model of accessibility, Higgins et al. (1985) proposed that the rate at which accessibility decays over time decreases with increases in the frequency or intensity of past priming. For competing accessible constructs, this model predicts a reversal of construct predominance as a function of priming-to-stimulus delay. Immediately after the priming of the most recently primed construct, the excitation level of this recently primed construct will be higher than the excitation level of the frequently primed or chronically accessible construct. The most recently primed construct will thus predominate at this point. But the frequently primed or chronically accessible construct has a slower rate of decay than this recently primed construct. Given sufficient priming-to-stimulus delay, therefore, the frequently primed or chronically accessible construct will predominate at a later point.

The fact that frequent priming in the Higgins et al. (1985) study functioned like chronic accessibility in the Bargh et al. (1988) study has an important implication. It suggests that frequency of priming could play an important role in the development of individual differences in chronic accessibility (see Higgins & King, 1981). Children whose parents strongly value certain attributes of people positively or negatively are more likely to have those attribute constructs primed frequently by their parents' evaluative remarks. More generally, children's exposure to a culture around them that communicates more regularly about some things than others are going to have the former constructs primed more frequently than the latter. This differential exposure during socialization could produce individual differences in chronic accessibility. Thus, priming as a situational variable could play a major role in the development of chronic accessibility as a personality variable. It should also be noted that, from this perspective, dispositional tendencies to use certain social constructs in interpreting social events would develop from exposure to one's culture rather than be inherited.

In sum, the answers to the questions raised in this section are that accessibility is a personality variable, but it is not just a personality variable, and it functions the same way as a "person" and a "situation" variable. Thus, both "persons" and "situations" are sources of variability for accessibility as a general principle of knowledge activation. The next section considers how "persons" and "situations" are also both sources of variability for regulatory focus as a general principle of self-regulation.

REGULATORY FOCUS AS A GENERAL PRINCIPLE OF SELF-REGULATION

People are motivated to approach pleasure and avoid pain. From the ancient Greeks, through 17th- and 18th-century British philosophers, to 20th-century psychologists, this hedonic or pleasure principle has dominated our understanding of people's motivation. The problem with the hedonic principle is not that it is wrong but, rather, that it is insufficient as an explanation for human behavior. How does the hedonic principle itself operate? What general principles underlie how people approach pleasure and avoid pain? This is a central question for psychologists because knowing alone that people approach pleasure and avoid pain is insufficient to account for the observed complexities of people's self-regulation.

There are three general answers to how people approach pleasure and avoid pain (for a fuller discussion of these answers, see Higgins, 1997). One is "regulatory anticipation." Freud (1920/1950) described self-regulation as a "hedonism of the future" in which behavior and other psychical activities are driven by anticipations of pleasure to be approached (wishes) and anticipations of pain to be avoided (fears). Mowrer (1960) proposed that the fundamental nature of self-regulation was to approach hoped-for end states and avoid feared end states. Atkinson's (1964) theory of achievement motivation distinguished between the approach tendencies of individuals with a "hope of success" and the avoidance tendencies of individuals with a "fear of failure."

A second general answer to how self-regulation approaches pleasure and avoids pain is "regulatory reference." Whereas regulatory anticipation concerns expectancies of pleasant versus painful outcomes, regulatory reference concerns desired end states versus undesired end states as the reference point for self-regulation. Thus, two people could both anticipate pleasure (hope), but for one it could be in reference to a desired end state (e.g., successfully attaining an "A" in a course), whereas for the other, it could be in reference to an undesired end state (e.g., successfully avoiding less than an "A" in a course). Regulatory reference is independent of whether pleasure or pain is anticipated. When people regulate in reference to a desired end state they want to approach or an undesired end-state they want to avoid, they might anticipate the pleasure of regulatory success, the pain of regulatory failure, or they might have no clear anticipation at all.

Distinguishing between self-regulation in relation to positive versus negative reference values also has a long history in psychology. Animal learning–biological models highlight the basic distinction between approaching desired end states versus avoiding undesired end states (e.g., Gray, 1982; Lang, 1995; Miller, 1944). Self theorists distinguish between good selves as positive reference values and bad selves as negative reference values (e.g., Erikson, 1963; Markus & Nurius, 1986; Sullivan, 1953). Social psychologists distinguish between positive reference groups and negative reference groups (e.g., Kelley, 1952; Merton, 1957; Newcomb, 1950; Sherif & Sherif, 1964). Self-regulatory systems that have positive versus negative reference values have also been distinguished in cybernetic and control process models (e.g., Miller, Galanter, & Pribram, 1960; Wiener, 1948). Regulatory reference as a principle of self-regulation is most developed in control process models (see Carver & Scheier, 1981).

A third general answer to how self-regulation occurs considers general differences in strategic inclinations for the same goal. "Regulatory focus" distinguishes between "promotion focus" versus "prevention focus." The same desired goal, such as receiving an "A" in a course, can be represented as an accomplishment (the presence of a positive) in a promotion focus or as security (the absence of a negative) in a prevention focus. People tend to use approach strategies for goal attainment when in a promotion focus (e.g., pursuing all means of advancement) and avoidance strategies when in a prevention focus (e.g., carefully avoiding any mistakes). Let us now consider the general principle of regulatory focus in more detail.

The Principle of Regulatory Focus

To illustrate the difference between a promotion focus and a prevention focus, it is useful to consider how their socialization would differ. Consider first caretaker–child interactions that involve a promotion focus. The child experiences the pleasure of the "presence of positive outcomes" when caretakers, for example, hug and kiss the child for behaving in a desired manner, encourage the child to overcome difficulties, or set up opportunities for the child to engage in rewarding activities. A child experiences the pain of the "absence of positive outcomes" when caretakers, for example, end a meal when the child throws some food, take away a toy when the child refuses to share it, stop a story when the child is not paying attention, or act disappointed in the child for failing to fulfill their hopes for him or her. The caretaker's message to the child in both cases is that what matters is attaining accomplishments or fulfilling hopes and aspirations, but that message is communicated in reference to either a desired or an undesired state of the child— either "This is what I would *ideally* like you to do" or "This is *not* what I would ideally like you to do." The regulatory focus is one of *promotion*, that is, a concern with advancement, growth, accomplishment.

Consider next caretaker–child interactions that involve a prevention focus. The child experiences the pleasure of the "absence of negative outcomes" when caretakers, for example, "child-proof" the house, train the child to be alert to potential dangers, or teach the child to "mind your manners." The child experiences the pain of the "presence of negative outcomes" when caretakers, for example, behave roughly with the child to get his or her attention, yell at the child when he or she doesn't listen, criticize the child when he or she makes a mistake, or punish the child for being irresponsible. The caretaker's message to the child in both cases is that what matters is insuring safety, being responsible, and meeting obligations, but that message is communicated in reference either to a desired or an undesired state of the child— either "This is what I believe you *ought* to do" or "This is *not* what I believe you ought to do." The regulatory focus is one of *prevention*, that is, a concern with protection, safety, responsibility.

These socialization differences illustrate how regulatory focus can be independent of regulatory reference. A promotion focus can be taken in reference to either a desired end state or an undesired end state, as can a prevention focus. It is also evident that regulatory focus distinguishes between two different kinds of desired end states: (1) aspirations and accomplishments and (2) responsibilities and safety. People are motivated to approach both kinds of desired end states, but regulatory focus theory proposes that the pleasurable experience of approach working or the painful experience of approach not working will be different for these two kinds of desired end states. In addition, by distinguishing between types of desired (and types of undesired) end states, regulatory focus distinguishes between approach and avoidance strategic means when approaching desired end states (or avoiding undesired end states).

Regulatory focus can induce approach or avoidance inclinations at the strategic level even within general approach movement in reference to "ideal" desired end states (hopes, wishes, aspirations) or "ought" desired end states (duties, obligations, responsibilities). Because self-regulation in relation to "ideal" self-guides is concerned with positive outcomes (their presence and absence), an inclination to approach matches to hopes and aspirations should be the natural strategy for ideal self-regulation. In contrast, because self-regulation in relation to "ought" self-guides is concerned with negative outcomes (their absence and presence), an inclination to avoid mismatches to "ought" duties and obligations should be the natural strategy for ought self-regulation (see Higgins, Roney, Crowe, & Hymes, 1994). Regulatory focus theory postulates, therefore, that people in a promotion focus strategically approach matches to desired end states represented as "ideals," aspirations, and accomplishments, whereas people in a prevention focus strategically avoid mismatches to desired end states represented as "oughts," responsibilities, and safety. Next we review research showing that regulatory focus varies as a function of both "persons" *and* "situations."

Regulatory Focus Effects as a Function of "Person" and "Situation" Variability

As for accessibility, there is evidence that regulatory focus varies across both persons and situations, and the effects of these two sources of variability are comparable. Evidence of such comparability will be presented for the effects of regulatory focus on memory, emotions, and decision making.

Memory Effects of Regulatory Focus as a "Person" and as a "Situation" Variable

The distinction between ideal and ought self-regulation in self-discrepancy theory concerns differences in the psychological situations represented by discrepancies and congruencies involving ideal versus ought self-guides. Actual self congruencies to hopes, wishes, or aspirations (ideals) represent the presence of positive outcomes, whereas discrepancies represent the absence of positive outcomes. Thus, the psychological situations involved in ideal self-regulation with its promotion focus are the presence and absence of positive outcomes. In contrast, discrepancies to duties, obligations, and responsibilities (oughts) represent the presence of negative outcomes, whereas congruencies represent the absence of negative outcomes. Thus, the psychological situations involved in ought self-regulation with its prevention focus are the absence and presence of negative outcomes.

This distinction between ideal and ought self-regulation suggests that sensitivity to events involving the presence and absence of positive outcomes should be greater when ideal concerns involving a promotion focus predominate, whereas sensitivity to events involving the absence and presence of negative outcomes should be greater when ought concerns involving a prevention focus predominate. To test these predictions, Higgins and Tykocinski (1992) selected undergraduate participants on the basis of their self-discrepancy scores using the Selves Questionnaire (see Higgins, Bond, Klein, & Strauman, 1986).

The Selves Questionnaire asks respondents to list up to 8 or 10 attributes for each of a number of different self states, including their actual self and their self guides. This questionnaire is a spontaneous, idiographic measure. On the first page of the questionnaire, the actual, ideal, and ought self states are defined. On each subsequent page, there is a question about a different self state, such as "Please list the attributes of the type of person *you* think you *actually* are" or "Please list the attributes of the type of person *you* would *ideally* like to be, that is, your hopes, wishes, and aspirations for yourself." The respondents are also asked to rate for each listed attribute the extent to which they actually possessed that attribute, ought to possess that attribute, or ideally wanted to possess that attribute. The procedure for calculating the magnitude of an actual–ideal or actual–ought self discrepancy involves comparing the actual self attributes to the attributes listed in either an ideal self guide or an ought self guide to determine which attributes in the actual self match or mismatch the attributes in that particular self guide. The self-discrepancy score is basically the number of mismatches minus the number of matches (see Higgins et al., 1986).

Using participants' responses to the Selves Questionnaire, median splits were performed on the actual–ideal discrepancy scores and on the actual–ought discrepancy scores. Participants were then selected who either were predominant actual–ideal discrepancy persons (i.e., possessed high actual–ideal discrepancies and low actual–ought discrepancies) or were predominant actual–ought discrepancy persons (i.e., possessed high actual–ought discrepancies and low actual–ideal discrepancies).

A few weeks after the selection procedure, all participants read the same essay about the life of a target person in which events reflecting the four different types of psychological situations occurred, such as (1) "I found a 20-dollar bill on the pavement of Canal Street near the paint store" (the presence of positive outcomes); (2) "I've been wanting to see this movie at the 8th Street Theater for some time, so this evening I went there straight after school to find out that it's not showing anymore" (the absence of positive outcomes);

(3) "I was stuck in the subway for 35 minutes with at least 15 sweating passengers breathing down my neck" (the presence of negative outcomes); and (4) "This is usually my worst school day. Awful schedule, class after class with no break. But today is Election Day—no school!" (the absence of negative outcomes).

Ten minutes after reading the essay, the participants were asked to reproduce the essay word-for-word. The study found, as predicted, that predominant actual–ideal discrepancy subjects tended to remember target events representing the presence and absence of positive outcomes better than did predominant actual–ought discrepancy subjects, whereas predominant actual–ought discrepancy subjects tended to remember target events representing the absence and presence of negative outcomes better than did predominant actual–ideal discrepancy subjects. No other interactions were significant, and the obtained interaction was independent of participants' premood, postmood, or change in mood.

The results of Higgins and Tykocinski's study indicate that people's free recall of events related to the absence or presence of positive or negative outcomes is influenced by regulatory focus as a "person" variable. A study by Stepper, Strack, and Higgins (1997) tested whether the same memory effects would occur for regulatory focus as a "situation" variable. Undergraduate participants arrived for a study supposedly testing physiological responses to different kinds of exercise, "physical" and "mental." They were told their physiological responses to different kinds of exercise would be measured by analysis of the saliva they excreted on cotton balls kept in their mouth during each type of exercise. The first exercise task was riding a stationary bicycle at a relatively easy pace. During this exercise the participants had a cotton ball in their mouths that was either *bitter* from a pure tea solution or *sweet* from a sugar solution. After completing this exercise, the cotton ball was removed ostensibly to analyze the saliva.

The second "mental" exercise task was reading the same kind of story used by Higgins and Tykocinski (1992) that contained events reflecting the presence of positives, the absence of positives, the presence of negatives, or the absence of negatives. Half of the participants performed this task with a cotton ball in their mouth that had the same solution as the first task and the other half now had a cotton ball with a neutral water solution. While reading the story events, therefore, participants were in one of four experimental conditions: $sweet_1$–$sweet_2$, $sweet_1$–$neutral_2$, $bitter_1$–$bitter_2$, and $bitter_1$–$neutral_2$.

It was predicted that the regulatory focus state that was situationally activated by the cotton balls would make the participants more sensitive to story events reflecting the same regulatory focus state. The results of the study supported this prediction. The percentage of participants who remembered more "presence of positive" story events than "absence of negative" story events was greater for participants in the "promotion–working" state ($sweet_1$–$sweet_2$) than participants in the "prevention–working" state ($bitter_1$–

neutral$_2$), whereas the reverse was true for those remembering more "absence of negative" story events than "presence of positive" story events. In addition, the percentage of participants who remembered more "absence of positive" story events than "presence of negative" story events was greater for participants in the promotion–not working state (sweet$_1$–neutral$_2$) than participants in the prevention–not working state (bitter$_1$–bitter$_2$), whereas the reverse was true for those remembering more "presence of negative" story events than "absence of positive" story events. Thus, the basic findings of the Higgins and Tykocinski (1992) study where regulatory focus was a "person" variable were replicated in this study where regulatory focus was a "situation" variable.

Emotional Effects of Regulatory Focus as a "Person" and as a "Situation" Variable

Attaining a goal with a promotion focus reflects the presence of positive outcomes underlying cheerfulness-related emotions such as feeling happy or satisfied, while not attaining a goal with a promotion focus reflects the absence of positive outcomes underlying dejection-related emotions such as feeling disappointed or discouraged. In contrast, attaining a goal with a prevention focus reflects the absence of negative outcomes underlying quiescence-related emotions such as feeling calm or relaxed, whereas not attaining a goal with a prevention focus reflects the presence of negative outcomes underlying agitation-related emotions such as feeling tense or uneasy.

Higgins, Shah, and Friedman (1997) hypothesized that stronger goals would relate to more intense emotional responses, and, more importantly, that strength of regulatory focus would determine the *type of emotional response* that was greater. They initially considered the implications of this hypothesis for regulatory focus as a "person" variable. As ideal mismatches increasingly predominate over ideal matches, dejection-related emotions should increase and cheerfulness-related emotions should decrease. As ought mismatches increasingly predominate over ought matches, agitation-related emotions should increase and quiescence-related emotions should decrease. In addition, strength of promotion focus increases as strength of ideal self guides increases, and strength of prevention focus increases as strength of ought self guides increases.

Consistent with previous work on attitude accessibility (e.g., Fazio, 1995), self-guide strength was conceptualized and operationalized in terms of self-guide accessibility, and self-guide accessibility was measured via individuals' response times to inquiries about their self-guide attributes. Accessibility is activation potential, and knowledge units with higher activation potentials should produce faster responses to knowledge-related inputs (see Higgins, 1996). A computer measure of actual self and self-guide attributes was developed that was similar to the original Selves Questionnaire. Self-guide strength was measured by response latencies in listing attributes and giving extent ratings. Actual–ideal and actual–ought discrepancies were measured by comparing the extent rating of each self-guide attribute with the extent rating of the actual self for that attribute (see Higgins et al., 1997).

This analysis leads to two specific predictions: (1) an interaction of ideal self-guide strength and actual–ideal discrepancy, such that the correlation between actual–ideal discrepancy and experiencing dejection-related emotions (or actual–ideal congruency and experiencing cheerfulness-related emotions) would increase as the accessibility of ideal self-guides increased; and (2) an interaction of ought self-guide strength and actual–ought discrepancy, such that the correlation between actual–ought discrepancy and experiencing agitation-related emotions (or actual–ought congruency and experiencing quiescence-related emotions) would increase as the accessibility of ought self guides increased.

Higgins et al. (1997) conducted three studies testing these hypotheses. Two studies tested the relation between self discrepancies (or congruencies) and the frequency that undergraduate participants experienced different kinds of emotions during the previous week. A third study tested the relation between self discrepancies (or congruencies) and the intensity of different kinds of emotions that undergraduate participants experienced before beginning a performance task. All three studies supported the predictions.

The results of these studies indicate that regulatory focus as a "person" variable combined with goal attainment predicts the intensity of different kinds of emotions that people will experience. Another study by Higgins et al. (1997) tested whether the same emotional effects would occur for regulatory focus as a "situation" variable. They used a framing technique to manipulate regulatory focus experimentally. The framing kept constant the actual consequences of attaining or not attaining the goal, as well as the criterion of success and failure, but varied the focus of the instructions.

The task involved memorizing trigrams. For the promotion focus, the participants began with 5 dollars, and the instructions were about gains and nongains: "If you score above the 70th percentile, that is, if you remember a lot of letter strings, then you will gain a dollar. However, if you don't score above the 70th percentile, that is, if you don't remember a lot of letter strings, then you will not gain a dollar." For the prevention focus, the participants began with 6 dollars, and the instructions were about losses and nonlosses: "If you score above the 70th percentile, that is, if you don't forget a lot of letter strings, then you won't lose a dollar. However, if you don't score above the 70th percentile, that is, if you do forget a lot of letter strings, then you will lose a dollar." Following performance of the task, the participants were given false feedback that they had either succeeded or failed on the task.

It was predicted that feedback-consistent emotional change, that is, increasing positive and decreasing negative emotions following success and decreasing positive and increasing negative emotions following failure, would be different in the promotion-framing versus prevention-framing conditions. Feedback-consistent change on the cheerfulness–dejection dimension should be greater for participants in the promotion- than the prevention-framing condition, whereas feedback-consistent change on the quiescence–agitation dimension should be greater for participants in the prevention-than the promotion-framing condition. This predicted two-way interaction was obtained. Thus, the same basic findings concerning the relations among regulatory focus, goal attainment, and intensity of different kinds of emotions were obtained when regulatory focus was a "situation" variable as when it was a "person" variable.

Decision-Making Effects of Regulatory Focus as a "Person" and as a "Situation" Variable

A basic assumption of expectancy-value models of motivation has been that both expectancy and value impact on goal commitment and that, in addition to their main effects, they combine multiplicatively (for a review, see Feather, 1982). The multiplicative assumption is that as either expectancy or value increases, the impact of the other variable on commitment increases. For example, it is assumed that the effect on goal commitment of a high versus a low likelihood of attaining the goal is greater when the goal is highly valued than when the goal has little value. This assumption reflects the notion that the goal commitment involves a motivation to *maximize* the product of value and expectancy.

Not all studies, however, have found the predicted positive interactive effect of value and expectancy. Shah and Higgins (1997) proposed that the inconsistencies in the literature might be due to differences in the regulatory focus of decision makers. They suggested that making a decision with a promotion focus is more likely to involve the motivation to maximize the product of value and expectancy. A promotion focus on goals as accomplishments might induce an "approach matches" strategic inclination to pursue highly valued goals with the highest expected utility, which maximizes value × expectancy. Thus, Shah and Higgins (1997) predicted that the positive interactive effect of value and expectancy assumed by classic expectancy-value models would increase as promotion focus increased.

But what about a prevention focus? A prevention focus on goals as security or safety might induce an "avoid mismatches" strategic inclination to avoid all unnecessary risks by striving to meet only responsibilities that are either clearly necessary (i.e., high-value prevention goals) *or* attainable with assurance (i.e., high expectancy of attainment). This strategic inclination creates a different interactive relation between value and expectancy. As the value of a prevention goal increases, the goal becomes a necessity, such as the Ten Commandments or the safety of one's child. When a goal becomes a necessity, one *must* do whatever one can to attain it regardless of the ease or likelihood of goal attainment. That is, expectancy information becomes less relevant as a prevention goal becomes more like a necessity. With prevention goals, motivation would still generally increase when the likelihood of goal attainment is higher, but this increase would be *smaller* for high-value, necessity goals than low-value goals. Thus, the second prediction is that the positive interactive effect of value and expectancy assumed by classic expectancy-value models would *not* be found as prevention focus increased. Specifically, as prevention focus increased, the interactive effect of value and expectancy would be *negative!*

Shah and Higgins (1997) first tested these predictions in studies of decision making in which regulatory focus was a "person" variable. In one study, for example, undergraduate participants were asked to evaluate the likelihood that they would take a course in their major for which the value of doing well and the expectancy of doing well in the course were experimentally manipulated, and participants' chronic regulatory focus was measured in terms of the strength of their ideal and ought self guides. High versus low value was established in terms of 95% versus 51% of previous majors being accepted into their honor society when they received a grade of B or higher in the course. High versus low expectancy was established in terms of 75% versus 25% of previous majors receiving a grade of B or higher in the course. As predicted, Shah and Higgins (1997) found that the contrast representing the expectancy × value effect on the decision to take the course was positive for individuals with a strong promotion focus (i.e., high chronic ideal strength) but was negative for individuals with a strong prevention focus (i.e., high chronic ought strength).

The results of this and another study by Shah and Higgins (1997) indicated that regulatory focus as a "person" variable influences how expectancy and value information interact in decision making. Another study by Shah and Higgins (1997) tested whether the same effects on decision making would occur for regulatory focus as a "situation" variable. They used a framing technique to manipulate regulatory focus experimentally. Participants in the promotion-framing condition were told to imagine that they want to maximize their chances of being accepted into their major's honor society, and their chances of being accepted are greater if they finish in the top half of the class taking the course than if they do not finish in the top half of the class. Participants in the prevention-framing condition were told to imagine that they want to minimize their chances of being rejected and that they are less likely to be rejected if they avoid finishing in the bottom half of the class than if they do finish in the bottom half of the class. Participants' subjective ratings of the value of finishing in the top half of the class taking the course and the likelihood that they would finish in the top half were also obtained.

The results of this framing study showed that the interactive effect of expectancy and value was significantly positive in the promotion-framing condition but was significantly negative in the prevention-framing condition.

Thus, the same basic findings concerning how expectancy and value information interact in decision-making were obtained when regulatory focus was a "situation" variable as when it was a "person" variable.

GENERAL DISCUSSION AND CONCLUSIONS

Historically, personality has been thought to have its own unique set of explanatory principles distinct from other areas of psychology. Personality principles have been distinguished from social psychological principles. What has varied among the classic perspectives on personality is how variability across "situations" is treated with respect to personality. The personality "traits" or "dimensions" perspective controls for or removes the influence of situations on behavior in order to study cross-situational effects of personality alone. The "psychoanalytic" perspective emphasizes the organization of interacting personality processes, such as characteristic conflicts and defenses, that reside within the person. The "interactionist" perspective considers variability across "persons" and across "situations" as reflecting separate principles whose functioning interacts to influence behavior. I have proposed an alternative, *"general principles" perspective* in this chapter in which psychological states reflect the functioning of general psychological principles, and personality as an area is concerned with a particular source of variability in the functioning of these general principles—variability across persons. Social psychology as an area is concerned with another source of variability in the functioning of the *same* general principles—variability across situations. The general explanatory principles are the same for both areas (and other areas of psychology as well). Only the source of variability to be investigated differs.

This chapter has examined general principles of knowledge activation (i.e., accessibility) and self-regulation (i.e., regulatory focus) to illustrate how "persons" and "situations" as sources of variability in psychological states can reveal the functioning of the same basic principle. The principles of accessibility and regulatory focus were each shown to have comparable effects when they varied as a function of "persons" and as a function of "situations." It is clear from these examples that it is possible to identify general psychological principles for which personality is one source, but not the only source, of variability. It would be fair to ask, however, whether the "general principles" perspective proposed in this chapter has implications for historical treatments of personality in which distinct personality principles have been identified. Although it is not possible here to provide an extensive review of classic explanatory principles in the personality area, some illustrations are provided.

One classic personality principle is Kelly's (1955) personal constructs. Kelly (1955) proposed that individuals varied in their viewpoints on the world as represented in the personal constructs they chronically used to encode events. This personality variable was the inspiration for one of Mischel's (1973) "person" variables in his social-cognitive learning reconceptualization of personality—individual differences in encodings or construals. This "person" variable remains as one of Mischel and Shoda's (1995) cognitive-affective units in their "personality system."

There are, unquestionably, stable individual differences in the constructs used to encode or categorize events. These differences can be understood in terms of individual differences in which constructs are available and/or have high chronic accessibility. But the accessibility of constructs is also influenced by contextual priming, and thus a person's encodings of events also vary as a function of the situation. In addition, high activation potential from chronic accessibility can work together with situational priming to produce such high levels of construct accessibility as to yield construct-related judgments of even extremely vague input (Higgins & Brendl, 1995). This possibility only emerges when accessibility is understood to be a general principle than varies across persons and situations. Moreover, accessibility, whether varying by "persons" or by "situations," not only influences encodings or categorizations. It can influence attention, memory, feelings, and problem solving as well (see Higgins, 1996). Therefore, it would seem better to identify accessibility as the general principle, rather than personal encodings or construals, and then examine the multiple effects of this principle as it varies across persons, situations, and their combinations.

Another classic personality principle is achievement motivation (e.g., Atkinson, 1964; McClelland et al., 1953; Murray, 1938). Beginning with Murray, need achievement was the need to accomplish or master something of value, to attain a high standard. This need is reflected in McClelland and Atkinson's "motive to succeed" personality variable, which also concerns a chronic motivation to attain a high standard and accomplish something of value, to approach the anticipated pleasure of success. The "motive to succeed" was distinguished from the "fear of failure," which concerns a chronic motivation to avoid the anticipated pain of failure. Reflecting their "interactionist" perspective, these theories included environmental forces or presses that provoked the achievement needs or motives, but these forces were treated as a set of "situation" variables distinct from the "person" variable of chronic individual differences in achievement motivation.

The distinction between individuals high in "motive to succeed" and individuals high in "fear of failure" can be reconceptualized as involving a comparison of two specific combinations of the general principles of regulatory anticipation, regulatory reference, and regulatory focus. Individuals high in "motive to succeed" anticipate pleasure, approach a desired end state, and have a promotion focus. Individuals high in "fear of failure" anticipate pain, avoid an undesired end state, and have a prevention focus. But regulatory anticipation, regulatory reference, and regulatory focus can also vary as a function of situations. Moreover, there are eight possible combinations of these three general principles rather than just the two identified by classic theories of achievement motivation. In addition, these general principles influence human motivation not only in the achievement domain but in other domains as well, such as influencing affiliation and attitudes. Thus, once again, it would seem better to identify regulatory anticipation, regulatory reference, and regulatory focus as the general principles, rather than chronic achievement needs or motives, and then examine the multiple effects of these principles as they vary across persons, situations, and their combinations.

"Authoritarianism" is another classic explanatory principle in the personality area (see Adorno, Frenkel-Brunswick, Levinson, & Sanford, 1950). High authoritarians have been described as having a rigid adherence to conventional values, intolerance of ambiguity, an attachment to "things as they are," obedience to moral authority, and a tendency to criticize and punish low-status individuals. These characteristics would be more common among individuals with a strong need for closure (Kruglanski, 1989) and a strong prevention focus. But Kruglanski (1989) reports that need for closure also varies as a function of situations, and we have already seen that there is situational variability in prevention focus as well. Thus, an authoritarian-like psychological state might also be induced by situational conditions. Moreover, both a need for closure and a prevention focus have effects on information processing and decision making beyond those described in the literature on authoritarianism as a personality variable. In this case as well, therefore, it would seem better to examine regulatory focus and closure motivation as general principles, rather than authoritarianism as a personality variable, and then examine the multiple effects of these principles as they vary across persons, situations, and their combinations.

These examples illustrate how a "general principles" perspective points to a different research enterprise than the traditional perspectives on personality. Rather than a concern with personality principles of psychology that provide unique "person" explanations for people's psychological states, general principles that explain variation across both persons and situations would be sought. Because it would be understood that both persons and situations can be sources of variability in the same principle, it would be natural to consider how "situation" and "person" sources of variability work together to influence the functioning of the same principle.

One way that "situation" and "person" sources of variability in the same principle can work together is for one source to compensate for the other. For example, increased accessibility from contextual priming can compensate for chronic accessibility, such that an individual with low chronic accessibility in a priming situation could function like an individual with high chronic accessibility in a no-priming situation (see Higgins & Brendl, 1995). Such compensation would be especially important when situations are themselves chronic or "institutionalized." Thus, an institution that chronically framed incentives

and feedback with positive anticipation, desired reference points, and a promotion focus could produce persistent "motive to succeed" psychological
states in its members. Similarly, an institution that chronically set prevention
goals (e.g., "putting out fires") and short deadlines, which induce a need for
closure (see Kruglanski, 1989), could produce persistent "authoritarian"
states in its members.

Another way that "situation" and "person" sources of variability in the
same principle can work together is for one source to inhibit the other. For
example, the functioning of chronic promotion or prevention focus associated
with ideal or ought self-regulation, respectively, can be inhibited by situationally framing outcomes in terms of the opposite regulatory focus.
Brendl, Higgins, and Lemm (1995), for instance, tested undergraduates' affective sensitivity to varying amounts of monetary gains and losses. The gains
and losses were framed with either a promotion focus or a prevention focus
(e.g., receive or not receive a $50 savings versus avoid or not avoid an addi-
tional $50 expense). Brendl et al. (1995) found that, controlling for the plea-
sure or pain of the outcome, affective discrimination was reduced (i.e., less
positive slope) when there was a mismatch between the participants' chronic
regulatory focus (ideal versus ought self-regulation) and the regulatory focus
of their framing condition (promotion versus prevention). Because promotion
focus and prevention focus are distinct self-regulatory systems, a momentary
situation activating one focus can inhibit a person's chronic predisposition for
the competing focus.

It should be noted that the search for general principles does not simply
translate well-known personality principles into a new language. It reconsid-
ers, for example, what it means to be a "moderate" on a personality dimension. How to conceptualize moderates has been a difficult problem for personality psychologists. It is well-known that moderates are not simply at the
middle level of some psychological dimension such as "motive to succeed,"
and individuals who score as moderates on some personality dimension are
often not the same psychologically (see Sorrentino & Short, 1977). A general
principles perspective could shed light on this issue. For instance, individuals
could be moderate on "motive to succeed" either because they are more motivated to avoid some undesired end state than to approach some desired end
state, or because they are motivated to approach some desired end state but
anticipate failing to attain it, or because the desired end state they anticipate
attaining successfully is represented as an obligation (prevention) rather than
as an accomplishment (promotion).

The search for general principles also emphasizes psychological states
and the principles underlying them rather than any particular source of variability in these states, such as personality. This naturally leads to considering
how "person" and "situation" sources of variability in the same principle
work together, as discussed earlier. More generally, it underscores why it is
unreasonable to explain people's responses to the world in terms of some

personality variable collapsed across situations. People's responses follow from their psychological states, and variability in these states is never just across persons. Why should one source of variability, such as personality, be given such explanatory status? Is it not more reasonable to give explanatory status to the general principles that underlie the psychological states?

It is not only the area of personality that could benefit by shifting attention from its own unique set of explanatory principles to general principles that vary across both persons and situations. Social psychology could benefit as well. Social psychologists have also emphasized their own unique set of explanatory principles with insufficient consideration of general principles that would vary across persons as well as situations.

One classic social psychological principle is cognitive dissonance. Dissonance has been characterized as "feeling responsible for an aversive event" (Cooper & Fazio, 1984) and has been related to self-evaluative processes involving a perceived discrepancy between one's actual behavior and the type of person one believes one should be (e.g., Aronson, 1969). As an experience, dissonance has been described as a state of unpleasant tension (see Festinger, 1957; Wicklund & Brehm, 1976). Dissonance, then, involves situations in which people experience tension because they feel responsible for having done something that is discrepant from the type of person they believe they should be.

Individuals with actual–ought discrepancies, however, also experience tension from chronic failure to meet what they believe to be their responsibilities (see Higgins, 1987). Thus, experiencing tension from failure to meet what one believes to be one's responsibilities can vary across situations *and* across persons. This personality perspective on dissonance is different from introducing separate personality variables, such as dogmatism or repression sensitization, as potential moderators of dissonance effects (see Wicklund & Brehm, 1976). What I am suggesting is that the *same* general principle concerning failure to meet what one believes to be one's responsibilities can be treated as a social psychological phenomenon varying across situations or as a personality phenomenon varying across persons.

Another classic explanatory principle in social psychology is obedience to authority made famous by Milgram (1974). People are assigned a role by an authority figure, such as the experimenter in Milgram's studies assigning participants the role of teacher, and the authority figure emphasizes the necessity of fulfilling the obligations of the role described in the instructions (e.g., "As teacher you must punish the learner when he makes a mistake"). What Milgram (1974) found was that people in this situation follow the instructions even when it involves hurting and even potentially harming another person. Thus, the situation makes people strongly motivated to avoid failing to meet their obligations as specified by the authority figure. It is clear from the literature on the authoritarian personality, however, that people differ chronically in how motivated they are to avoid failing to meet obligations prescribed by authority figures. Once again, the *same* general principle concerning a strong prevention motivation to avoid failing to meet significant others' prescriptions can be treated as a social psychological phenomenon varying across situations or as a personality phenomenon varying across persons.

Accessibility and regulatory focus have each been used in this chapter to illustrate that "person" variables and "situation" variables can concern the functioning of the same general principle. I have used these examples to argue that personality concerns how the functioning of general principles underlying people's psychological states varies across persons but that the functioning of the *same* general principles also varies across situations. I have proposed that the area of personality is unique within psychology with respect to its concern with a particular source of variability in underlying principles but not with respect to the nature of the principles themselves.

Some psychologists might question whether the "person" variables serving as illustrations in this chapter are true *personality* principles. They might argue that variability across persons in the relative accessibility of different kinds of knowledge or in the relative strength of promotion focus versus prevention focus is better characterized as *individual differences*. Personality, they might argue, concerns different kinds of predispositions that are somehow more basic to a person's self-regulatory style or self-control in responding to situations generally. Classic personality principles of this sort are rigidity or overcontrol and lack of willpower or undercontrol (e.g., Adorno et al., 1950; Block & Block, 1980; Lewin, 1935; Mischel, Shoda, & Peake, 1988). These personality principles concern how people control themselves and make choices in the face of situational pressures. They concern the classic conflict between personal needs and situational demands. By capturing the classic notion of person–situation conflict, they highlight the notion that persons and situations are *not* the same. Surely, then, unique psychological explanations are provided by these true personality principles.

What is evident from the literature is that even these kinds of personality principles reflect general principles whose functioning varies across situations as well. As mentioned earlier, rigid adherence to a restricted set of goals, beliefs, or strategies can be increased or decreased situationally by inducing a need for closure versus a need to avoid closure, respectively (Kruglanski, 1989) or by inducing a prevention focus versus a promotion focus, respectively (Higgins, 1997). Willpower or resistance to goal disruption can be increased situationally by inducing elaborations of task-facilitating plans (Mischel, 1996) or implementation intentions (Gollwitzer, 1996). The general principles are need for closure, regulatory focus, and implementation plans. The functioning of these principles does vary across persons, and such variability has been captured by classic personality concepts such as rigidity and willpower. But the underlying principles are not unique to personality and thus are not personality principles per se. They are general principles of psychological functioning. Because the

functioning of each principle can vary across situations as well as persons, a sit
uation variable can inhibit the influence of a person variable on the functioning
of a principle, as described earlier for regulatory focus. But such person–situation relations involve the *same* principle rather than a conflict between separate
person and situation principles.

It is time for psychologists in personality and social psychology, as well
as in other areas of psychology such as abnormal, developmental, and cross-
cultural, to emphasize their own unique explanations for their own distinct
phenomena less, and emphasize general principles of psychology more. It is
time to seek and examine general principles that underlie different phenomena across areas and that vary as a function of both "persons" and "situations," including mental health status, age, culture, and other sources of variability. These general principles can be at different levels of analysis
providing different levels of explanation, but levels of analysis are not the
same as areas of psychology. The area of social psychology, for example, has
principles at the biological, cognitive, interpersonal, and cultural levels of
analysis (see Higgins & Kruglanski, 1996), as does personality (see Pervin,
1990). Discovering and examining general principles at different levels of
analysis will benefit all areas of psychology by providing a deeper understanding of the phenomena in each area. It will also create bridges across
areas and increase the coherence of psychology as a discipline. Personality
and the others areas would continue to play a critically important role in psychology because of what they tell us about different sources of variability in
the general principles. Psychology, however, would become a science of principles rather than a confederation of separate areas.

REFERENCES

Adorno, T. W., Frenkel-Brunswick, E., Levinson, D. J., & Sanford, R. N. (1950). *The authoritarian personality.* New York: Harper.

Aronson, E. (1969). The theory of cognitive dissonance: A current perspective. In L. Berkowitz (Ed.), *Advances in experimental social psychology* (Vol. 4, pp. 1–34). New York: Academic Press.

Atkinson, J. W. (1964). *An introduction to motivation.* Princeton, NJ: Van Nostrand.

Bandura, A. (1986). *Social foundations of thought and action: A social cognitive theory.* Englewood Cliffs, NJ: Prentice-Hall.

Bargh, J.A. (1982). Attention and automaticity in the processing of self-relevant information. *Journal of Personality and Social Psychology, 43,* 425–436.

Bargh, J. A., Bond, R. N., Lombardi, W. J., & Tota, M. E. (1986). The additive nature of chronic and temporary sources of construct accessibility. *Journal of Personality and Social Psychology, 50,* 869–878.

Bargh, J. A., Lombardi, W. J., & Higgins, E. T. (1988). Automaticity of chronically accessible constructs in person × situation effects on person perception: It's just a matter of time. *Journal of Personality and Social Psychology, 55,* 599–605.

Bargh, J. A., & Pietromonaco, P. (1982). Automatic information processing and social perception: The influence of trait information presented outside of conscious awareness on impression formation. *Journal of Personality and Social Psychology, 43,* 437–449.

Bargh, J. A., & Pratto, F. (1986). Individual construct accessibility and perceptual selection. *Journal of Experimental Social Psychology, 22,* 293–311.

Bargh, J.A., & Thein, R.D. (1985). Individual construct accessibility, person memory, and the recall–judgment link: The case of information overload. *Journal of Personality and Social Psychology, 49,* 1129–1146.

Bartlett, F. C. (1932). *Remembering.* Cambridge, England: Cambridge University Press.

Block, J. H., & Block, J. (1980). The role of ego-control and ego-resiliency in the organization of behavior. In W. A. Collins (Ed.), *Minnesota symposium on child psychology* (Vol. 13, pp. 39–101). Hillsdale, NJ: Erlbaum.

Brendl, C. M., Higgins, E. T., & Lemm, K. M. (1995). Sensitivity to varying gains and losses: The role of self-discrepancies and event framing. *Journal of Personality and Social Psychology, 69,* 1028–1051.

Bruner, J. S. (1951). Personality dynamics and the process of perceiving. In R. R. Blake & G. V. Ramsey (Eds.), *Perception: An approach to personality.* New York: Ronald Press.

Bruner, J. S. (1957a). Going beyond the information given. In H. Gruber, G. Terrell, & M. Wertheimer (Eds.), *Contemporary approaches to cognition.* Cambridge, MA: Harvard University Press.

Bruner, J. S. (1957b). On perceptual readiness. *Psychological Review, 64,* 123–152.

Cameron, N. (1963). *Personality development and psychopathology.* Boston: Houghton Mifflin.

Carver, C. S., & Scheier, M. F. (1981). *Attention and self-regulation: A control-theory approach to human behavior.* New York: Springer-Verlag.

Cantor, N., & Zirkel, S. (1990). Personality, cognition, and purposive behavior. In L. A. Pervin (Ed.), *Handbook of personality: Theory and research* (pp. 135–164). New York: Guilford Press.

Cooper, J., & Fazio, R.H. (1984). A new look at dissonance theory. In L. Berkowitz (Ed.), *Advances in experimental social psychology* (Vol. 17, pp. 229–265). New York: Academic Press.

Endler, N. S. (1982). Interactionism comes of age. In M. P. Zanna, E. T. Higgins, & C. P. Herman (Eds.), *Consistency in social behavior: The Ontario Symposium* (Vol. 2, pp. 209–249). Hillsdale, NJ: Erlbaum.

Epstein, S. (1979). The stability of behavior: On predicting most of the people much of the time. *Journal of Personality and Social Psychology, 37,* 1097–1126.

Erikson, E. H. (1963). *Childhood and society* (Rev. ed.). New York: Norton. (Original work published 1950).

Fazio, R. H. (1995). Attitudes as object–evaluation associations: Determinants, consequences, and correlates of attitude accessibility. In R. E. Petty & J. A. Krosnick (Eds.), *Attitude strength: Antecedents and consequences* (pp. 247–282). Mahwah, NJ: Erlbaum.

Feather, N. T. (1982). Actions in relation to expected consequences: An overview of a research program. In N. T. Feather (Ed.), *Expectations and actions: Expectancy–value models in psychology* (pp. 53–95). Hillsdale, NJ: Erlbaum.

Festinger, I.. (1957). *A theory of cognitive dissonance.* Evanston, IL: Row, Peterson.

Freud, S. (1950). *Beyond the pleasure principle.* New York: Liveright. (Original work published 1920)

Gollwitzer, P. M. (1996). The volitional benefits of planning. In P. M. Gollwitzer & J. A. Bargh (Eds.) *The psychology of action: Linking cognition and motivation to behavior* (pp. 287–312). New York: Guilford Press.

Gray, J. A. (1982). *The neuropsychology of anxiety: An enquiry into the functions of the septohippocampal system.* New York: Oxford University Press.

Higgins, E. T. (1987). Self-discrepancy: A theory relating self and affect. *Psychological Review, 94,* 319–340.

Higgins, E. T. (1990). Personality, social psychology, and person–situation relations: Standards and knowledge activation as a common language. In L. A. Pervin (Ed.), *Handbook of personality: Theory and research* (pp. 301–338). New York: Guilford Press.

Higgins, E. T. (1996). Knowledge activation: Accessibility, applicability, and salience. In E. T. Higgins & A. W. Kruglanski (Eds.), *Social psychology: Handbook of basic principles* (pp. 133–168). New York: Guilford Press.

Higgins, E. T. (1997). Beyond pleasure and pain. *American Psychologist, 52,* 1280–1300.

Higgins, E. T., & Bargh, J. A. (1987). Social cognition and social perception. *Annual Review of Psychology, 38,* 369–425.

Higgins, E. T., Bargh, J. A., & Lombardi, W. (1985). The nature of priming effects on categorization. *Journal of Experimental Psychology: Learning, Memory and Cognition, 11,* 59–69.

Higgins, E. T., Bond, R. N., Klein, R., & Strauman, T. (1986). Self-discrepancies and emotional vulnerability: How magnitude, accessibility, and type of discrepancy influence affect. *Journal of Personality and Social Psychology, 51,* 5–15.

Higgins, E. T., & Brendl, M. (1995). Accessibility and applicability: Some "activation rules" influencing judgment. *Journal of Experimental Social Psychology, 31,* 218–243.

Higgins, E. T., & King, G. (1981). Accessibility of social constructs: Information processing consequences of individual and contextual variability. In N. Cantor & J. Kihlstrom (Eds.), *Personality, cognition, and social interaction* (pp. 69–121). Hillsdale, NJ: Erlbaum.

Higgins, E. T., King, G. A., & Mavin, G. H. (1982). Individual construct accessibility and subjective impressions and recall. *Journal of Personality and Social Psychology, 43,* 35–47.

Higgins, E. T., & Kruglanski, A. W. (Eds.). (1996). *Social psychology: Handbook of basic principles.* New York: Guilford Press.

Higgins, E. T., Rholes, W. S., & Jones, C. R. (1977). Category accessibility and impression formation. *Journal of Experimental Social Psychology, 13,* 141–154.

Higgins, E. T., Roney, C., Crowe, E., & Hymes, C. (1994). Ideal versus ought predilections for approach and avoidance: Distinct self-regulatory systems. *Journal of Personality and Social Psychology, 66,* 276–286.

Higgins, E. T., Shah, J., & Friedman, R. (1997). Emotional responses to goal attainment: Strength of regulatory focus as moderator. *Journal of Personality and Social Psychology, 72,* 515–525.

Higgins, E. T., & Tykocinski, O. (1992). Self-discrepancies and biographical memory: Personality and cognition at the level of psychological situation. *Personality and Social Psychology Bulletin, 18,* 527–535.

John, O. P. (1990). The "big five" factor taxonomy: Dimensions of personality in the natural language and in questionnaires. In L. A. Pervin (Ed.), *Handbook of personality: Theory and research* (pp. 66–100). New York: Guilford Press.

Kelley, H. H. (1952). Two functions of reference groups. In G. E. Swanson, T. M. Newcomb, & E. L. Hartley (Eds.), *Readings in social psychology* (2nd ed., pp. 410–420). New York: Holt, Rinehart & Winston.

Kelly, G. A. (1955). *The psychology of personal constructs.* New York: Norton.

Kruglanski, A. W. (1989). *Lay epistemics and human knowledge: Cognitive and motivational bases.* New York: Plenum Press.

Lang, P. J. (1995). The emotion probe: Studies of motivation and attention. *American Psychologist, 50,* 372–385.

Lau, R. R. (1989). Construct accessibility and electoral choice. *Political Behavior, 11,* 5–32.

Lewin, K. (1935). *A dynamic theory of personality.* New York: McGraw-Hill.

Lombardi, W. J., Higgins, E. T., & Bargh, J. A. (1987). The role of consciousness in priming effects on categorization. *Personality and Social Psychology Bulletin, 13,* 411–429.

Magnusson, D. (1990). Personality development from an interactional perspective. In L. A. Pervin (Ed.), *handbook of personality: Theory and research* (pp. 193–222). New York: Guilford Press.

Magnusson, D., & Endler, N. S. (Eds.). (1977). *Personality at the crossroads: Current issues in interactional psychology.* Hillsdale, NJ: Erlbaum.

Markus, H. (1977). Self-schemata and processing information about the self. *Journal of Personality and Social Psychology, 35,* 63–78.

Markus, H., & Nurius, P. (1986). Possible selves. *American Psychologist, 41,* 954–969.

Martin, L. L. (1986). Set/reset: Use and disuse of concepts in impression formation. *Journal of Personality and Social Psychology, 51,* 493–504.

Martin, L. L., & Achee, J. W. (1992). Beyond accessibility: The role of processing objectives in judgment. In L. L. Martin & A. Tesser (Eds.), *The construction of social judgments* (pp. 195–216). Hillsdale, NJ: Erlbaum.

McClelland, D. C., & Atkinson, J. W. (1948). The projective expression of needs: I. The effect of different intensities of the hunger drive on perception. *Journal of Psychology, 25,* 205–232.

McClelland, D. C., Atkinson, J. W., Clark, R. A., & Lowell, E. L. (1953). *The achievement motive.* New York: Appleton-Century-Crofts.

Merton, R. K. (1957). *Social theory and social structure.* Glencoe, IL: Free Press.

Milgram, S. (1974). *Obedience to authority.* New York: Harper & Row.

Miller, G. A., Galanter, E., & Pribram, K. H. (1960). *Plans and the structure of behavior.* New York: Holt, Rinehart, & Winston.

Miller, N. E. (1944). Experimental studies of conflict. In J. M. Hunt (Ed.), *Personality and the behavior disorders* (Vol. 1, pp. 431–465). New York: Ronald Press.

Mischel, W. (1973). Toward a cognitive social learning reconceptualization of personality. *Psychological Review, 80,* 252–283.

Mischel, W. (1996). From good intentions to willpower. In P. M. Gollwitzer & J. A. Bargh (Eds.), *The psychology of action: Linking cognition and motivation to behavior* (pp. 197–218). New York: Guilford Press.

Mischel, W., & Shoda, Y. (1995). A cognitive-affective system theory of personality: Reconceptualizing situations, dispositions, dynamics, and invariance in personality structure. *Psychological Review, 102,* 246–268.

Mischel, W., Shoda, Y., & Peake, P. K. (1988). The nature of adolescent competencies predicted by preschool delay of gratification. *Journal of Personality and Social Psychology, 54,* 687–699.

Mowrer, O.H. (1960). *Learning theory and behavior.* New York: Wiley.

Murray, H.A. (1938). *Exploration in personality.* New York: Oxford University Press.

Newcomb, T. M. (1950). *Social psychology.* New York: Dryden Press

Pervin, L. A. (Ed.). (1990). *Handbook of personality; Theory and research.* New York: Guilford Press.

Rotter, J. B. (1954). *Social learning and clinical psychology.* Englewood Cliffs, NJ: Prentice-Hall.

Sarbin, T. R., Taft, R., & Bailey, D. E. (1960). *Clinical inference and cognitive theory.* New York: Holt, Rinehart & Winston.

Shah, J., & Higgins, E. T. (1997). Expectancy × value effects: Regulatory focus as a determinant of magnitude *and* direction. *Journal of Personality and Social Psychology, 73,* 447–458.

Sherif, M., & Sherif, C. W. (1964). *Reference groups.* New York: Harper.

Smith, E. R., & Branscombe, N. R. (1987). Procedurally mediated social inferences: The case of category accessibility effects. *Journal of Experimental Social Psychology, 23,* 361–382.

Smith, E. R., Stewart, T. L., & Buttram, R. T. (1992). Inferring a trait from a behavior has long-term, highly specific effects. *Journal of Personality and Social Psychology, 62,* 753–759.

Sorrentino, R. M., & Higgins, E. T. (1986). Motivation and cognition: Warming up to synergism. In R. M. Sorrentino & E. T. Higgins (Eds.), *Handbook of motivation and cognition: Foundations of social behavior* (pp. 3–19). New York: Guilford Press.

Sorrentino, R. M., & Short, J. C. (1977). The case of the mysterious moderates: Why motives sometimes fail to predict behavior. *Journal of Personality and Social Psychology, 35,* 478–484.

Srull, T.K., & Wyer, R. S. (1979). The role of category accessibility in the interpretation of information about persons: Some determinants and implications. *Journal of Personality and Social Psychology, 37,* 1660–1672.

Srull, T. K., & Wyer, R. S., Jr. (1980). Category accessibility and social perception: Some implications for the study of person memory and interpersonal judgments. *Journal of Personality and Social Psychology, 38,* 841–856.

Stepper, S., Strack, F., & Higgins, E. T. (1997). *The memory system: A self-regulatory perspective.* Unpublished manuscript, Wurzburg University.

Sullivan, H. S. (1953). *The collected works of Harry Stack Sullivan: Vol. 1. The interpersonal theory of psychiatry* (H. S. Perry & M. L. Gawel, Eds.). New York: Norton.

Tulving, E., & Pearlstone, Z. (1966). Availability versus accessibility of information in memory for words. *Journal of Verbal Learning and Verbal Behavior, 5,* 381–391.

Wertheimer, M. (1923). Untersuchunger zur Lehre van der Gestalt: II. *Psychologische Forschung, 4,* 301–350.

Westen, D. (1990). Psychoanalytic approaches to personality. In L. A. Pervin (Ed.), *Handbook of personality: Theory and research* (pp. 21–65). New York: Guilford Press.

Wicklund, R.A., & Brehm, J.W. (1976). *Perspectives on cognitive dissonance.* Hillsdale, NJ: Erlbaum.

Wiener, N. (1948). *Cybernetics: Control and communication in the animal and the machine.* Cambridge, MA: MIT Press.

4

Personality Development from the Bottom Up

ARNALDO ZELLI
KENNETH A. DODGE

Twelve-year-old Andrew is riding home on the school bus when a peer begins to say something about his short hair cut. Andrew sees the other boys on the bus laugh. In a rash moment, he punches the peer in the nose, thereby getting himself into trouble with the school principal, yet another time. Although Andrew is fairly intelligent and good looking, this scenario is a common one for him, and he can't seem to resist these fights. Andrew's principal calls him a "bad apple." His teacher asks him why he has "a chip on [his] shoulder." His mother just worries what will happen to him when he grows up. Everyone wonders how he got this way. And yet, Andrew gets along well with his cousin, who teases him unmercifully, and his kindergarten teacher would not recognize him today, because when he was in her classroom, Andrew never got into fights.

If one sought a psychological account for Andrew's behavior, one strategy would be to turn toward the models of personality functioning that contemporary personality psychology has to offer. Upon undertaking this task, one would certainly notice that trait theories have a seemingly undisputed edge in the field and would be eager to consider the fundamental hypothesis that personality trait theorists (e.g., Goldberg, 1993; McCrae & Costa, 1997) would put forward in Andrew's case: Andrew fights because he has a trait called "disagreeableness." It is one of the five basic tendencies that constitute the taxonomy of traits at the highest level of personality organization, according to the five-factor model of personality (Costa & McCrae, 1988). This explanation would suit many people very well, including Andrew's teachers who are perplexed by his behavior. They would be comforted in the knowledge that Andrew's behavior is a recognizable personality pattern called disagreeableness. They would be even more comforted if his "condition" could be given a label called conduct disorder, and they could conclude that conduct disorder caused his conduct-disordered behavior.

There are major problems with the trait explanation, however. Andrew's cousin is never the object of Andrew's fighting or "disagreeableness," and Andrew did not fight in his younger years. Thus, Andrew's aggressive behavior seems rather confined within the bounds of specific contexts, whether one thinks of these circumstances in terms of certain social encounters or particular periods in Andrew's development. The five-factor model captures neither of these possibilities or tendencies. Nonetheless, the notion of context-bound phenomena is critical as it forces one to reevaluate the scientific merits of general (trait) tendencies as one form of explanation for personality. We return to this issue at a later point.

GOALS AND ORGANIZATION OF THIS CHAPTER

Context, and the psychological processes it possibly elicits or with which it covaries, do not merely challenge trait explanations. These processes provide the basic grammar of an utterly different conception of personality functioning (Cervone, 1997; Mischel & Shoda, 1995). Throughout this chapter, we endorse a contemporary approach to the field of personality that has its foundations in the "dynamic" principles and hypotheses emerging from a social-cognitive theory of human functioning (Bandura, 1986; Cervone, 1991). The pivotal principle of this theory is that of reciprocal determinism (Cervone & Williams, 1992). Persons and situations do not merely *interact* in a statistical sense to predict behaviors; rather, they *transact over time* in mutually influential ways. Contexts do not act merely as restrictions on the generalization of empirical relations; rather, they are part of the fabric of behavior and provide the "ground" for the "figure" of personality. The persistent behavior of Andrew in the example above can be understood as an emerging pattern of interaction between himself and his social world. He is influenced by early experiences, perhaps of chronic peer rejection, and he exerts an influence on others, perhaps in leading others to identify him as an easy "mark" for teasing. The goal of this chapter is to enrich the social-cognitive theory of personality by articulating the importance of context and development.

This chapter is organized into five sections. First, trait psychology and social-cognitive theory are briefly contrasted in terms of their approaches to discovery. We draw upon key distinctions between trait theories and social-cognitive personality theories in an attempt to recast the utility of a trait approach, to argue that it falls short of providing a valid form of explanation for personality and human functioning and to introduce the guiding principles of a social-cognitive approach to the study of personality and personality development.

Fundamentally, trait and social-cognitive approaches differ in how they operate as strategies to scientific explanation (also see Cervone, Chapter 9, this volume). Trait psychology is characterized as a "top-down" approach because it assumes a structure that is universal, its units are hypothetical and very broad, and its methods are nomothetic. Social-cognitive personality theory is described as a "bottom-up" approach because its structure is idiosyncratically dependent on time and context, its units are discrete, and its methods include both nomothetic and idiographic descriptions. Trait psychology and social-cognitive theory also differ in their descriptions of how personality itself develops. Trait theory posits little or no development; rather, traits unidirectionally influence behaviors, events, and outcomes, "from the top down." In contrast, according to social-cognitive theory, discrete events and operations occur, these operations persist over time within situations, and they begin to provide an organizing influence on future events, "from the bottom up."

In the second section, we describe the basic building-block units of social-cognitive personality theory in terms of social information-processing mechanisms that operate mostly within classes of stimulus conditions. Personality is not merely conceived as an organized reactive system, however. Rather, it is a system of mental operations that dynamically represent, accommodate, and respond to a constantly mutable environment. Despite a clear emphasis on "process" mechanisms, we do not intend to reduce personality to mere "action" either. Social-cognitive mechanisms operate within a system that develops and that may forge highly enduring, and relatively stable, personality structures that guide one's functioning. To this end, we draw distinctions between patterns in social cognitions (e.g., attributional tendencies) and knowledge mechanisms (e.g., schemas and scripts) in a variety of research domains.

In the third section, we attempt to describe how styles of processing social information develop and how they typify the operating mechanisms through which a variety of ecological and life experiences exert an influence on behavioral development. Examples are provided from recent empirical research on the development of chronically aggressive behavior.

The important role of situational context in constraining, enabling, and conditionalizing behavior is described and synthesized in the fourth section. We draw upon research on aggressive behavior and patterns of processing current social cues and review work demonstrating that child-processing biases and incompetent behavior vary across a variety of problematic situations and child characteristics. We also highlight how relatively narrow social-cognitive mechanisms or processes may contribute to "broad" effects or consistencies in thought and action across seemingly diverse circumstances. Finally, the last section integrates concepts of development across time and differences across situations through the concept of personality coherence.

APPROACHES TO DESCRIPTION, PREDICTION, AND EXPLANATION IN PERSONALITY THEORY

We already have alluded to the shortcomings of a trait approach to personality functioning with respect to an analysis of one's context or development. At an even more basic level, trait explanations are tautological formulations that offer little insight into how one's behavior occurs. Let us turn again to the opening example. Andrew hits others because he is disagreeable, and we call him disagreeable because he hits others. Trait theory offers few insights into the causes of behavior, other than hints at nonspecified heritable characteristics. Essentially, Andrew is endowed with a dose of "disagreeableness." As he goes through life, this dose does not change. Traits can be hidden, but only partially. They can be perturbed, but only slightly. Their essence is that of an "enduring characteristic" (McCrae & Costa, 1996): "*Personality traits are endogenous basic tendencies.* There is considerable evidence that traits are substantially heritable (Tellegen et al., 1988) but unaffected by shared environmental influences (Plomin and Daniels, 1987); any influence of nonshared environment is hypothetical at this time, and most parsimoniously omitted. Arrows . . . lead out from personality traits, but not in" (McCrae & Costa, 1996, p. 72).

According to this perspective, traits do not develop. In fact, according to trait theory, the concept of personality development is an oxymoron. As McCrae and Costa (1996) stated, "Personality development is not a focus of interest" (p. 76). Traits do not change; they unfold. Traits are not altered by experience; they are unearthed. The rhetoric given by trait theorists to concepts of "dynamic processes," "adaptation," and "external influences" (McCrae & Costa, 1996) applies only to the appearances of behaviors. The concept of reciprocal determinism between the individual and the environment (a concept that is central to biological theories of symbiosis and ecological theories of balance) is rejected in trait theory. Ironically, the figure offered by McCrae and Costa (1996, p. 73) as proof of dynamic processes in trait theory includes an arrow (labeled "dynamic processes") emanating from "Basic Tendencies" (i.e., traits) toward "characteristic adaptations" (i.e., attitudes and habits, partly derived from culture and external influences). In turn, there is an arrow emanating from "characteristic adaptations" toward "basic tendencies," but the arrow stops before it reaches "basic tendencies" and instead circles back onto itself! Nothing influences basic tendencies. They endure, and they influence everything else.

Thus, traits are static constructs that are offered as hypothetical entities to be inferred rather than operationalized in overt phenomena. In fact, the typical measurement of traits presumes a static structure. In measuring traits, the self (or others) are explicitly induced to characterize a person according to the way that he or she usually behaves (McCrae & Costa, 1989). Differences across situations or across time are regarded as error, to be smoothed over either by statistical modeling or by experimenter induction. Only after this "error" is corrected can the analysis commence. Of course, if one defines cross-situation and cross-time variance as error to be purged, then what remains is static and enduring.

In contrast, the units of personality in social-cognitive theory are defined by actions, albeit often cognitive operations. Personality units include operations such as pessimistic attributions (Cantor, Norem, Niedenthal, Langston, & Brower, 1987), self-efficacy judgments (Bandura & Cervone, 1983), and hostile attributions (Dodge, 1980). The units of personality for the boy Andrew are not dispositions of disagreeableness; rather, they are social-cognitive operations, such as persistent patterns of attributing hostile intent to peers upon provocation and expectancies for the outcomes of social events. Furthermore, these social-cognitive units are dynamic operations in symbiotic relation to one's social ecology. The challenge for the study of personality in social-cognitive theory is thus to understand how the boy Andrew can persistently respond to teasing by classroom peers with aggression while also persistently responding to his cousin with nonaggression. The challenge for inquiry in personality development is to understand how this pattern evolved.

Despite the above considerations, trait accounts undoubtedly pervade communication and characterize "explanations" in both social and nonsocial arenas. Any world traveler readily understands the urge to characterize the cultural climate and ambience of various cities in terms of personality-like traits. New Orleans is bawdy. New York is rude. Paris is sophisticated. Venice is romantic. And San Francisco is . . . "flaky." These traits describe a (perceived) central tendency that is consistent across time and circumstances and is readily apparent to most observers. Disagreements about the most accurate trait for a city (e.g., is New York really rude or simply busy?) merely reinforce the notion that cities do, indeed, have personalities. Anecdotes of exceptions (e.g., "She lost her purse in New York, and a stranger actually returned it to her!") only prove the rule. Like stereotypes, these traits cause sharp retort from dissenters, but even dissenters often acknowledge the kernel of truth in these terms.

However, one must question what function the application of a trait term to a city really serves. As a descriptor, it summarizes the speaker's perceptions and evaluations, crossed across multiple individual experiences, and as a predictor, it has practical value (e.g., "Be wary of strangers in New York, find a love affair in Venice, and let your hair down in San Francisco"). But does it have scientific explanatory value? Does the trait of a city cause its people to behave in particular ways? Perhaps a latent feature of a city (e.g., its geographic location, the density of its population, or the diversity of its economy) exerts an exogenous influence on certain outcomes (e.g., the number of encounters with strangers per day), but in most respects the trait term is only a descriptive summary and reflection of multiple overlapping events rather than a cause of those events. Proof of the causal status of traits of cities inevitably ends up in tautological statements (e.g., "New York's rudeness causes people to act rudely"). The trait term is a useful heuristic device for communication, but it has no scientific explanatory value because the entity being characterized by the trait plays no causal role in outcomes. The construct can be described, but it exerts no unitary force in a scientific sense.

Similar functions of descriptions are served, and problems are apparent, in the attempted use of trait terms to characterize "behavior" in some other domains as well, including the average weather of a city (e.g., "The dry desert climate keeps it from raining"), the trends of an economy (e.g., "The bull market is leading investors toward stocks"), and the actions of groups (e.g., "The unruliness of soccer crowds inevitably leads to fights").

The problem with all these trait applications can be represented as one of "top-down" versus "bottom-up" explanation in science (Salmon, 1989). In top-down phenomena, a single overarching force exerts uniform pressure on multiple individual events, possibly with some error or additional forces also exerting pressure on those events. For example, a mathematical model of the amount of daylight present at any location on earth at a particular point in time would start with a general, overarching factor of "orientation to the sun at that moment." The orientation to the sun is a top-down factor that exerts a constant pressure on the phenomenon of daylight, which is then modified by additional factors such as local cloud movements, humidity levels, and latitude. In bottom-up phenomena, each event is caused by a confluence of microforces, without an overall causal factor. Consider the phenomenon of the average number of sunny days per year in any given city, averaged across all years in this century. The amount of sunshine in a city on any single day in any given year is a function of top-down and bottom-up forces that include air pressure, humidity, cloud movements, and other forces. One could sum this value across all days in a year and average this score across all years in a century. The resulting score would have great heuristic value in characterizing a city ("San Diego is sunny, whereas Seattle is rainy"), and this score could prove valuable in predicting the weather in the future, at a gross level. Thus, this score has trait-like features. However, this score has no top-down causal status. The average "sunniness" of a city does not cause that city to be sunny. Rather, the degree of sunniness of a city is indicated by the average of daily, bottom-up factors that determine a city's sunshine on a given day.

The distinction between top-down and bottom-up phenomena is captured in the psychometric distinction between a scale and an index. A scale is a set of items that presumably reflect a single, underlying characteristic (i.e., a "trait"), with the only determinants of the total score being the trait and error. All items in a scale are presumed to measure the trait, and the trait presumably causes item scores. Classic scales include the intelligence quotient and personality traits such as the Big Five. In contrast, an index is a set of items with no presumed underlying common cause. Items can be summed for heuristic value, and the sum score may have predictive value as well; however, it is not presumed that the sum score is a single construct exerting unitary causal force. Examples of indices in psychological research include total stress scores from a daily hassles instrument and total phobia scores from a list of possible phobias. The total stress score is derived from a list of stressors (e.g., marital trouble, death in the family, monetary woes), but it is not presumed that each stressor has the same underlying cause. Likewise, a total phobia score is derived from a list of phobias (e.g., snakes, high places, open spaces), but it is not presumed that a phobia trait causes all phobias. In a scale, all items are significantly correlated, but in an index, no such covariation of items is necessary.

Yet one more example of the same distinction is captured by the direction of arrows in a structural equation model. When the arrows point away from one circle (called the "latent construct") toward several boxes (called "indicators"), the figure depicts a single underlying trait "causing" its expression in measurable items of a scale. When the arrows from multiple boxes point instead toward a common circle, the circle represents a heuristic summary of the indexed boxes, without a presumed single underlying trait. Both kinds of models are statistically useful, with the theoretical assumptions of the model differing.

Applied to individual persons, trait terms, like scales and structural models with arrows pointed toward circles, have the scientific advantage of parsimony; however, the theoretical burdens of proving a single underlying causal structure without tautology are often too great to be supported by empirical study. Nonetheless, indices, such as "aggressive behavior levels" and "degree of optimism," are heuristically useful in identifying groups of individuals for further inquiry, as long as the inquirer does not make the error of metamorphosizing the index score into a causal factor. Aggressive behavior levels are relevant scores for psychological researchers, but they do not reflect a trait of "aggressiveness."

Does this line of argument reduce the concept of "personality" to one of heuristic importance with no scientific coherence? At the level of cities, trait concepts will not weather the onslaught of rigorous science. At the level of individuals, the constructionist social-cognitive perspective of this chapter is that personality coherence does evolve across development, from a set of reciprocally influential behavior experiences, each of which is determined by both top-down and bottom-up factors. At the heart of each behavior experience is the information-processing system, which forms the foundation for personality development. This system consists of a set of brain processes that occur during social exchanges; thus, personality is described by a set of mental operations rather than a static set of traits.

SOCIAL COGNITION AND SOCIAL INFORMATION
PROCESSING AS BUILDING BLOCKS OF PERSONALITY

As we have seen, trait formulations conceive personality as an array of behavioral dispositions that predispose individuals to engage in trait-relevant behaviors. One's characteristic traits, and their magnitude relative to trait levels in a population of individuals, are assumed to be the invariant and distinctive qualities of one's personality and functioning (Mischel & Shoda, 1995).

Alternatively, in a social-cognitive conception of personality (Bandura, 1986; Cervone & Williams, 1992; Mischel & Shoda, 1995), specific environment–person relations and psychological processes are hypothesized to give rise to relatively stable and distinctive patterns of functioning and behavior. For example, the theoretical account of one's typical level of conscientious behavior resides in the *social settings* in which one selectively acts in a conscientious way, in the specific *social skills, capabilities, or competencies* that enable the individual to act conscientiously, and in the *personal goals or standards* through which one "self-regulates," and constantly scrutinizes, his or her conscientious conduct (Bandura, 1996; Cervone & Williams, 1992).

Thus, one's behavior has social foundations, arises in particular and contingent psychological conditions, and depends upon what a person does cognitively and affectively in the process of coping with the environment (Higgins, 1996; Mischel, 1990). Upon encountering a stimulus event (e.g., being rejected by a lover), one must actively attend to, comprehend, elaborate upon, and respond to that event. Furthermore, the social repercussions of an individual's responses acquire their own stimulus status, thus contributing to an ongoing cycle of processing, and responding to, social information.

From this perspective, there are two critical—and complementary—levels of analysis. One's behavior in any given event occurs as a result of processing, and making decisions upon, current social cues that are salient or meaningful to the self. Humans however are also capable of mentally utilizing linguistic symbols in order to elaborate, reflect upon, and summarize past events, as well as to give form to future goals and choices (Cantor & Kihlstrom, 1987; Markus & Nurius, 1986; Nelson, 1993). To the extent that one repeatedly encounters or experiences a given class of behaviors, self- and social knowledge may arise that increasingly foster coherent patterns of responses in one's social action and social environment (Cervone, 1997; Fuhrman & Funder, 1995; Smith, 1994).

In the end, information-processing models are formulations linking specific stimulus circumstances to specific behaviors, thus describing how a particular behavior comes about (or the "phenomenology" of social interaction; Dodge, 1993). Models of knowledge acquisition and use, on the other hand, are learning formulations that describe the assumptions, belief systems, and goals or strategies one may hold for oneself and that represent the link between one's typical experiences and coping with future demands and tasks (see Cervone & Williams, 1992; Higgins, 1996; Kihlstrom & Klein, 1994; Mischel & Shoda, 1995, for extensive reviews).

Social Information-Processing Theories

Social information-processing theories are formal hypotheses about the sequence of mental activities or decisions regulating one's response to a stimulus event (Crick & Dodge, 1994; Huesmann, 1998; Rubin, Bream, & Rose-Krasnor, 1991; Weary & Edwards, 1994). From the standpoint of situational specificity, differences in one's processing across stimuli covary with differences in the nature of eliciting cues. From the standpoint of personality functioning, differences in processing patterns across persons covary with differences in behavior within a given domain of stimulus situations (Crick & Dodge, 1994; Dodge, 1993; Huesmann, 1998).

In response to a social stimulus (e.g., peers teasing the boy Andrew), one must first attend to the stimulus situation and *encode* its most relevant features in working memory. Differences in social cues prompt differences in one's attention and encoding. For instance, an academic situation may alert one to focus on any minimal sign of personal failure or struggle, whereas a social encounter may relieve the same individual from attending to cues pertinent to one's own performance (Dweck & Leggett, 1988). Alternatively, a novel situation may well appear complex and overwhelming in many respects and limit one's ability to comprehend it. Thus, a relatively healthy person may attend to an unexpected medical check-up somewhat anxiously and have difficulty in attending to, and evaluating, what a doctor is saying (Clark, 1994). Encoding also varies in systematic ways across individuals and social experiences. Repeated experiences with depression seemingly predispose one to direct attention toward the self and away from environmental information and circumstances (Ingram, 1990; Pyszczynsky, Greenberg, Hamilton, & Nix, 1991) or to access depressogenic information over other types of information in the context of a personal analysis but not necessarily in evaluating others (Bargh & Tota, 1988; see also Ingram & Reed, 1986; Weary & Edwards, 1994a). Likewise, aggressive children who have had experience with social conflict search for fewer cues or relevant information upon encountering problematic peer situations (Dodge & Newman, 1981; Slaby & Guerra, 1988). They are also overly sensitive to social cues conveying hostile or malevolent intent and have difficulties in evaluating the value of alternative or positively valued information (Dodge & Frame, 1982).

Any further elaboration upon encoded cues (e.g., interpretation of one's facial expression, inferences about others' dispositions) may affect how one mentally represents the stimulus situation (Tulving & Thomson, 1973), which constitutes the second step of social information processing. Again, contextual factors may partially govern this process. An instance of clearly reckless behavior may momentarily prompt one to categorize others' behaviors as reckless rather than as other applicable dispositions (Bargh, Lombardi, & Higgins, 1988; Higgins, Bargh, & Lombardi, 1985; Higgins, Rholes, & Jones, 1977). Likewise, one who is habitually depressed may (unsolicitedly, or with no apparent conscious intention) assign negative qualities to oneself but not to other people (Bargh & Tota, 1988). Idiosyncracies in people's goals moderate individuals' interpretations and representations. Individuals who have a heightened motive to seek structure and understanding in their social world, draw inferences about others' qualities and dispositions routinely (Anderson & Deuser, 1993; Moskowitz, 1993). Similarly, people who are characteristically outgoing, may readily think of gregariousness qualities when observing others' behavior (Bargh et al., 1988). Individual differences in chronically accessible (Higgins & King, 1981) social constructs characterize clinical phenomena or populations, as well. For instance, it is quite clear that chronically aggressive children characteristically process, and mentally represent, potentially problematic interactions in terms of others' hostile motives, especially when the self is the explicit target of another person's provocative behavior (Dodge & Frame, 1982; see also Crick & Dodge, 1994; Dodge, 1993, for an extensive review of over 25 independent studies on this issue).

The mere exposure in one context to stimulus material comprising clear behavioral configurations or stereotypes (e.g., rudeness, or the elderly) may—in a seemingly unrelated and subsequent context—evoke stimulus-consistent behaviors (e.g., impatience, slow walking) in participants who have no awareness of the links between prior stimulus and following response (Bargh, Chen, & Burrows, 1996, study 1 and study 2). Thus, the next step of processing is a mental search for a response option among an array of responses available in long-term memory. Different people routinely access different types of responses or vary in the ease of accessing certain responses instead of others (Higgins & King, 1981). Furthermore, these individual differences in mental accessing predict differences in maladaptive behaviors. For example, highly aggressive persons access more incompetent, action-oriented solutions to a variety of interpersonal situations than nonaggressive persons (see Dodge, 1993, for a review; Rubin et al., 1991). Also, in situations of direct provocation, aggressive persons readily generate solutions of immediate retaliation (Slaby & Guerra, 1988; Waas, 1988), whereas in situations of threat to social status or of open conflict with peers, they tend to consider coercion or adult punishment responses, respectively (Dodge, Pettit, McClaskey, & Brown, 1986).

Accessing a behavioral response from memory is not tantamount to enactment of that response, however. The next step of processing is a response evaluation and decision step. Responses that are *evaluated* as appropriate to a current situation are more likely to be enacted. Several mechanisms may regulate one's responding at this processing step. For instance, in the domain of moral agency, one may counteract internal sanctions against aggressing another individual by consciously construing ways of disengaging oneself from the conduct being considered or evaluated (Bandura,

Barbaranelli, Caprara, & Pastorelli, 1996). Thus, one may actively minimize the consequences to others of detrimental social conduct (Bandura et al., 1996) as well as misconstrue the benefits associated with acting aggressively (Dodge, 1993). For instance, habitually aggressive persons tend to praise the high instrumental value of aggression by believing it leads to more material gain; they do not foresee or they dismiss the negative sanctions aggression may lead to; and they feel overconfident in their ability to behave aggressively (Crick & Dodge, 1996; Crick & Ladd, 1990; Perry, Perry, & Rasmussen, 1986). Thus, a sequence of decision-making tasks logically define one's processing of social cues, and this processing significantly regulates one's behavioral responding within specific stimulus situations (see also Feldman & Dodge, 1987).

Knowledge Mechanisms Regulating Processing Patterns

Even seemingly identical events may elicit different responses in the same person. Individuals are sensitive to differences among eliciting situations, and their responses only cohere across situations that are perceived as similar, that is, situations that acquire similar "psychological meaning" and that elicit in turn similar cognitive, affective, and behavioral responses (Higgins, 1996; Mischel & Shoda, 1995).

At this stage of analysis, consistency or coherence in one's responding critically depends upon one's knowledge of specific person–environment relations (Fiske & Taylor, 1991; Kihlstrom & Klein, 1994). This knowledge can affect social phenomena such as one's dispositional judgments about others (Shoda & Mischel, 1993; Shoda, Mischel, & Wright, 1993). Thus, rather than mentally averaging over multiple instances of behavior, one's judgment about a peer's aggressive disposition seems to arise from an analysis of contingencies between specific situations and specific behaviors (e.g., acting aggressively in situation A but not in situation B). Likewise, knowledge of person–environment relations shapes thought and action concerning the self. One who is shy and knows he or she becomes anxious in making public stands may view two different situations (e.g., giving a business presentation, telling a joke at a party) as equally challenging, and in turn express low confidence in performing in both settings. Such a consistency across situations in self-confidence (i.e., efficacy) judgments, however, may not readily appear for one who, although shy, sees this personal "weakness" as only affecting his or her performance in work situations (Cervone, 1997). Importantly so, cross-situational coherence in efficacy self-appraisals is not found if its assessment dismisses either highly salient (i.e., schematic) personal attributes or the sets of situations that one categorizes as relevant to one's own strengths or weaknesses (Cervone, 1997). In addition to personal knowledge, person–environment relations are also critical with respect to personal goals and standards through which people organize and motivate their course of action (see

Pervin, 1989). For instance, in academic settings, which inherently challenge one's performance and success, persistent maladaptive behavior seemingly arises only in people who are chronically concerned with documenting their level of competence and who, in turn, are particularly sensitive to self-appraisals of incompetence (Dweck & Leggett, 1988).

The influence of knowledge mechanisms is pervasive in several research domains. Chronic individual differences in uncertainty beliefs (i.e., one's perceived ability to understand the causal conditions of personal or social events) are closely tied to differences in extensive processing of social information and to differences in personal judgment confidence. However, these linkages appear solely in the context of situations that call upon personal control (Weary, Marsh, Gleicher, & Edwards, 1993) or in the context of tasks of causal analysis (Weary & Edwards, 1994b, study 4), respectively. One's experience of personal and social events can also explicitly call upon "relational schemas," that is, one's understandings and expectations about interpersonal experiences (see Baldwin, 1992 and Chapter 5, this volume, for a review). For instance, one may chronically expect that interpersonal rejection or acceptance is contingent upon personal failure and success, respectively (e.g., "If I fail the exam, my friends will not talk to me"), and these expectations seem to exert a significant influence on one's self-esteem appraisals (Baldwin & Sinclair, 1996). Likewise, people's relationship experiences in domains such as interpersonal trust, dependency, and closeness clearly depend upon specific relational expectations (e.g., "If I trust others, they will hurt me") that shape one's interpretations and responses to interpersonal encounters (Baldwin, Fehr, Keedian, Seidel, & Thompson, 1993; Baldwin, Keelan, Fehr, Enns, & Koh-Rangarajoo, 1996).

Thus, one need not describe and explain personality organization and functioning by positing high-level dispositional variables or traits. Instead, this organization and functioning can be understood in terms of basic psychological processes, operations, and structures that manifest themselves as individuals interact with their social environment. Implicit in this view is the notion that one's personal ways to respond to, select, or alter his or her social environment have their foundations in one's own unique life experiences. It is thus critical to discuss, albeit briefly, the paths of development that can give rise to one's own styles of processing social information and learning experiences.

THE DEVELOPMENT OF SOCIAL-COGNITIVE STYLES IN PERSONALITY

Sources of Influence on Personality Development

Most theories of social development (e.g., Coie & Dodge, 1998) acknowledge three sources of influences on the development of social behaviors such as aggression. The first influence is the array of biologically based response tendencies that derive from genes or in utero experiences. For a behavior pattern such as aggressiveness, early factors such as serotonin metabolites (5-HIAA), resting heart rate, and attention deficits have all been linked empirically to later individual differences in aggressiveness. Although these factors might well form the biological basis for patterns that some researchers would call traits, these factors are not behavior patterns in and of themselves, and their empirical links to behavior patterns are not very strong and are very indirect. Furthermore, empirical studies have begun to identify changes in these biologically based factors as a function of life experiences (Coie & Dodge, 1998). Thus, these factors do not fit the pattern of traits as articulated in trait theory. Nonetheless, almost every theory of social personality development starts with the biological organism.

A child is born into a social culture, and so contextual factors constitute the second source of influence on personality development. Children born into poverty, neighborhoods characterized by high rates of violence, or families filled with stress are relatively likely to develop patterns of aggressive behavior as they grow older (Guerra, Huesmann, Tolan, Van Acker, & Eron, 1995).

Of course, personality development is not fully determined by birth, so life experiences constitute the third kind of influence. For aggressive behavior, numerous early life experiences have been correlated empirically with later enduring patterns of aggressive behavior, including harsh parenting, peer social rejection, exposure to aggressive role models, and academic failure (Coie & Dodge, 1998).

Biological factors, sociocultural context, and life experiences all provide significant predictive relations with the emergence of personality characteristics and individual differences in social behavior. Few critics would argue the empirical literature. The crucial developmental questions, however, concern (1) the way in which these factors relate to each other across time, and (2) the mechanisms through which these factors lead to social behavior patterns.

Aggregating Biological Factors, Sociocultural Context, and Life Experiences

Without refuting the empirical relations between each of these factors and later personality characteristics, we recognize that the important questions concern the way in which these factors relate to each other in their empirical predictions. The most obvious way to combine these factors is through an additive model, in which each factor increments the contribution made by other factors. Empirical analyses have demonstrated that aggregation of factors, either through a simple summing of the number of factors present or through multiple regression techniques, leads to stronger predictions of personality than does any single factor (Deater-Deckard, Dodge, Bates, & Pettit, 1998).

Even stronger predictions can be made by considering the moderating effects of one factor on the prediction afforded by another factor, as in interaction effects. For example, the type and magnitude of effect of restrictive parenting on the development of aggressiveness depends on the parent's perception of the temperament of the child (Bates, Pettit, Dodge, & Ridge, in press). That is, a resistant temperament in infancy is more strongly correlated with later aggressive behavior under conditions in which the child experiences very little restrictiveness during socialization by parents; under conditions in which parents exert relatively greater restrictiveness, the correlation between early temperament and later aggressive behavior is weak. Thus, the prediction of individual differences in aggressive behavior is significant from early markers of resistant temperament and restrictive parenting (in an additive model), but the strength of this prediction is magnified by consideration of the interaction of these factors as well.

Additive and interactive models can provide powerful predictions of personality development, but these models fail to consider that these factors might be correlated with each other or even causal of one another. In fact, staunch theorists of biological determinism argue that life experiences can be predicted from biological factors, even to the point where the life experience factors are merely outcomes of biological factors with no causal role in personality development. Consider the difficult-temperament child who leads his or her parents to "burn a short fuse" and become harsh and abusive in parenting. In this case, the life experience of harsh parenting is predictable from the child's constitution. Such a model does not mean that the life experience factor plays no role in personality development, however. It might well be that some life experiences are predictable from child factors, but the life experiences still play a crucial role in mediating the effect of the child factor. Perhaps the difficult-temperament child grows into an aggressive adolescent *only if* the parents respond to the child's difficultness with rejection and anger. Mediational models can test these developmental theories.

Mechanisms of Effect on Behavioral Development

Study of the role of biological factors, sociocultural context, and life experiences in personality development provides evidence of empirical prediction of individual differences in behavior, but this inquiry tells us little about how these effects operate. Understanding of the mechanisms of personality development is perhaps the strongest potential appeal of social-cognitive theories of personality. Social cognition offers a theory for how these predictive factors exert their influence on personality development.

Consider the effect of early harsh parenting and physical abuse on the development of aggressive behavior styles in children. This effect has been demonstrated through prospective inquiry with large community samples of children, even after statistical control of a variety of other factors, including child temperament, socioeconomic status, and exposure to marital conflict (Dodge, Bates, & Pettit, 1990). But how does such an effect operate? Dodge, Pettit, Bates, and Valente (1995) found that the life experience of physical abuse by a parent leads a child to process information in particular ways. Specifically, abused children become hypervigilant to hostile cues, biased toward attributing hostile intent to others during provocation situations, likely to access aggressive responses from memory, and likely to evaluate the consequences of aggressing as favorable. Furthermore, each of these patterns of social information processing has been shown in other studies to predict individual differences in aggressive behavior (Crick & Dodge, 1994). Finally, these acquired social information-processing patterns have been found to mediate partially the effect of early physical harm on the later development of aggressive behavior. That is, these processing patterns assessed at time 2 account for statistically significant portions of the correlation between physical harm at time 1 and aggressive behavior at time 3 (about half of the effect) (Dodge et al., 1995).

Social-cognitive theories, then, have the potential to account for the effects of biological, sociocultural, and life experience factors in social development. Patterns of social cognitions are acquired as a function of these factors and account for the effects of these factors on important outcomes. These social-cognitive patterns *are* the building blocks of personality itself.

CONTEXT SPECIFICITY IN BEHAVIOR AND PROCESSING PATTERNS

Thus far, we have endorsed two guiding assumptions. First, personality and its functioning can be understood in terms of a system of cognitive-affective elements and operations that dynamically mediate an individual's exchanges with his or her social environment. Second, one's life events and circumstances influence, and find expression in, one's unique ways of learning about, comprehending, and coping with the surrounding world.

In this conceptual approach, social behavior, functioning, and context become inseparable referents to an individual's "invariant" personality characteristics (Mischel & Shoda, 1995). For instance, consistency in one's behavior across a variety of situations may well attest to personality coherence, but only when it is evaluated among situations that acquire a similar *psychological* meaning (see Higgins, 1996, for the notion of applicability; Mischel, 1990). One who fears "audiences" might knowingly avoid speaking about his work in a public forum and joining a crowded social party, because both situations bring to mind this personal "weakness" and elicit similar levels of anxiety (Cervone, 1997). Note that the same person also might be professionally capable of expressing his work in writing as well as gregarious and jovial in face-to-face encounters. Thus, neither incompetence nor shyness would seem to be viable descriptions or explanations of the person's withdrawal from "public" arenas as an extension of trait models would suggest.

One's behavior does not vary *randomly* across situations, however. A tenet of this perspective is that the same person-variables that generate behavioral consistency should also regulate how behavior varies across (psychologically) different types of situations (Higgins, 1990; Mischel & Shoda, 1995). "Variability" in one's characteristic behavioral responses thus becomes an important part of an individual's personality and its coherence, insofar as it signifies organization in one's cognitive (and affective) responses to varying significant events.

A child might act (consistently) aggressively in provocations arising from dyadic exchanges, since this context typically provides a clear target for drawing judgments of peer malintention and for retaliation. The same child might also act (consistently) less aggressively in situations of peer group-entry failures, since these events typically lack single social referents for blame and aggression. Finally, a second child could show opposite patterns (e.g., more aggression in group-entry confrontations relative to aggression in dyadic provocations), thus virtually ruling out explanations calling for mere generalized situational effects (Dodge, McClaskey, & Feldman, 1985). If the focus were only on one's characteristic level of behavior, both children would be assigned an aggression score averaged across the two situations and, as a result, appear equally aggressive on this criterion. This conclusion, of course, would be misleading. It would not be acceptable to contrast the two children's aggression scores only within one type of situation given that neither domain alone is exhaustive of the universe of situations children encounter. Thus, both procedures seem inherently limited and would inevitably lead to an incomplete description (or explanation) of our fictitious characters. Instead, the most promising inquiry would be to evaluate each child's characteristic level of aggression *both within and across* different domains of situations.

In sum, both behavioral stability and cross-situational variability are critical facets of the reliable set of relations among one's environment, cognition, and behavior. Both stability and variability define personality coherence. Neither can be detected apart from the particular circumstances or events that engage one's stable psychological system and organization. Furthermore, consistency (or variability) in one's behavior necessarily reflects corresponding consistency (or variability) in psychological, cognitive-affective, responses.

Undoubtedly, then, personality is inherently "contextual." It finds expression in the psychological events (e.g., self-evaluations, intent attributions) linking specific stimulus situations to specific behaviors. This conditional nature of personality does not necessarily interfere with an assessment of personality coherence, nor does it penalize its detection. However, it warns a researcher to formulate hypotheses about regularities in social behavior that inherently attend to individual differences in the personal relevance of vary-ing stimulus situations and circumstances and to the multiplicity in one's cognitive (and affective) responses to seemingly similar events.

The fundamental hypothesis that deviant processing of current social cues regulates the expression of aggressive behavior has generated several lines of inquiry that are consistent with, and confirm the utility of, this condi-tional model of personality coherence. One important aspect of this research developed in response to those who argued that processing at any single step (e.g., hostile attributional biases) did not predict much of the variance in aggressive behavior (see Dodge, 1993). A processing theory of aggression describes a logical sequence of mental activities or judgments leading one to act aggressively (Dodge, 1993). In this sense, each instance of aggression is directly linked to one or more ill decisions an individual makes along this sequence (e.g., a hostile intent attribution, or a positive evaluation of the con-sequences of aggression, or both). Across individuals, however, the relative value of each processing task or decision-making point varies, and the theory thus provides multiple "loci" for individual differences in the *magnitude* of the relations linking any deviant processing step to aggression. For instance, one aggressive child might regularly make hostile interpretations in judging others' motives and react aggressively in a variety of situations, whereas another aggressive child might regularly evaluate favorably the instrumental benefits seemingly associated with acting aggressively. Yet a third aggressive child might regularly act aggressively as a result of both perceiving hostile motives in others and overestimating the benefits that come with enacting aggressive behaviors. In this hypothetical sample of children, interpretation biases and response evaluation patterns would separately predict variance in aggression only to some small degree (i.e., each processing step elicited only some of the aggression in the sample). Alternatively, the best prediction of variance in aggression should accrue from considering interpretation errors and aggressive endorsement *together*. Over the years, several studies have confirmed that an aggregated assessment of deviant processing patterns through multiple correlation yields a larger improvement in the prediction of aggression than an assessment of any single step (Dodge et al., 1986; Dodge, Bates et al., 1990; Dodge et al., 1995; Slaby & Guerra, 1988).

Situation Specificity in Processing and Behavior

Within the same conceptual approach, another critical research theme has revolved around methods of situational assessment and the possibility of identifying stimulus situations capable of eliciting deviant processing and aggressive behavior. Situational taxonomies generated a priori on the basis of "objective" qualities of stimulus situations are ill-defined, as many have rec-ognized early on (Goldfried & d'Zurilla, 1969; McFall, 1982). Instead, one must recognize that individuals actively construe situations (Higgins, 1990;

Mischel, 1990). That is, the same stimulus event may acquire a very different meaning for two different individuals, activate distinctly different elaborations and processing, and trigger different behavioral responses.

Research on social adjustment status in childhood has supported this basic hypothesis (Dodge et al., 1985; Dodge & Feldman, 1990; Feldman & Dodge, 1987). In this work, the initial hypothesis was that child social status (i.e., whether a child is regularly rejected by peers) is not a generalized construct that implies a generalized condition but, rather, emerges from personal elaborations and behaviors that unfold within specific social settings and situations. The research task was to identify the types of social contexts or situations that could lead various incompetent children to experience social difficulties. In a two-study investigation (Dodge et al., 1985), school teachers were asked to generate several situations that they thought would be particularly problematic for elementary school students of different ages. Each situation was then classified (by clinical psychologists) as belonging to one of several domains of problematic situations (e.g., failures to enter a peer group activity, situations of peer provocations). In the next step, the authors identified two groups of children, one socially rejected, the other socially adjusted, on the basis of sociometric peer ratings (e.g., peers' nominations of classmates they liked and disliked). Their teachers were then provided with a subset of the problematic situations identified early on and were asked to indicate the extent to which each situation was problematic for their students. Analysis of the teacher ratings clearly indicated that situations converged on a cluster of dimensions that substantially mapped onto the original taxonomy. Additionally, each situation could reliably distinguish between "socially rejected" and "average" children (Dodge et al., 1985, study 1). In study 2, independent samples of aggressive-rejected and nonaggressive children were presented with a subset of the problematic situations, and were asked to role-play what they would do in these situations (Dodge et al., 1985, study 2). As expected, aggressive children as a group responded less competently than nonaggressive children to each type of social situation, thus obtaining further evidence for the validity of the situational taxonomy developed in study 1.

More importantly, however, the analysis of behavioral teacher ratings (from study 1) as well as the analysis of role-play behavioral observations (from study 2) clearly suggested that there is both overall *coherence* and *cross-situational variation* in children's behaviors. There were multivariate main effects for group status on both measures, thus suggesting that rejected children, overall, acted less competently than adjusted children. The magnitude of these effects was not uniform across situations, however, and univariate effects clearly showed that peer provocations or social expectations (i.e., violation of group norms) elicited or were associated with the largest differences between groups with respect to competent behavior.

Another study (Dodge et al., 1986) demonstrated that some children show a reliable pattern of behaving aggressively in response to peer provocations, whereas other children show a pattern of responding aggressively in peer group-entry situations. Furthermore, these situational differences in behavior are highly predictable from situational differences in how these children process information about the two types of situations. That is, patterns of encoding peer-provocation cues, attributing hostile intent to peer provocateurs, accessing aggressive responses to peer provocations, and evaluating aggressive retaliation as leading to favorable outcomes significantly predicted aggressive behavioral responding to a laboratory-induced peer provocation. These processing patterns in the peer-provocation situation did not predict aggressive behavior in the peer group-entry situation, however. In contrast, patterns of processing peer group-entry information (i.e., encoding, attribution of intent, response generation, and response evaluation) significantly predicted aggressive behavior in the peer group-entry situation but not in the peer-provocation situation. Thus, the relation between processing patterns and aggressive behavior was found to be remarkably strong (with multiple correlations of up to .75) but equally situation-specific.

Interactional Partners as Distinct "Situations"

The content of different situations (i.e., peer provocation vs. failure to enter a peer group) is not the only aspect of social situations to influence people's cognition. People with whom one typically interacts come to represent the defining and salient features of an individual's social context, and different relationships may represent the source of differences in cognition and behavior. In this regard, different social partners may represent different situations for a person. These themes were investigated in a series of studies designed to understand the processes that foster and sustain aggressive dyadic relationships in childhood (Dodge, Price, Coie, & Christopoulos, 1990; Hubbard, Coie, Dodge, Cillesson, & Schwartz, 1998). In these studies, dyads were observed *in vivo*. Each child had a chance to interact with five same-age peers during five play-group sessions distributed over the course of a week or so. Their behaviors were recorded and coded for aggression.

In one of these investigations (Dodge, Price, et al., 1990), children were not acquainted with each other when the observations began. The authors nevertheless found evidence of situational (dyadic) specificity in aggression. Nearly 50% of aggressive behavior occurred within a relatively small (i.e., 20%) fraction of the dyads suggesting that, indeed, some dyads were relatively more aggressive than others. This distribution of dyadic aggression was not merely a reflection of child effects (i.e., some children were generally more aggressive than others), however, and it held even within a subgroup of "most aggressive" children. Another finding was that aggressive behavior in children's exchanges produced—or was associated with—different types of dyadic relationships. Children who displayed high rates of aggression were involved in dyadic relationships in which either a peer partner was regularly bullied and victimized, or both members exchanged high rates of aggression toward each other. Furthermore, once established, this dyad status persisted across time (i.e., the classification of a child's dyad status did not vary much over the course of most or all sessions) (Dodge, Price, et al., 1990).

Finally, highly aggressive children also displayed different types of aggressive behavior in different types of dyadic relationships. A traditional distinction in the aggression literature is between aggression that is unprovoked, premeditated, and utilized to achieve some external goal, or "instrumental–proactive" aggression, and aggression that is affectively charged, and that occurs in retaliation to some real or perceived provocation or threat from the environment, or "hostile–reactive" aggression (Bandura, 1986; Berkowitz, 1993; Hartup, 1974). Empirical evidence shows that this distinction is a meaningful and valid one. Reactive and proactive aggression in children and young adolescents can be measured reliably on teacher rating scales (Dodge & Coie, 1987). These rating measures converge with natural observations of reactively and proactively aggressive behaviors (Dodge & Coie, 1987; Price & Dodge, 1989). Also, differences in reactive and proactive aggression are distinctively associated with differences in deviant processing, namely, differences in hostile attributional biases in the case of reactive aggression (Dodge & Coie, 1987; Crick & Dodge, 1996) and differences in biased positive endorsement of aggressive solutions in the case of proactive aggression (Crick & Dodge, 1996; Dodge, Lochman, Harnish, Bates, & Pettit, 1997). In the dyad investigation we reviewed above (Dodge, Price, et al., 1990), authors observed differential rates of reactive and proactive aggression in aggressive children. In those dyads characterized by a clear aggressor and a clear victim, highly aggressive children displayed significantly higher rates of proactive or coercive aggression than did highly aggressive individuals involved in mutually aggressive dyads. On the other hand, relative to bully–victim dyads, high-conflict dyads were predominantly characterized by reactively aggressive exchanges (Dodge, Price, et al., 1990).

In sum, one's aggression unfolds within a few ongoing dyadic relationships, and these relationships influence the type and rate of aggression that is observed. Aggression does not reside merely within the individual (i.e., those with the highest rates of aggression displayed their aggression selectively). Nor does it merely reflect rigid patterns of behavior. Rather, highly aggressive individuals are sensitively tuned to their partners' characteristics or behaviors and display aggressive behaviors that vary according to the opportunities they foresee (as in the case of acting proactively aggressively especially toward peers who are potential victims), and according to the challenges to personal status they encounter in their immediate social environment (as in the case of acting reactively aggressively toward peers who are similarly aggressive).

A recent study (Hubbard et al., 1998) extended these conclusions even further. The authors examined *both* dyadic aggression *and* dyadic social cognition, thus seeking correspondence between dyadic effects on aggression and dyadic effects on one's processing. The study also provided statistical estimates of the variance in behavior and cognition that actor, partner, and dyadic relationship uniquely account for, thus providing a formal test of the hypothesis that aggression unfolds and develops in the context of specific relationships. The authors also pursued a third objective, namely, the analysis of whether the linkages between reactive aggression and hostile biases, and between proactive aggression and biased outcome expectations, are a reflection of (general) child effects versus (specific) dyadic effects. The authors hypothesized that a child's hostile intent attributions about a peer will be associated with his or her reactive aggression (but not proactive aggression) toward that particular peer. Likewise, they also hypothesized that to the extent a child would evaluate positively the possibility to aggress toward a peer, he or she would also act proactively aggressively (but not reactively aggressively) toward that particular peer (Hubbard et al., 1998). The authors collected daily (videotaped) behavioral data from 66 children distributed in 11 experimental playgroups of six familiar boys each. Children in each group interacted for 45 minutes once a day, over the course of 5 consecutive days. In 2 of these days (the 2nd and 4th days), children in each group were also individually interviewed to measure each child's dyadic social cognitions. Stimuli were hypothetical scenarios depicting ambiguous peer provocations in which each member of their group alternated as actor. Dyadic hostile intent attributions and dyadic outcome expectations were collected. This assessment led to a data set with 330 records of direct observations of dyadic behavior and dyadic social cognition responses. Each child appeared five times as a dyad's actor, and five times as a dyad's partner. Mixed-model hierarchical linear modeling analyses controlled for interdependencies in the data set and sorted out actor, partner, and dyadic relationship effects.

The findings (Hubbard et al., 1998) supported a conceptual model in which deviant processing of current social cues (and aggressive behavior) is organized and develops within specific dyadic relationships. A child's hostile intent attributions (or his or her positive evaluations of aggressive solutions) toward a particular peer were not merely a result of *child effects* (i.e., one's deviant processing is not manifested indiscriminately toward most of or all available peers). Nor were they merely a reflection of *partner effects* (i.e., a child elicited negative judgments indiscriminately from most of or all available peers). Rather, the results showed that nearly 20% of the variance in deviant social cognition was uniquely accounted for by *relationship effects* (e.g., a child's specific relationship with a particular peer partially elicited deviant processing). Findings also strongly suggested that hostile attributions (and reactive aggression) unfold within specific dyadic exchanges. At least in terms of regression effects, a child's hostile attributions toward a particular peer contributed to the level of child's reactive aggression toward that particular peer. This basic effect held even after controlling for other critical sources of influence such as the child's generalized tendencies to make hostile attributions and to display reactive aggression and his or her partner's generalized attribute to elicit reactive aggression from peers (Hubbard et al., 1998).

Thus, neither deviant processing patterns nor different forms of aggression can be thought of solely as generalized, trait-like, attributes producing generalized phenomena. Rather, both processing patterns and aggressive behavior seemingly acquire specific social referents and develop within the dynamic exchanges of particular relationships. Thus, for instance, a child may realize that his or her aggression is often highly effective against one child and seldom effective against another, and ultimately revise his or her behavior to conform with these different realizations.

Idiographic Analysis of Behavior and Processing Profiles

In the end, the specificity of children's responses may be so great that the most informative level of assessment is (or should be) the individual child (Dodge et al., 1985). Inherently, this statement calls upon a researcher's ability to model within-subject variability in one's functioning and to obtain a direct estimate of its stability and value. We recently reanalyzed the dyadic relationship dataset of Hubbard et al. to conform with this possibility. In line with much work on idiographic methods of analysis conducted by Shoda, Mischel, and colleagues (Shoda, Mischel, & Wright, 1994), we reasoned that children's characteristic responses toward their peers (i.e., differences across dyads) should be reliably indexed by (temporally) stable "profiles." Illustratively, let us assume that a boy shows his highest level of reactive aggression toward a first peer, no aggression at all toward a second peer, and a moderate amount of reactive aggression toward a third peer. If we could observe the same child interacting with the same three peers a second time, a perfect reactive aggression "stability" profile for this child would be confirmed if he still displayed the most reactive aggression toward the first peer, no reactive aggression toward the second peer, and a moderate level of reactive aggression toward the third peer.

We followed this conceptual approach in examining whether dyadic relationships represent "situations" across which one could reliably measure systematic "intraindividual" variation in children's behavior and cognition. We first indexed profile stability separately for reactive aggression, proactive aggression, hostile biases, and outcome expectations. We then tested whether there is correspondence between behavior profiles and cognition profiles (e.g., between reactive profile and hostile bias profile). Again, each child was "actor" in five dyads and "partner" in five dyads (Hubbard et al., 1998). For each of the four variable scores, we first converted the five child-as-actor scores into deviation unit scores to rescale his or her responses relative to normative group responses (e.g., a child's standardized score for his or her reactive aggression toward a particular peer was calculated with respect to the total amount of reactive aggression displayed by the entire group toward the same peer over the course of the five play-group sessions). We adopted this procedure in order to define intraindividual "profiles" that did not merely reflect "partner" effects. Thus, a child's profile represented the variation across his or her (five peer) deviation unit scores and could have been drawn for any one of the five play-group sessions. We estimated "profile stability" by correlating variability "profiles" computed at two different time points.

There were substantial individual differences in the level of stability in children's intraindividual profiles. Illustratively, Figure 4.1 shows two quite different cases of profile stability estimated for hostile attribution responses (i.e., day 2 profile correlated with day 4 profile). Relative to normative levels, child 18 displayed similar average levels of hostile biases toward his peers at both time points, and this similarity (stability) in profiles was estimated to be quite high, $r = .90$. On the contrary, the profile stability correlation for child 26 was only .40 and was seemingly due to very different judgments of hostile intent the child made toward one of his or her peers on the two occasions (i.e., for peer 2, the child was nearly two standard deviations above the group mean at day 2, but near the norm at day 4).

Despite a wide range of individual differences in profile stability, systematic variability in children's own responses is a reliable phenomenon, on the whole. After transforming each variable's stability profile scores to z-scores, we tested whether profile stability coefficients averaged across the entire sample were reliably different from zero, and we obtained significant results for proactive aggression and outcome expectations (sample $r = .21$ and $r = .27$, respectively, each $p < .05$) and marginally significant results for reactive aggression and hostile intent attributions (sample $r = .15$ and $r = .11$, respectively, each $p < .10$).

We also found some evidence for an "idiographic" (i.e., within-subject) correspondence between subject variability in behavior and subject variability in cognition. To the extent that a child shows, for instance, relatively high levels of reactive aggression toward a particular peer over the course of several play sessions, we would expect that he or she would also make relatively strong hostile attributions about the same peer's motives. Figure 4.2 summarizes the findings on the correspondence between hostile attribution profiles and reactive aggression profiles. Interestingly, we found that this correspondence increases with subjects' relative use of reactive aggression. Children who were relatively more reactive than proactive over the course of five sessions (i.e., indicated by the right bar in Figure 4.2) showed a greater profile correspondence than those children who were relatively less reactive than proactive (i.e., indicated by the left bar). The zero-order sample correlation between subjects' relative frequency of reactive aggression and the magnitude of correspondence between profiles was $r = .31$, $p < .05$.

Thus, even when we examined possible dyadic effects on one's cognition

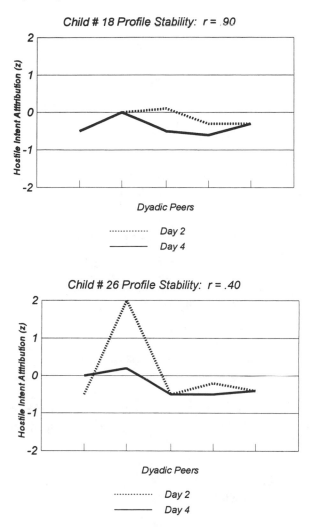

FIGURE 4.1. Illustrative intraindividual profile stabilities in hostile intent attributions across five dyadic relationships. The two lines indicate the profiles based on two different occasions (i.e., two 2-day-apart interview sessions).

and behavior with respect to more direct indices of intraindividual variability profiles, we were able to support the conclusions reached in previous studies (Dodge, Price, et al., 1990; Hubbard et al., 1998). Aggression is not a phenomenon that is regulated by a single generalized tendency or high-level disposition exerting an indiscriminate influence on one's behavior. Rather, both aggression and its associated cognitions unfold within the context of different relationships a child experiences. Thus, a child's characteristic *modus operandi*

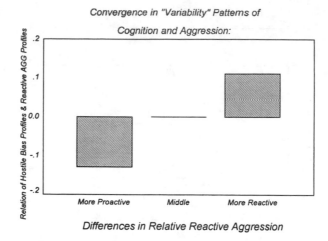

FIGURE 4.2. The relation between intraindividual variability profiles for reactive aggression and intraindividual variability profiles for hostile intent attributions is moderated by the relative frequency with which children enact reactive aggression.

in his or her social world must be understood with respect to *consistency* in *both* how he or she responds to specific situations *and* how he or she meaningfully modifies or modulates responding to changing circumstances in his or her social environment. Both levels of analysis are needed to fully appreciate and understand the coherent organization of a child's personality, and a social-cognitive perspective can adequately provide the means for such a comprehensive analysis.

Chronic Accessibility of Knowledge and Its Relation to Behavior and Experience

In addition to the types of social information-processing mechanisms reviewed thus far (e.g., hostile biases), mechanisms such as "chronic accessibility" of one's knowledge structures (Higgins, 1996) may exert pervasive effects on how one encodes and responds to stimulus situations. Aggressive and socially rejected children who have little or no (experimental) opportunity for reflective reasoning readily access ineffective social problem solving such as conflict-escalating responses (Rabiner, Lenhart, & Lochman, 1990). This effect tends however to disappear or be substantially reduced when incompetent social solutions are generated in conditions in which a child has time to reflect and, seemingly, more control over his or her response options (Rabiner et al., 1990).

A variety of input situations may readily elicit or call upon one's most chronically accessible response patterns, especially when the circumstances call for one's quick responding rather than careful consideration (as often happens in actual social interactions). In a series of recent social inference studies, Zelli and colleagues collected evidence supporting this claim (Zelli, Cervone, & Huesmann, 1996; Zelli, Huesmann, & Cervone, 1995). The authors hypothesized that individual differences in aggressive experiences would be associated with differences in "spontaneous" hostility trait inferences, that is, inferences that are unsolicited and outside of one's awareness (see Uleman, Newman, & Moskowitz, 1996, for an extensive review on spontaneous trait inferences). In both investigations, the authors utilized a cued-recall paradigm in which adults were presented sentences implying either a hostile or a nonhostile dispositional interpretation (e.g., "The policeman pushes Dave out of the way") and then aided in sentence recall by means of varying recall dispositional cues. The thrust of both investigations was that aggressive adults would spontaneously encode the sentences in hostility terms and be relatively more effective in sentence recall when aided by hostility cues than by other types of recall cues. The findings of both studies supported these hypotheses. College students who were assigned to the "spontaneous" processing condition (i.e., received no instruction to engage in inference processing) and who reported frequent experiences in which they punched, kicked, or threatened others showed relatively stronger sentence recall in the presence of hostility recall cues than either semantic (Zelli et al., 1995) or nonhostility (Zelli et al., 1996) recall cues.

Together, these findings suggest that salient social experiences foster knowledge structures that may become so highly accessible as to pervasively influence one's social thinking. They further suggest that knowledge may exert this influence in situations that are relatively unrelated to the original contexts in which the experiences occurred. Aggressive subjects' spontaneous hostility inferences appeared in a context seemingly lacking of any element of interpersonal threat, physical challenge, or state of high arousal that probably characterized their prior aggressive experiences. Nonetheless, individual differences in spontaneous hostility inferences were readily apparent (Zelli et al., 1996). Knowledge accessibility, then, is a social-cognitive mechanism that may directly contribute to broad consistencies in thought and action across relatively diverse circumstances and situations.

CONCLUSION: THE CONCEPT OF PERSONALITY COHERENCE

In this chapter, we endorsed a general view of personality as a complex, adaptive system in which cognitive (and affective) mechanisms of personality can attain a high degree of organization and can give rise to personality coherence. As individuals interact with their social environment, they develop and consolidate idiosyncratic ways to perceive, interpret, and respond to social challenges, and these patterns become the defining features of what make individuals unique.

The richness and organization of one's functioning and personality would be defamed if one merely had to posit high-level dispositional variables to explain them away, as trait approaches would argue. Instead, one can do justice to this richness only by taking a bottom-up perspective and investigating basic psychological processes and structures, the patterns of interaction among these mechanisms as they unfold throughout one's development, and the unique ways organized personality structures find expression in one's thought and action.

A social-cognitive analysis of personality functioning does not reduce individuality to a rigid system responding to context contingencies. It, rather, recognizes the plasticity of personality development and the ever-evolving organizing features that ultimately define one's unique personality. The conditional nature of personality does not render the outcomes of personality assessment into a noncoherent whole across one's life span. In contrast, personality can be and is indeed coherent. Stability in behavior is readily observable as long as it is measured within contexts. For instance, the remarkable stability of aggressive behavior patterns stands as a striking example that can be understood within a theory of social-cognitive personality development (Huesmann & Moise, 1998). Intraindividual stability in the patterning of behavior is observed regularly as long as one adopts methods of analysis that are sensitive and tuned to the inherently idiographic nature of the phenomena being observed (Shoda et al., 1994).

Importantly, a social-cognitive perspective demands that coherence is not sought merely at the level of behavioral manifestations. To the extent that personality is a dynamic system encompassing a highly organized pattern of psychological responses operating at multiple levels of functioning, one must instead conceive that *the personality system* is coherent as a whole and that one's scientific quest is to discover the principles and psychological mechanisms that explicate and give rise to this personality coherence at any level of one's functioning. For instance, as we have shown, a child seemingly modulates and enacts his or her aggression toward peers in ways that are highly sensitive to the dynamic qualities and defining features of the dyadic exchanges he or she experiences.

In the context of that example, averaging a child's aggression across dyads would not only undermine the search for coherence, but it would also instigate a process of analysis that would likely lead to fundamentally wrong conclusions. Instead, we have attempted to show how a social-cognitive analysis of dyadic aggressive behavior would seek and predict both consistency and variability in behavioral patterns, and how consistency and variability can effectively index coherence in one's functioning. Moreover, we have also shown how reliable and identifiable patterns in behavioral manifestations must correspond—in ultimate analysis—to reliable and identifiable patterns in clearly enunciated social-cognitive operations or mechanisms.

In conclusion, the bottom-up approach to personality theory, with its emphasis on reciprocal determinism and repeated transactions across development and different contexts, provides a rich source of understanding, explanation, and prediction of behavior. It provides theoretical mechanisms for behavior in a way that trait approaches cannot. Finally, it offers an understanding of behavioral change mechanisms as well, thus guiding systematic efforts at intervention.

ACKNOWLEDGMENT

We are grateful to John Coie for sharing the data of the peer-group project and to Robert Laird for his many constructive suggestions and creative input into the idiographic analyses reported here.

REFERENCES

Anderson, C. A., & Deuser, W. E. (1993). The primacy of control in causal thinking and attributional style: An attributional functionalism perspective. In G. Weary, F. Gleicher, & K. L. Marsh (Eds.), *Control motivation and social cognition* (pp. 94–121). New York: Springer-Verlag.

Baldwin, M. W. (1992). Relational schemas and the processing of social information. *Psychological Bulletin, 112,* 461–484.

Baldwin, M. W., Fehr, B., Keedian, W., Seidel, M., & Thompson, D. W. (1993). An exploration of the relational schemas underlying attachment styles: Self-report and lexical decision approaches. *Personality and Social Psychology Bulletin, 19,* 746–754.

Baldwin, M. W., Keelan, J. P. R., Fehr, B., Enns, V., & Koh-Rangarajoo, E. (1996). Social-cognitive conceptualization of attachment working models: Availability and accessibility effects. *Journal of Personality and Social Psychology, 71*(1), 94–109.

Baldwin, M. W., & Sinclair, L. (1996). Self-esteem and "if . . . then" contingencies of personal acceptance. *Journal of Personality and Social Psychology, 71*(6), 1130–1141.

Bandura, A. (1986). *Social foundations of thought and action: A social cognitive theory.* Englewood Cliffs, NJ: Prentice-Hall.

Bandura, A., Barbaranelli, C., Caprara, G. V., & Pastorelli, C. (1996). Mechanisms of moral disengagement in the exercise of moral agency. *Journal of Personality and Social Psychology, 71*(2), 364–374.

Bandura, A., & Cervone, D. (1983). Self-evaluative and self-efficacy mechanisms governing the motivational effects of goal systems. *Journal of Personality and Social Psychology, 45,* 1017–1028.

Bargh, J. A., Chen, M., & Burrows, L. (1996). Automaticity of social behavior: Direct effects of trait construct and stereotype activation on action. *Journal of Personality and Social Psychology, 71*(2), 230–244.

Bargh, J. A., Lombardi, W. J., & Higgins, E. T. (1988). Automaticity of chronically accessible constructs in person × situation effects on person perception: It's just a matter of time. *Journal of Personality and Social Psychology, 55*(4), 599–605.

Bargh, J. A., & Tota, M. E. (1988). Context-dependent processing in depression: Accessibility of negative constructs with regard to self but not others. *Journal of Personality and Social Psychology, 54,* 924–939.

Bates, J. E., Pettit, G. S., Dodge, K. A., & Ridge, B. (in press). The interaction of temperamental resistance to control and restrictive parenting in the development of externalizing behavior. *Developmental Psychology.*

Berkowitz, L. (1993). *Aggression: Its causes, consequences, and control.* New York: Academic Press.

Cantor, N., & Kihlstrom, J. F. (1987). *Personality and social intelligence.* Englewood Cliffs, NJ: Prentice-Hall.

Cantor, N., Norem, J. K., Niedenthal, P. M., Langston, C. A., & Brower, A. M. (1987). Life tasks, self-concept ideals, and cognitive strategies in a life transition. *Journal of Personality and Social Psychology, 53,* 1178–1191.

Cervone, D. (1991). The two disciplines of personality psychology. *Psychological Science, 2,* 371–377.

Cervone, D. (1997). Social-cognitive mechanisms and personality coherence: Self-knowledge, situational beliefs, and cross-situational coherence in perceived self-efficacy. *Psychological Science, 8,* 43–50.

Cervone, D., & Williams, S. L. (1992). Social cognitive theory and personality. In G. V. Caprara & G. L. Van Heck (Eds.), *Modern personality psychology: Critical reviews and new directions* (pp. 200–252). New York: Harvester Wheatsheaf.

Clark, L. F. (1994). Social cognition and health psychology. In R. S. Wyer & T. K. Srull (Eds.), *Handbook of social cognition* (Vol. 2, pp. 239–288). Hillsdale, NJ: Erlbaum.

Coie, J. D., & Dodge, K. A. (1998). Aggression and antisocial behavior. In W. Damon (Series Ed.) & N. Eisenberg (Vol. Ed.), *Handbook of child psychology: Vol. 3. Social, emotional, and personality development* (5th ed., pp. 779–862). New York: Wiley.

Costa, P. T., Jr., & McCrae, R. R. (1988). From catalog to classification: Murray's needs and the five-factor model. *Journal of Personality and Social Psychology, 55,* 258–265.

Crick, N. R., & Dodge, K. A. (1994). A review and reformulation of social-information processing mechanisms in children's social adjustment. *Psychological Bulletin, 115,* 74–101.

Crick, N. R., & Dodge, K. A. (1996). Social-information-processing mechanisms in reactive and proactive aggression. *Child Development, 67,* 993–1002.

Crick, N. R., & Ladd, G. W. (1990). Children's perceptions of the outcomes of aggressive strategies: Do the ends justify being mean? *Developmental Psychology, 26,* 612–620.

Deater-Deckard, K., Dodge, K. A., Bates, J. E., & Pettit, G. S. (1998). Multiple risk factors in the development of externalizing behavior problems: Group and individual differences. *Development and Psychopathology, 10,* 469–493.

Dodge, K. A. (1980). Social cognition and children's aggressive behavior. *Child Development, 51,* 162–170.

Dodge, K. A. (1993). Social-cognitive mechanisms in the development of conduct disorder and depression. *Annual Review of Psychology, 44,* 559–584.

Dodge, K. A., Bates, J. E., & Pettit, G. S. (1990). Mechanisms in the cycle of violence. *Science, 250,* 1678–1683.

Dodge, K. A., & Coie, J. D. (1987). Social information processing factors in reactive and proactive aggression in children's peer groups. *Journal of Personality and Social Psychology, 53,* 1146–1158.

Dodge, K. A., & Feldman, E. (1990). Issues in social cognition and sociometric status. In S. R. Asher & J. D. Coie (Eds.), *Peer rejection in childhood: Origins, consequences, and intervention* (pp. 119–155). New York: Cambridge University Press.

Dodge, K. A., & Frame, C. L. (1982). Social cognitive biases and deficits in aggressive boys. *Child Development, 53,* 630–635.

Dodge, K. A., Lochman, J. E., Harnish, J. D., Bates, J. E., & Pettit, G. S. (1997). Reactive and proactive aggression in school children and psychiatrically-impaired chronically assaultive youth. *Journal of Abnormal Psychology, 106,* 37–51.

Dodge, K. A., McClaskey, C. L., & Feldman, E. (1985). A situational approach to the assessment of social competence in children. *Journal of Consulting and Clinical Psychology, 53,* 344–353.

Dodge, K. A., & Newman, J. P. (1981). Biased decision making processes in aggressive boys. *Journal of Abnormal Psychology, 90,* 375–379.

Dodge, K. A., Pettit, G. S., Bates, J. E., & Valente, E. (1995). Social-information processing patterns partially mediate the effect of early physical abuse on later conduct problems. *Journal of Abnormal Psychology, 104,* 632–643.

Dodge, K. A., Pettit, G. S., McClaskey, C. L., & Brown, M. (1986). Social competence in children. *Monographs of the Society for Research in Child Development, 51* (2, Serial No. 213).

Dodge, K. A., Price, J. M., Coie, J. D., & Christopoulos, C. (1990). On the development of aggressive dyadic relationships in boys' peer groups. *Human Development, 33,* 260–270.

Dweck, C. S., & Leggett, E. L. (1988). A social-cognitive approach to motivation and personality. *Psychological Review, 95,* 256–273.

Feldman, E., & Dodge, K. A. (1987). Social information processing and sociometric status: Sex, age, and situational effects. *Journal of Abnormal Child Psychology, 15,* 211–227.

Fiske, S. T., & Taylor, S. E. (1991). *Social cognition* (2nd ed.). New York: McGraw-Hill.

Fuhrman, R. W., & Funder, D. C. (1995). Convergence between self and peer in the response-time processing of trait-relevant information. *Journal of Personality and Social Psychology, 69,* 961–974.

Goldberg, L. R. (1993). The structure of phenotypic personality traits. *American Psychologist, 48,* 26–34.

Goldfried, M. R., & d'Zurilla, T. J. (1969). A behavioral-analytic model for assessing competence. In C. D. Spielberger (Ed.), *Current topics in clinical and community psychology* (Vol. 1, pp. 151–196). New York: Academic Press.

Guerra, N. G., Huesmann, L. R., Tolan, P. H., Van Acker, R., & Eron, L. D. (1995). Stressful events and individual beliefs as correlates of economic disadvantage and aggression among urban children. *Journal of Consulting and Clinical Psychology, 63*(4), 518–528.

Hartup, W. W. (1974). Aggression in childhood: Developmental perspectives. *American Psychologist, 29,* 336–341.

Higgins, E. T. (1990). Personality, social psychology, and person–situation relations: Standards and knowledge activation as a common language. In L. A. Pervin (Ed.), *Handbook of personality: Theory and research* (pp. 301–338). New York: Guilford Press.

Higgins, E. T. (1996). Knowledge activation: Accessibility, applicability, and salience. In

E. T. Higgins & A. E. Kruglanski (Eds.), *Social psychology: Handbook of basic principles* (pp. 133–168). New York: Guilford Press.

Higgins, E. T., Bargh, J. A., & Lombardi, W. (1985). The nature of priming effects on categorization. *Journal of Experimental Psychology: Learning, Memory, and Cognition, 11,* 59–69.

Higgins, E. T., & King, G. A. (1981). Accessibility of social constructs: Information-processing consequences of individual and contextual variability. In N. Cantor & J. F. Kihlstrom (Eds.), *Personality, cognition, and social interaction* (pp. 69–122). Hillsdale, NJ: Erlbaum.

Higgins, E. T., Rholes, W. S., & Jones, C. R. (1977). Category accessibility and impression formation. *Journal of Experimental Social Psychology, 13,* 141–154.

Hubbard, J. A., Dodge, K. A., Coie, J. D., Cillessen, A. H. N., & Schwartz, D. (1998). *The dyadic nature of social-information-processing in children's reactive and proactive aggression.* Unpublished manuscript, University of Delaware.

Huesmann, L. R. (1998). The role of social information processing and cognitive schema in the acquisition and maintenance of habitual aggressive behavior. In R. G. Geen & E. Donnerstein (Eds.), *Human aggression: Theories, research, and implications for social policy* (pp. 73–109). New York: Academic Press.

Huesmann, L. R., & Moise, J. F. (1998). Stability and continuity of aggression from early childhood to young adulthood. In D. J. Flannery & C. R. Huff (Eds.), *Youth violence: Prevention, intervention, and social policy* (pp. 73–95). Washington, DC: American Psychiatric Press.

Ingram, R. E. (1990). Self-focused attention in clinical disorders: Review and a conceptual model. *Psychological Bulletin, 107,* 156–176.

Ingram, R. E., & Reed, M. J. (1986). Information encoding and retrieval processes in depression: Findings, issues, and future directions. In R. E. Ingram (Ed.), *Information processing approaches to clinical psychology* (pp. 131–150). Orlando: Academic Press.

Kihlstrom, J. F. & Klein, S. B. (1994). The self as a knowledge structure. In R. S. Wyer & T. K. Srull (Eds.), *Handbook of social cognition* (Vol. 1, pp. 153–208). Hillsdale, NJ: Erlbaum.

Markus, H., & Nurius, P. (1986). Possible selves. *American Psychologist, 41,* 954–969.

McCrae, R. R., & Costa, P. T., Jr. (1989). The structure of interpersonal traits: Wiggins' circumplex model and the five-factor model. *Journal of Personality and Social Psychology, 56,* 586–595.

McCrae, R. R., & Costa, P. T., Jr. (1996). Toward a new generation of personality theories: Theoretical contexts for the five-factor model. In J. S. Wiggins (Ed.), *The five-factor model of personality: Theoretical perspectives* (pp. 51–87). New York: Guilford Press.

McCrae, R. R., & Costa, P. T., Jr. (1997). Personality trait structure as a human universal. *American Psychologist, 52,* 509–516.

McFall, R. M. (1982). A review and reformulation of the concept of social skills. *Behavioral Assessment, 4,* 1–33.

Mischel, W. (1990). Personality dispositions revisited and revised: A view after three decades. In L. A. Pervin (Ed.), *Handbook of personality: Theory and research* (pp. 111–164). New York: Guilford Press.

Mischel, W., & Shoda, Y. (1995). A cognitive-affective system theory of personality: Reconceptualizing situations, dispositions, dynamics, and invariance in personality structure. *Psychological Review, 102,* 246–286.

Moskowitz, G. B. (1993). Individual differences in social categorization: The influence of personal need for structure on spontaneous trait inferences. *Journal of Personality and Social Psychology, 65*(1), 132–142.

Nelson, K. (1993). Developing self-knowledge from autobiographical memory. In T. K. Srull & R. S. Wyer (Eds.), *Advances in social cognition* (Vol. 5, pp. 111–122). Hillsdale, NJ: Erlbaum.

Perry, D. G., Perry, L. C., & Rasmussen, P. (1986). Cognitive social learning mediators of aggression. *Child Development, 57,* 700–711.

Pervin, L. A. (Ed.). (1989). *Goal concepts in personality and social psychology.* Hillsdale, NJ: Erlbaum.

Plomin, R., & Daniels, D. (1987). Why are children in the same family so different from one another? *Behavioral and Brain Sciences, 10,* 1–16.

Price, J. M., & Dodge, K. A. (1989). Reactive and proactive aggression in childhood: Relations to peer status and social context dimensions. *Journal of Abnormal Child Psychology, 17,* 455–471.

Pyszczynsky, T., Greenberg, J., Hamilton, J. & Nix, G. (1991). On the relationship between self-focused attention and psychological disorder: A critical reappraisal. *Psychological Bulletin, 110,* 538–543.

Rabiner, D. L., Lenhart, L., & Lochman, J. E. (1990). Automatic versus reflective social problem solving in relation to sociometric status. *Developmental Psychology, 26*(6), 1010–1016.

Rubin, K. H., Bream, L. A., & Rose-Krasnor, L. (1991). Social problem solving and aggression in childhood. In D. J. Pepler & K. H. Rubin (Eds.), *The development and treatment of childhood aggression* (pp. 219–246). Hillsdale, NJ: Erlbaum.

Salmon, W. C. (1989). Four decades of scientific explanation. In P. Kitcher & W. C. Salmon (Eds.), *Minnesota studies in the philosophy of science: Vol. 3. Scientific explanation* (pp. 3–219). Minneapolis: University of Minnesota Press.

Shoda, Y., & Mischel, W. (1993). Cognitive social approach to dispositional inferences: What if the perceiver is a cognitive social scientist? *Personality and Social Psychology Bulletin, 19*(5), 574–585.

Shoda, Y., Mischel, W., & Wright, J. C. (1993). Links between personality judgments and contextualized behavioral patterns: Situation-behavior profiles of personality prototypes. *Social Cognition, 4,* 399–429.

Shoda, Y., Mischel, W., & Wright, J. C. (1994). Intraindividual stability in the organization and patterning of behavior: Incorporating psychological situations into the idiographic analysis of personality. *Journal of Personality and Social Psychology, 67*(4), 674–687.

Slaby, R. G., & Guerra, N. G. (1988). Cognitive mediators of aggression in adolescent offenders: I. Assessment. *Developmental Psychology, 24,* 580–588.

Smith, E. R. (1994). Procedural knowledge and processing strategies in social cognition. In R. S. Wyer, Jr., & T. K. Srull (Eds.), *Handbook of social cognition* (2nd ed., vol. 1, pp. 99–152). Hillsdale, NJ: Erlbaum.

Tellegen, A., Lykken, D. T., Bouchard, T. J., Jr., Wilcox, K. J., Segal, N. L., & Rich, S. (1988). Personality similarity in twins reared apart and together. *Journal of Personality and Social Psychology, 54,* 1031–1039.

Tulving, E., & Thomson, D. M. (1973). Encoding specificity and retrieval processes in episodic memory. *Psychological Review, 80,* 352–373.

Uleman, J. S., Newman, L. S., & Moskowitz. G. B. (1996). People as flexible interpreters:

Evidence and issues from spontaneous trait inference. In M. P. Zanna (Ed.), *Advances in experimental social psychology* (Vol. 28, pp. 211–279). San Diego, CA: Academic Press.

Waas, G. A. (1988). Social attributional biases of peer-rejected and aggressive children. *Child Development, 59,* 969–992.

Weary, G., & Edwards, J. A. (1994a). Social cognition and clinical psychology: Anxiety, depression and the processing of social information. In R. S. Wyer & T. K. Srull (Eds.), *Handbook of social cognition* (Vol. 2, pp. 289–338). Hillsdale, NJ: Erlbaum.

Weary, G., & Edwards, J. A. (1994b). Individual differences in causal uncertainty. *Journal of Personality and Social Psychology, 67*(2), 308–318.

Weary, G., Marsh, K. L., Gleicher, F., & Edwards, J. A. (1993). Social-cognitive consequences of depression. In G. Weary, F. Gleicher, & K. L. Marsh (Eds.), *Control motivation and social cognition* (pp. 255–287). New York: Springer-Verlag.

Zelli, A., Huesmann, L. R., & Cervone, D. (1995). Social inference and individual differences in aggression: Evidence for spontaneous judgments of hostility. *Aggressive Behavior, 21,* 405–417.

Zelli, A., Cervone, D., & Huesmann, L. R. (1996). Behavioral experience and social inference: Individual differences in aggressive experience and spontaneous versus deliberate trait inference. *Social Cognition, 14*(2), 165–190.

5

Relational Schemas
Research into Social-Cognitive Aspects
of Interpersonal Experience

MARK W. BALDWIN

Nowhere is the influence of personality, and the social-cognitive processes contributing to it, more evident than in the dynamics of people's interpersonal relationships. A person who has repeatedly been abandoned by romantic partners may find it difficult to form new attachments with others and may tend to interpret any ambiguous behavior of a new partner in a negatively biased way. A person raised by domineering, hypercritical parents may adopt a correspondingly harsh self-evaluative stance when contemplating his or her performance outcomes. Conversely, a person with a history of warm, supportive relationships may automatically anticipate pleasant interactions with others and act in ways that actually bring about positive interchanges.

Over the past decade my collaborators and I have been developing a social-cognitive model of how people think about their significant relationships and the effects this thinking has on their interactions and sense of self. The central construct is the relational schema, or cognitive structure representing regularities in patterns of interpersonal relatedness (Baldwin, 1992). Our research has explored how relational schemas shape expectations, social behavior, and the interpretations people make of their interpersonal experiences.

In a sense, the work discussed in this chapter represents an attempt to integrate social-cognitive models of personality with models drawn from interpersonal, attachment, symbolic interactionist, and object relations psychodynamic traditions. As such, the theoretical background encompasses some of the classic ideas from social and personality psychology, including "working models" (Bowlby, 1969), "transference" (Freud, 1912/1958), the "looking-glass self" (Cooley, 1902), and so on. As outlined elsewhere (Baldwin, 1992), the relational schemas framework also draws heavily from other recent efforts at integration (e.g., Fiske, 1992; Horowitz, 1988; Mitchell, 1988; Planalp, 1985; Safran, 1990; Stern, 1985). A priority of the current research program has been to link the model carefully to specific research findings and predictions on the assumption that theoretical progress will be greatly facilitated by keeping close ties to the rapidly developing social-cognitive literature.

Some of the research we have done has examined social-cognitive factors contributing to a number of trait-like variables, such as adult attachment style, self-esteem, and social anxiety. At the same time, the guiding assumption (following Mischel, 1973, among others) has been that the very same cognitive processes that support these chronic tendencies also underlie the meaningful situational variability of people's behavior. Indeed, we have invested much of our efforts in using experimental manipulations to study variability in these basic processes as a way of exploring the social-cognitive underpinnings of personality coherence. In what follows, I outline the core principles of the relational schemas approach and then survey research that has been conducted in my lab and elsewhere on the measurement, activation, and influence of relational schemas.

BASIC PRINCIPLES OF THE RELATIONAL SCHEMAS APPROACH

The elements of the model are consistent with those of various social learning models of personality (e.g., Bandura, 1986; Cantor & Kihlstrom, 1985; Mischel, 1973; Rotter, 1954) and the social-cognitive literature generally (Higgins & Bargh, 1987; Markus & Zajonc, 1985; Smith, 1984). The building blocks of social cognition are assumed to be declarative knowledge structures— schemas—consisting of descriptive knowledge about the people and situations that make up the social world. It is usually assumed that memories of specific stimuli or experiences become linked together with memories of other similar or related stimuli either through a kind of resonance among their shared features, or because one has explicitly considered them as exemplars of some larger category. Thus, memories of specific schoolteachers might become organized into a schoolteacher stereotype; similarly, information about specific forms of "kind" behavior become organized into a trait category for "kindness." Often, this exemplar knowledge is linked to generic category knowledge that includes abstracted or generalized expectancies about the characteristics of typical category members. One can think of a schema, then, as a "chunk of associative network" (Carlston & Smith, 1996, p.

196) with links connecting informational nodes that represent exemplar and generic knowledge about some element or aspect of the social world.

A relational schema is a cognitive structure representing interpersonal information and is hypothesized to be made up of three interrelated components: a self-schema, an other-schema, and an interpersonal script. Self-schemas (Markus, 1977) represent information about the self and are thought to be organized in much the same way as information about other people with links between episodic and generic knowledge, and so on. People are assumed to have multiple self-schemas, and the particular subset that is activated in working memory at any given time defines the "working self-concept" (Markus & Kunda, 1986) of the moment. In this way, the experience of self can shift, so a person might feel like a psychologist at one moment, a chocolate aficionado the next, and a hard worker the next.

Specific self-schemas are hypothesized to be associated with representations of specific other people, or types of people. The sense of self as "teacher" is associated with an other-schema for a "learner," for example, just as the self-schema "rebellious, put-upon teenager" is associated with the complementary role "overbearing parent." Ogilvie and Ashmore (1991) discussed this sort of self-with-other unit, defined as "a mental representation that includes the set of personal qualities (traits, feelings, and the like) that an individual believes characterizes his or her self when with a particular other person" (p. 290).

Central to the current model of relational schemas is the assumption that the critical link between self and other is an interpersonal script or event schema (see, e.g., Abelson, 1981) representing the typical interaction patterns occurring in that relationship. One might, for example, have had many experiences of asking one's graduate advisor a question, with the advisor responding in a positive, impressed manner. If so, one might develop a script that "I ask a question then my advisor responds positively." Associated with this script will be the self-with-other schema of "bright student" and the other-schema of "impressed advisor." Interpersonal scripts can include numerous specific tracks (Abelson, 1981) representing different behavior-outcome, or *"if...then..."* contingencies: For example, the student might also learn that "If I offer my own opinions then my advisor will respond critically and dismissively" (see Mischel, 1973; Safran, 1990, for other discussions of *if...then...* contingencies).

In terms of declarative knowledge, then, individual differences in relational schemas involve differences in what kinds of information are available in memory due to a person's learning history and also which schemas the person typically uses to encode social information. One person might tend to see interpersonal experiences in terms of the honesty of others, for example, whereas another might attend to people's intelligence or status. In some respects at least, people's typical, or "chronically accessible" schemas reflect the effects of practice: Over time, perceivers simply get better at making judgments in certain content domains and develop tendencies to think in certain ways (e.g., Smith & Branscombe, 1987). This is the procedural knowledge aspect of schematic processing, whereby social perceivers learn inference rules for going beyond the information given in a social situation. Consider a woman who is inclined to interpret people's behavior in terms of how kind or unkind they are, for example. Each time she draws an inference that "Since so-and-so helped a stranger with her groceries, he is kind," she establishes a link between that behavior and trait that can assist her in making a future judgment of similar information. Such links make up her expertise at making inferences in that domain, allowing her to make snap judgments about people's kindness. One way to conceptualize such judgments is as the result of spreading activation from a node representing the behavior to a node representing the trait label linked to it in the associative network. Spreading activation thereby increases the trait label's accessibility, or activation readiness; as such it comes to mind easily or "fluently" (e.g., Jacoby, Toth, Lindsay, & Debner, 1992).

A parallel analysis can be made of other effects of schematic processing. "Stereotyping," for example, presumably involves spreading activation from a group label to a specific characteristic associated with that group so that the characteristic is then judged more likely or accurate because of its cognitive fluency. Gap-filling effects in memory (e.g., for self-relevant information; Rogers, 1977) may also reflect the misattribution of fluency as a feeling of familiarity, leading to the erroneous conclusion that schema-consistent information has been seen before. When interpretive processes operate automatically in this fashion, "their products are experienced as direct or 'true' perceptions rather than as consciously mediated interpretations" (Jacoby et al., 1992, p. 89).

Similar dynamics apply to spreading activation across elements of an interpersonal script, as the activation of the "if" part of an overlearned script automatically increases the fluency of the associated "then." This fluency can then be experienced as an automatic expectancy: The possible outcome comes to mind easily, as the person thinks, "I can easily imagine that happening" (Anderson & Godfrey, 1987; Cervone, 1989). Because that possible outcome can be a desired or undesired state (e.g., affection, respect, rejection), interpersonal scripts have direct motivational and behavioral implications, with if...then... contingencies functioning according to the principles described in expectancy–value models of behavior.

As Mischel and Shoda (1995) have demonstrated, the result is often that people display an if...then... "behavioral signature" from one situation to the next, such as "If he is in an achievement situation, he is dominant; however if he is with a romantic partner, he is submissive." The relational schema approach reinforces the point that this cross-situational variability is coherent, psychologically meaningful, and derived from if...then... outcome expectancies (Mischel, 1973), particularly expectancies regarding the environmental contingencies of valued interpersonal goals. For example, a person who believes that "If I am dominant, opponents respect me" but also "If I am submissive, my romantic partner is more affectionate" will act quite differently depending on competitive versus romantic possibilities in the current interpersonal situation!

The relational schema approach also introduces another source of meaningful variability in interpersonal behavior by noting that, although people may have a general orientation to or expectancy about a given type of situation, such as competition or intimacy, in some sense every different relationship presents a specific subset of psychological situations. A man who has learned that "If I am dominant, opponents respect me" might also have specific relational knowledge that "If I am dominant with my father, he will humiliate me" and will be predictably different in his behavior with his father than with others. As I discuss below, the fact that people have multiple relational schemas available to them serves as a powerful principle for experimental research into these cognitive mediators of people's "behavioral signatures."

RESEARCH

Over the past decade, my collaborators and I have conducted research based on this core set of theoretical constructs, employing a few standard empirical methods to examine the content, structure, and function of relational schemas across a number of interpersonal contexts. Often the focus has been on people's schemas for their closest significant relationships, particularly in work in the adult attachment domain conducted with Beverley Fehr and others. Other studies have focused on the influence relational schemas have on the construction of the sense of self, especially on evaluation of self in ego-threatening contexts. In reviewing some of this research, I group studies according to the theoretical issues addressed and methods used, rather than according to specific research domains.

Assessing the Content and Structure of Relational Schemas

Self-Reports

Perhaps the most straightforward way to investigate the content of people's interpersonal models is simply to ask them. In the adult attachment literature, for example, it is now generally acknowledged that people's views of their close relationships vary widely, with some people feeling relatively secure, others feeling very anxious about their relationships, and others tending to avoid close relationships altogether. Research has shown that these orientations predict a wide range of, not only affective and behavioral responses, but also significant relationship outcomes such as breakups or divorce (see, e.g., Hazan & Shaver, 1994, for a review). Theoretically, the causal construct has been assumed to be expectations about relationship partners' emotional availability, dependability, trustworthiness, and so on, and some (e.g., Bretherton, 1990; Collins & Read, 1994) have framed these expectations in terms of the kinds of interpersonal scripts being discussed here.

In our research (Baldwin, Fehr, Keedian, Seidel, & Thomson, 1993) we have asked participants to consider a number of possible behaviors (e.g., "If I depend on my partner") and then to rate the likelihood of various potential outcomes (e.g., "then my partner will leave me," or "then my partner will support me"). We found meaningful relations between such *if...then...* expectancies and the basic attachment orientations (Hazan & Shaver, 1987). For example, people who said they tended to be anxious in close relationships were more likely than others to endorse a script in which depending on a partner led to a negative outcome.

In a later set of studies (Baldwin, Keelan, Fehr, Enns, & Koh-Rangarajoo, 1996), we examined the foundation of generalized social expectations on specific exemplar knowledge. First, in a study of knowledge availability, we established that people's self-reported general attachment orientations (i.e., secure, avoidant, or anxious–ambivalent) corresponded to the number of specific relationships they could think of in which they tended to relate to another in that way. Next, we used a self-report method to study the cognitive fluency of such exemplar knowledge. As mentioned earlier, it is now well established that the ease of activation of social information can influence people's judgments; for example, numerous studies have shown that the ease with which information about some type of event (e.g., airplane crashes) comes to mind affects people's estimates of the event's probability (e.g., Tversky & Kahneman, 1973). Some researchers (e.g., Anderson & Godfrey, 1987; Cervone, 1989) have studied this phenomenon as it applies to social events and have shown that, if a particular social script comes to mind easily (e.g., because it was recently thought about), people judge that event as much more likely to occur in the future. Extending this principle to relational knowledge, we reasoned that people's beliefs about the prevalence of a certain relational pattern might be a function of the accessibility of examples of that pattern. We asked individuals of different self-rated attachment styles to try to think of relationships that matched the prototypes of secure, avoidant, and anxious relationships. We found that, indeed, participants' reports of the ease with which secure and insecure types of relationships came to mind predicted their overall style. Fluency phenomena such as this are closely related to the availability of information, of course, as the more examples one has of something, the easier it will be to bring an example to mind. The implications go beyond that, however: As I will discuss shortly, various factors other than sheer availability—recent experiences, for example, or motivational relevance—can influence fluency and social expectations.

We have used this type of self-report research in a number of domains other than adult attachment to reveal the *if...then...* social expectations that correlate with specific individual differences in social behavior. We studied gender differences in expectancies of friendliness and dominance, for example, drawing on earlier work by Hill and Safran (1994) on the interpersonal circle and found that women in our sample tended to anticipate that submissive behavior would lead to positive, affiliative responses from others (Baldwin & Keelan, 1998). In a study of anger in close relationships (Fehr, Baldwin, Collins, Patterson, & Benditt, in press), we found that men anticipated that expressing anger directly would lead to withdrawal and rejection by a partner, but women were more likely to expect their partner to mock them and deny responsibility. Finally, a study of social anxiety showed that people prone to this disorder were particularly likely to endorse the expectancy that acting in a warm and friendly manner toward others would result in being dominated and rejected by them (Baldwin & Fergusson, 1998). In these domains, as well as the adult attachment domain, it is not surprising that people with divergent expectations about social outcomes often approach their interactions with different strategies.

Spreading Activation Paradigms and the Examination of Cognitive Structure

As reviewed earlier, a critical assumption of schema models of knowledge representation is that there is a degree of interconnection or association among the elements of a schema. For example, people might expect that someone who smokes a pipe and wears a tweed jacket with elbow patches also is probably intelligent and somewhat pedantic. It is because of this associative structure that schemas function as modular units, as demonstrated when informational gaps in perception and memory are filled in with whatever would be expected on the basis of past experience. A collection of promising methods for more directly examining the structure of schemas is based on the principle of spreading activation (Collins & Loftus, 1975), that once one element of a schema is primed, activation will spread through associative links to other elements of the schema. This "wakening of associations" (James, 1890) can be studied using procedures whereby one element of a hypothesized schema (e.g., "smokes a pipe") is activated, and measures are taken to see if activation spreads to other elements (e.g., "pedantic"). Dependent measures can assess the activation of these other elements using reaction-time tasks, impression formation, and so on. A number of writers have argued that this kind of evidence of spreading activation is required before one can confidently claim the existence of a schema (e.g., Higgins & Bargh, 1987; Segal, Hood, Shaw, & Higgins, 1988).

This logic has been used in some creative research into the structure of the self-schema, which is thought to consist in large part of an associative network of self-descriptive traits (e.g., images of self as introverted, generous, and clumsy). In an adaptation of the well-known Stroop task, participants are instructed to name the color of ink in which various self-descriptive adjectives are printed. Before each color-naming trial, subjects are shown a prime: either another self-descriptive adjective, or a non-self-relevant adjective. If self-descriptive traits are in fact associated with each other in an organized self-schema, then priming one trait descriptor in this way should activate the other traits as well, via spreading activation. Thus, evidence of structure would consist of a priming effect whereby presentation of one self-descriptive term (e.g., "generous"), as a prime, produced interference when the subject tried to color-name a second self-descriptive term (e.g., "introverted"). Research has shown that while results on this spreading-activation task are not as robust as one might anticipate, the effect is most evident in domains where people have particularly well-organized evaluative structures relating to traits in which they feel they are falling short of standards (Higgins, Van Hook, & Dorfman, 1988; Segal et al., 1988).

My colleagues and I have used this logic to examine the *if...then...* structure of interpersonal scripts using an adaptation of the "lexical decision paradigm," another reaction-time procedure for assessing spreading activation. In the basic lexical decision task (Meyer & Schvaneveldt, 1971), subjects read letter-strings on a computer screen and attempt to judge as quickly as possible whether they are words (e.g., "nurse") or nonwords (e.g., "sernu"). Reaction times are quicker if a context related to the target word has just been provided. For example, subjects recognize "nurse" as a word more quickly if they have just read "doctor," compared with an unrelated word such as "bread." This method can be adapted to investigate the associative links hypothesized to characterize various types of schemas. In their research on stereotyping, for example, Gaertner and McLaughlin (1983) found that white subjects identified "ambitious" as a word more quickly if they had been primed with "Whites" than if they had been primed with "Blacks."

We reasoned that the lexical decision task could be adapted to reveal the *if...then...* structure of interpersonal expectations. That is, priming the "if" element in the contingency should, by virtue of spreading activation, increase the accessibility of the "then" expected outcome as well (Baldwin, 1992). Baldwin et al. (1993) used this logic to examine relational expectations in adult attachment styles. We first had subjects read a sentence fragment such as "If I trust my partner, then my partner will . . . " to establish a specific interpersonal context. Immediately after reading this sentence, they were to make a word–nonword response for interpersonal target words such as "care" and "hurt." We found that, consistent with the principle of spreading activation, avoidantly attached individuals were faster to recognize "hurt" after reading a sentence that described trusting a romantic partner. If thinking about trusting their partner automatically activates an expectation of being hurt, it is not surprising that these individuals avoid becoming vulnerable to relationship partners.

We took a similar approach in a related set of studies into the link between low self-esteem and expectations about contingencies of interpersonal acceptance (Baldwin & Sinclair, 1996). It often has been noted that a belief that acceptance by others is conditional on successful performances appears to play a role in depression and self-esteem disturbances (e.g., Deci & Ryan, 1995; Kuiper & Olinger, 1986; Rogers, 1959). Anticipating that "If I succeed people will accept me," but "If I fail people will reject me" gives performance outcomes an obvious importance and emotional impact. From the current perspective, the sense of contingent acceptance arises from associative *if...then...* links between success and acceptance, and failure and rejection. In our lexical decision task, therefore, undergraduate participants made word–nonword judgments on letter strings that included social outcome words such as "respect," "cherished," "despised," and "criticism." Each trial was preceded by a performance context word, representing either success or failure. Consistent with the hypothesis that self-esteem problems are related to such conditions of worth, we found that people with insecure self-esteem were faster to identify positive interpersonal outcomes such as "cherished" as words when given the context of success (rather than failure), and faster to identify negative targets such as "despised" when given the context of failure (rather than success). Additional analyses confirmed that this spreading activation was not simply due to mood or valence congruency: trials with positive and negative—but not interpersonal—words (e.g., "vomit," "tranquil") showed very different effects. The information processing of low-self-esteem people showed links specifically between success and acceptance, and failure and rejection: This explains why their level of momentary self-feelings often fluctuates in response to performance outcomes, as their self-worth and social acceptability are always "on the line" (Kernis & Waschul, 1995).

Reaction-time methods complement self-report approaches by sidestepping some of the thornier problems inherent in asking people to introspect about their cognitive processes. Lexical decision and Stroop methods can provide a window into a person's automatic assumptions, as revealed in spreading activation across an associative network, even when the person might be unwilling or unable to report on those assumptions. Indeed, recent research on stereotypes is showing that people's split-second reaction times may in some cases predict behavior even better than do self-reports (Dovidio, Kawakami, Johnson, Johnson, & Howard, 1997).

Temporary Accessibility

From the social-cognitive perspective, stable individual differences largely reflect the chronic accessibility of certain cognitive structures. At the same time, as has been argued elsewhere, variability in people's thought and behavior should not be dismissed as some kind of error or unpredictability, but rather can be seen as reflecting the temporary or situated accessibility of cognitive structures (e.g., Baldwin & Fehr, 1995; Mischel & Shoda, 1995). That is, although most people have a repertoire of constructs or schemas available to guide attention, interpretation, and memory, such information-processing effects are particularly likely to occur for those structures that are currently the most accessible. There are a number of sources of temporary accessibility that have been studied (e.g., Higgins, 1996), such as context effects (e.g., perceiving a yellow car as a taxi because one is in Manhattan) and current goals (e.g., perceiving a yellow car as a taxi because one needs to get somewhere fast). The most straightforward source, however, is recent experience: Schemas activated in the recent past (e.g., by the taxi that almost ran one down a few minutes ago) are more likely to be used when processing novel information.

This basic principle of temporary accessibility, that simply priming or activating a construct in one context makes it more accessible, and so more likely to be applied in a later unrelated context, underlies dozens of priming studies in the social-cognition literature. In an early priming study, Higgins, Rholes, and Jones (1977) first exposed subjects to either the term "adventurous" or the term "reckless" during a bogus perception task in which the subjects were to hold these words in memory for a few moments. In a later, ostensibly unrelated task, subjects read a story about a man who shot rapids and planned to learn skydiving, and they were asked to evaluate this person. Impressions showed the effect of the previously activated construct on the interpretation of the current ambiguous behavior: Subjects interpreted the target person's behavior more positively, for example, and liked the target person more, if they had been primed with "adventurous" rather than "reckless." Similar results have been obtained using a host of different priming techniques. Most of these techniques involve subtly presenting the priming stimulus during a task that is portrayed as unrelated to a later impression-formation task. Srull and Wyer (1979), for example, primed the construct of hostility by having subjects construct sentences out of groups of words, some of which were hostility-related (e.g., leg–break–arm–his). Herr (1986) primed hostility by briefly exposing subjects to the names of hostility-related people (e.g., boxer Joe Frazier). As in the Higgins et al. (1977) study, these incidental exposures to the construct of hostility left subjects more likely to apply it in a later impression-formation task.

The principle of temporary accessibility applies to relational schemas also, as is well-recognized in clinical psychology. For example, whereas an individual might typically perceive interpersonal experiences in a reasonably veracious, undistorted way, some minor event—such as a holiday dinner with the extended family—can activate or "trigger" a schema representing distorted views of self and other. In order to understand the way individuals construe and navigate their world, then, one needs to know not only the nature of the cognitive maps they have available to them, but also which maps they tend to use most often and in which situations they use them.

Priming procedures have been used in a series of experimental studies of relational schema activation. In one experiment (Baldwin & Holmes, 1987, study 1), we had undergraduate women perform a guided-imagery exercise in which they spent a few moments imagining being with specific significant others. Some subjects were instructed to imagine being with their parents, while others were told to imagine being with two friends from campus. During this exercise, they closed their eyes and were given the following instructions:

> Focus your attention on this person. . . . Picture the person's face. Really try to get an experience of the person being with you. . . . You may want to remember a time you were actually with the person, or you may already have a clear experience of what this person is like. . . . Just try to get a good image of this person. You may find that you can see the color of their eyes or their hair, or maybe hear their voice. . . . Imagine that this person is right there with you. . . . Now once you have an image of the person, try to zoom in and get a close-up, focused impression. . . . Hold this image for a little while. . . . Imagine talking with the person. . . . Try to feel them there with you. (Baldwin & Holmes, 1987, p. 1089)

Our prediction was that this priming procedure would produce a state of mind representing a specific sense of self-with-other—either "me-with-my-family" or "me-with-my-friends." Ten minutes later in a different context, the subjects were asked to rate their enjoyment of a number of written passages, one of which was a sexually permissive story taken from a popular women's magazine. This story described a young woman contemplating having sex with a good-looking man whom she did not know well. As we anticipated, women who had visualized their parents in the first phase of the experiment rated the later passage as less enjoyable and exciting than did those who had visualized their (presumably more permissive) college friends. Thus, the primed relational schema apparently shaped their sense of what kinds of behavior are acceptable. There was also some anecdotal evidence for the activation of specific relational states of mind: At the end of the experiment, one woman said that she had felt embarrassed that it was taking her so long to fill out the rating scale for the sexual passage. She reported that as she was trying to answer the questions about how exciting she had found the passage, she noticed herself carrying on, in fantasy, an intense argument with her mother about which number to circle. When asked, she said that it had not occurred to her that the earlier guided visualization of her parents might have been the source of her later conflictual fantasy.

Priming studies similar to this one, conducted in a variety of domains, have shown clearly that activated relational schemas can have an impact on feelings of self-evaluation, attachment, and social anxiety, as well as on interpersonal behavior. I review some of these findings below, organizing the studies under some of the major themes that have emerged in this research.

Implicit Priming

We have conducted a number of studies showing that people's sense of self is very much tied to the imagined reactions and evaluative styles of others, consistent with the symbolic interactionist notion of the "looking glass self" (Cooley, 1902). In these studies, we have found that relational priming manipulations influence people's momentary views of self. People show heightened self-criticism, for example, after visualizing a judgmental significant other (Baldwin & Holmes, 1987), reading that judgmental other's name (Baldwin, 1994), or being exposed to that other's scowling face (Baldwin, Carrell, & Lopez, 1990). Conversely, self-evaluations are more positive after individuals receive primes of unconditionally accepting others (Baldwin & Holmes, 1987; Baldwin, 1994; Baldwin & Main, 1998).

As the notion of processing fluency suggests, the influence of a knowledge structure depends partly on whether it becomes activated but also partly on how the person interprets that activation; accordingly, a number of writers (e.g., Bargh, 1992; Jacoby et al., 1992) have characterized the typical priming effect as a two-stage phenomenon. First, activation of the construct leads to a greater fluency with which an ambiguous stimulus can be categorized in terms of that construct. That is, the categorization of a target person's ambiguously adventurous behavior as "reckless," for example, occurs automatically and effortlessly, resulting in the "reckless" interpretation of the behavior coming to mind easily. Second, the subject misattributes the fluency of this interpretation to qualities of the information itself ("he is clearly reckless") rather than to the influence of the prime. Thus, priming typically leads to assimilation effects, in which ambiguous stimuli are interpreted in a way consistent with the accessible schema. Assimilation effects, while the rule, do not always occur, however, as in other circumstances they can be overridden or even reversed to produce a contrast effect. A number of studies in the impression-formation literature (e.g., Lombardi, Higgins, & Bargh, 1987; Newman & Uleman, 1990), for example, have shown that if people surmise that a recent prime might be affecting their thoughts and feelings about some person, they will attribute their current judgment to the prime and adjust their impression of the person accordingly.

Consistent with this reasoning, a number of our studies have identified an important boundary condition of relational priming effects: It seems clear that experimental primes need to be quite subtle, or even subliminal, in order to produce assimilation effects. In our research with relational primes, we often have delivered primes in a separate context, as in the "two study" format described earlier, in order to keep them unobtrusive. In studies where these precautions were not taken, there have occasionally been contrast effects where, for example, subjects receiving a critical-other prime actually reported more positive self-evaluations (e.g., Baldwin, 1994, study 2). The normal assimilation effect holds even with relatively obtrusive primes, however, so long as the participant's attention is directed away from thinking about the primed significant other and directed toward thinking about the self. If experimental participants are confronted with their reflection in a mirror, for example, which increases their tendency to focus on themselves (Duval & Wicklund, 1972), the contrast effect disappears, and they again think about themselves in a manner consistent with the primed relational schema (Baldwin, 1994, study 2; Baldwin & Holmes, 1987, study 2).

Subliminal Priming. If schemas are influential because they work outside of awareness, it is perhaps not surprising that recent research sometimes involves the use of subliminal exposure techniques to present stimuli below the threshold of conscious perception. Research into subliminal perception, once judged to be confounded by serious methodological flaws (e.g., Holender, 1986), is once again gaining scientific respectability due to recent developments in cognitive theory and methodology. Some researchers have used subliminal primes to activate trait categories, for example, making it more likely that these constructs will be used in forming impressions. Bargh and Pietromonaco (1982) gave some subjects brief exposures of hostility-related words during a bogus reaction-time task. As in other priming studies, when these subjects later read a description of a person acting in an ambiguously hostile way, they were more likely than subjects in a control condition to see this person as angry or aggressive. Subliminal primes also can produce affective responses (see, e.g., Murphy & Zajonc, 1993; Robles, Smith, Carver, & Wellens, 1987), which can be transferred to other, neutral, material. Krosnick, Betz, Jussim, and Lynn (1992) found that subjects formed more positive impressions of a target person if pictures of her were preceded by subliminally exposed, positive-affect-arousing photos, such as of a pair of kittens or of a couple in a romantic setting, than if preceded by negative-affect-arousing photos, such as of a skull or a bucket of snakes.

In our lab, we have used subliminal priming techniques to activate relational schemas that are particularly relevant to our subjects' sense of self. We have focused primarily on the psychological situation of being evaluated negatively by an authority figure. Subjects in an early study (Baldwin et al., 1990) were social psychology graduate students at the University of Michigan. Coincidentally, the Director of their department was Robert Zajonc, known in the literature for his influential work on subliminal perception (e.g., Zajonc, 1980) and known among the students for his unnerving ability to ask them difficult questions that identified serious shortcomings in their work. In designing this study, we decided to use photographs as our primes on the assumption that imagery-based stimuli might tap most directly into affect-laden interpersonal representations involving authority and criticism. Professor Zajonc agreed to pose for a photograph looking directly into the camera and scowling in disgust in order to prepare a sufficiently evocative stimulus. In the experiment, this superego-like slide was flashed subliminally at the graduate student subjects four times during a bogus reaction-time task, for which they were to press a button as soon as they saw "a flash of light." Immediately following these exposures, subjects were asked to rate the quality of one of their own research ideas, a highly ego-involving exercise for students enrolled in this empirically oriented graduate program. As predicted, they tended to give lower self-ratings for their idea following the negative prime than following a positive, smiling prime or no prime at all.

In our second study, we wished to replicate and extend this finding with a different subject population. We asked Roman Catholic undergraduate women to first read the sexually permissive passage we had used in previous research (Baldwin & Holmes, 1987, study 1). Shortly after they had read the passage, we asked them to perform a bogus reaction-time task. During this task, we exposed some of them to the disapproving face of Pope John Paul II, which we surmised might produce some strong self-evaluative effects, especially given the context of permissive sexuality. Indeed, following this prime, participants' ratings of self-esteem were lower, and their ratings of anxiety were higher when compared to a no-prime control condition. Thus, as in the previous study, the subliminal prime was effective in shaping participants' self-evaluative reactions. Additionally, the prime had an impact to the extent it represented a personally significant authority figure. The Pope stimulus was most effective for participants who considered themselves practicing Catholics; also a third group that was shown the disapproving picture of a total stranger gave self-ratings that were no different from those of the control participants who were shown no picture at all. The subliminal prime had a self-evaluative effect, then, only if it activated personally important knowledge structures.

We are continuing this line of research into the priming of evaluative relational schemas. In one study (Baldwin, 1994, study 1), we used the name of a significant other, rather than a picture, as the stimulus. Participants who were subliminally exposed to the name of a judgmental significant other were more self-critical about their performance on a difficult task than those who were exposed to the name of an accepting significant other.

Elsewhere (Baldwin, 1994, study 1) I proposed that the kinds of findings obtained in assimilation–contrast and subliminal-priming studies may speak to the types of issues often raised in psychodynamic discussions of personality. Breuer and Freud (1895/1955) argued that it is because repressed desires are unconscious that they are particularly difficult to defend against or counteract. A similar account could be given of schematic processing: Information is automatically processed in line with the schematic representation, and the resultant thoughts appear in consciousness with no awareness of the inference processes that produced them. This point was argued by cognitive therapists Moretti and Shaw (1989), who suggested that a major problem in overcoming depression, for example, may be that depressive thoughts about self arise automatically and uncontrollably, with the person unable to detect the source of their negative cognitions. They contrast this with other types of activities where overriding errors is more straightforward: "For example, a a [*sic*] typist who strikes the wrong key can often determine the source of error in performance" (p. 388). In depressive cognition, however, negative thoughts arise with great fluency, and it may be difficult for the depressed individual to identify them as errors and discount them, particularly without some model of where they derive from. As Horowitz (1988; also Barber & DeRubeis, 1989) has argued, successful therapy may therefore involve a process of recognizing and overriding the automatic processing influences of accessible relational schemas, just as avoiding the assimilation effects of a prime involves first recognizing it as the source of one's interpretation. This suggests that priming paradigms might offer a reasonable experimental analogue to some of the processes involved in overcoming unconscious influences. Procedures involving the priming of dysfunctional schemas might be useful in this endeavor, as well as in establishing paradigms for studying this component of therapy.

Behavior and Behavioral Intentions

In studying the activation of relational knowledge structures, there is the assumption, of course, that people's thoughts about themselves and others can have an enormous effect on their behavior. A man discussing a stressful issue with his relationship partner might act very differently, for example, depending on whether he was recently reminded of his unfailingly supportive mother versus his unfailingly excoriating ex-wife! Activated relational schemas can define what kinds of interpersonal states seem possible, or even likely, yielding approach or avoidance intentions depending on how the expected states are valued.

Much evidence for the behavioral effects of activated relational structures has been generated by other researchers. Neuberg (1988), for example, flashed competition-relevant words such as "enemy" and "combative" to subjects right before they engaged in a laboratory game in which players could act either cooperatively or competitively. The primes affected how people interacted, and there was an intriguing effect of premeasured personality dispositions: People who were already predisposed to be competitive became significantly more competitive if they were shown the words, whereas people who were predisposed to be noncompetitive actually behaved slightly less competitively when primed.

A clever study by Lewicki (1985) provided another example of how interpersonal expectations learned about one person can be transferred or applied to a new person. In the first phase of one of his experiments, some subjects had an unpleasant interaction with a short-haired female experimenter who wore thick-rimmed glasses. A short time later, subjects walked down the hall into another room where they were to approach one or the other of two experimenters seated there, to begin the second part of the study. One of these new experimenters resembled the woman in the first phase, in that she also had short hair and thick glasses. Subjects' spontaneous choices about which woman to approach strongly suggested that they were transferring their expectations from the first woman: Whereas in the control condition roughly 57% of participants approached the short-haired woman, in the negative-interaction condition only 20% did.

Other researchers have examined in more detail the processes whereby knowledge about a person's characteristics can activate expectations about how the person is likely to act, which can, in turn, influence interpersonal motives and behaviors. In a sophisticated transference paradigm developed by Andersen and her colleagues (Andersen, Glassman, Chen, & Cole, 1995; Andersen & Cole, 1990), participants first describe in some detail someone they know. Weeks later, ostensibly in a different experiment, they are presented with a set of statements supposedly about a new person they are about to meet, and they are asked what they think the person is like, how much they think they will like the person, and so on. For some participants these statements actually have been drawn from their earlier description of their own significant other, and results show they often go beyond the information given to infer characteristics about the new person that are in no way justified by the data. In one study (Andersen, Reznik, & Manzella, 1996), participants transferred expectations about how accepting versus rejecting the person would be and also reported greater motivation to interact with someone who reminded them of a well-liked significant other.

Finally, in an earlier study, White and Shapiro (1987) had male participants choose from a set of pictures a woman who most "closely resembles a good friend." The researchers then arranged for a telephone interaction in which the man thought he was speaking with this woman—in fact, the woman on the other end of the line was also a naive research participant. By the end of the 8-minute conversation, however, there was evidence of a self-fulfilling prophecy: When the female participant's behavior was rated on a number of trait dimensions by independent judges, she was rated in ways that lined up with the male participant's views of his own good friend! Thus, his interpersonal expectations, transferred from a significant relationship into a new acquaintanceship, led him to behave in ways that produced expectancy-confirming feedback from the new person.

My collaborators and I have examined behavioral intentions as a function of activated attachment orientation. The adult attachment literature is based on an assumption of chronic individual differences, with the notion that people have one attachment "style," thought to derive from a stable working model laid down in childhood. We found much evidence for intrasubject variability: First we found that when people filled out attachment measures on two separate occasions, approximately 30% of the sample gave different self-descriptions at different times (Baldwin & Fehr, 1995; see also Davila, Burge, & Hammen, 1997). Next, we found that when asked to characterize their important relationships, fully 88% of the sample described different orientations with different people, showing that they had multiple models of attachment available in memory (Baldwin et al., 1996). Based on the notion of temporary accessibility, we then hypothesized that many of the behavioral correlates of chronic attachment orientation that have been established in the literature, such as choosing a dating partner or communicating with partners in intimate or stressful contexts, should also show intrasubject variability as a function of priming effects.

We conducted a study in which we attempted to prime attachment-relevant relational schemas by having participants visualize a person with whom they felt secure, avoidant, or anxious. Then, we asked them to indicate how willing they would be to meet various potential dating partners, whose descriptions depicted them as having one of the three attachment orientations; Frazier, Byer, Fischer, Wright, and DeBord (1996) had already shown that these target people were found differentially attractive by people of different chronic attachment orientations. In our study, people who, in a different context, had spent a few moments imagining someone they knew who made them feel anxious and unsure, were now particularly drawn to a potential partner who was likely to desire a high level of closeness and intimacy. Their interpersonal motives, then, were shaped by the temporary activation of working models and, in fact, were very similar to the motives of those for whom those models are chronically accessible.

Activation of Procedural Knowledge

While much of the focus of relational schemas research has been on the activation of declarative knowledge structures—views of self and other, and interpersonal scripts—it is also possible to view many of the findings primarily in terms of the activation of procedural knowledge, or the rules people use for drawing conclusions from social information. In cognitive models of depression, for example, a central issue involves the individual's procedures for drawing inferences about self from various types of information. Depression is hypothesized to involve self-evaluative styles in which people overgeneralize from single failures to infer global negative traits (Beck, 1967; Kernis, Brockner, & Frankel, 1989) or take responsibility for all manner of negative events (Peterson & Seligman, 1984). It has become apparent to many, however, that such self-evaluative phenomena cannot be fully understood without reference to internalization processes and the influence of past and present relationships, such as with a highly critical spouse or parent (Safran

& Segal, 1990). Indeed, Hooley and Teasdale (1989) reported that the best predictor of relapse for remitted depressives was the perceived criticalness of the person's spouse.

In a relational schemas view of internalization, the *if...then...* scripts for communicating with a significant other come to define the *if...then...* inference processes one uses in thinking about oneself (Baldwin, 1997). As discussed earlier, lexical decision studies have shown that negative self-evaluations correlate with the interpersonal expectation that "If I fail, then he or she will criticize and reject me." A follow-up study (Baldwin & Sinclair, 1996, study 3) showed that this contingency script can be activated by the type of guided visualizations used in other priming studies: Subjects who visualized a judgmental significant other, and shortly thereafter performed the lexical decision task, were more likely than controls to show the *if... then...* reaction time pattern that was consistent with contingency expectations.

One study (Baldwin & Holmes, 1987, study 2) gave a particularly clear demonstration of how this kind of contingency or conditional acceptance schema can influence procedures of self-evaluation. We first used a guided visualization procedure to prime nondepressed male undergraduates with either a supportive, unconditionally accepting relationship or else an evaluative, highly conditional relationship. The accepting person was a friend who "would accept you no matter what," whereas the conditional person was someone who seemed to like the subject primarily because of some talent or ability he had. We then had subjects carry out an extremely difficult task on which they performed quite poorly to see if their style of self-evaluation would be shaped by the earlier prime. While they were engaged in this task, half the subjects were exposed to their mirror image, in order to promote self-awareness and the attendant self-evaluation process (and, as mentioned earlier, to reduce the likelihood that they would attribute their self-feelings to the prime). As predicted, subjects who were made self-aware tended to evaluate themselves according to the inference rules embodied in the interpersonal context that had been primed. For example, those who had been primed with a conditional, evaluative relationship were particularly likely to say their failure was due to "something about me." Also, on a questionnaire measuring general social orientations, these subjects were more likely to overgeneralize from a single negative behavior or outcome (e.g., "If I told someone something that was untrue") to global conclusions about self (e.g., "That would mean I was a liar"). Thus, a depressive-like style of self-construal was engendered by the activation of a hypercritical relational schema.

As discussed earlier, once a contingency schema is accessible, activation should spread easily from the "if" (e.g., "If I fail") to various "thens" (e.g., "then people will criticize me and think I am inadequate"). Phenomenologically, this will be experienced automatically as a sense of being inadequate or unworthy of social acceptance. So long as the person is not able to attribute his or her negative self-feelings to the primed relational schema, he or she will experience negative self-evaluations. I have suggested that this can be conceptualized in terms of the tacit or implicit use of social knowledge (Baldwin, 1994), as the person's self-construal is shaped by the *if...then...* inference rules embodied in a relational script. One way to conceptualize internalization, then, is that it involves an error in monitoring the source of various thoughts and feelings: People evaluate themselves as worthy or unworthy of love, attributing these judgments to their own standards and reasoning processes rather than to the interpersonal knowledge structures that produce them (see Jacoby & Kelley, 1987, for a similar argument).

This analysis returns self-evaluative procedures to their interpersonal roots. Some theorists studying self-construal have argued that stability in the sense of self may derive primarily from stability and coherence in procedural knowledge, that is, in the way people tend to draw inferences from new information about themselves (e.g., Strauman, 1996). The results of the kinds of priming studies reviewed here make it clear that, since this procedural knowledge may be represented as interpersonal scripts, self-evaluative stability ultimately is grounded in the stable activation of the relational schemas that define the inference rules.

Cued Activation

In day-to-day life, relational schemas presumably can become activated in a host of different ways, including by characteristics of an interaction partner or by recent thoughts and experiences, as demonstrated in the research already reviewed. Our most recent research has examined indirect, or cued activation, such as occurs when a whiff of a familiar perfume or a few bars of a favorite song serve to activate a network of memories, thoughts, and emotions. In several studies, we have examined whether conditioning paradigms could be used to lead people to associate specific relational schemas with previously neutral stimuli. In these studies, participants heard distinctive tones on a computer while they were thinking about either critical, judgmental people or very accepting people. They later performed difficult tasks and/or filled out self-evaluation scales while tones—either the conditioned tones or some other tone sequence—were played repeatedly in the background. Results showed that self-evaluations were very different depending on which tone was played.

In one of the paradigms we have used, participants complete a bogus questionnaire on a computer, answering multiple-choice questions about their favorite flavor of ice cream, their preferences for social activities, and other mundane topics. They are told that these questions have already been pretested with a large sample of their peers, who have given their preferences for which response to each question would be the most socially desirable. The reason for collecting the participant's data is supposedly to see the extent to which real people actually live up to the ideals of their peers. While they answer the questions, participants are given feedback, consisting of a row of smiling faces (indicating desirability) or frowning, disgusted faces (indicating undesirability) to indicate to them the degree to which their answers are matching the desired alternatives. This feedback is entirely bogus: In fact, every subject receives 10 exposures of smiles and 10 exposures of frowns in the same random order irrespective of the answers he or she gives. The faces are merely to serve as unconditioned stimuli representing approval and disapproval. Each presentation is signaled by a tone sequence generated by the computer, with one sequence always signaling approval and another always signaling disapproval (the specific tone sequences are, of course, counterbalanced across participants). Shortly after this conditioning experience, participants are placed in some self-evaluative context such as performing a difficult task. While they are in this context, one of the conditioned tone sequences (i.e., the CS-approval or the CS-disapproval) is presented repeatedly in the background on a computer across the room that is ostensibly unrelated to the experiment.

Several studies now have shown an impact of such cued structures. In a study of social anxiety (Baldwin & Main, 1998), undergraduate women underwent the conditioning procedure and then interacted for 5 minutes with a cool, aloof male experimental confederate posing as a research assistant. Participants who heard the CS-approval playing in the background while they carried on this interaction reported more positive, relaxed feelings than those in the CS-disapproval condition. The CS-approval was particularly influential in reducing the anxiety of people who were typically very uncomfortable in social situations. Chronically high-social-anxious participants in the CS-approval condition felt they were viewed more positively by the confederate, compared with their counterparts in the control or CS-disapproval conditions. And, indeed, they were: In the CS-approval condition, the confederate rated chronically high-anxious people as appearing just as confident and relaxed as chronically low-anxious people.

Other experiments have shown similar cued-activation effects. People trying to solve difficult anagrams under time pressure, for example, report more interfering, self-critical thoughts (Baldwin, Granzberg, & Pippus, 1997) when a CS-disapproval tone is played in the background. Recently, we used the lexical decision task to examine more directly the *if...then...* structures that are activated, and we found an interesting interaction effect with participants' attachment orientations (Baldwin & Meunier, in press). Computer tones were conditioned to visualizations of either contingently accepting or noncontingently accepting significant others. When the CS-contingent tone was played during the lexical decision task, chronically secure individuals showed an activation of success–acceptance contingencies, whereas preoccupied individuals showed an activation of failure–rejection contingencies. For both types of individuals, the CS activated a contingent relational schema, but while some people focused on contingencies of earning acceptance, others focused on contingencies of being rejected.

PERSONALITY COHERENCE: STABILITY AND VARIABILITY

I have reviewed some research methods and findings from studies on the information-processing effects of relational schemas, primarily in the cognitive-affective domains of self-esteem, social anxiety, and adult attachment in close relationships. I now briefly reexamine some of this work, particularly in the attachment domain, insofar as it pertains to issues of personality stability and variability.

Adult attachment orientations have generally been treated as nomothetic, trait-like "styles," typically measured using categorical scales where subjects characterize themselves as secure, avoidant, or anxious–ambivalent (e.g., on the Hazan & Shaver, 1987, three-category measure). Indeed, research into the correlates of attachment styles (see, e.g., Hazan & Shaver, 1994, for a review) supports the idea that there are important individual differences in how people orient to their close relationships. Self-reported styles may reflect a self-perceived "average" orientation across relationships and situations, or perhaps a "default" orientation adopted in the absence of specific relational information (Collins & Read, 1994). From a relational schema perspective, such fairly stable individual differences in social behavior result in large part from chronically accessible knowledge structures that shape and define the way a person typically construes self, others, and interpersonal situations. These chronic views of the world can be assessed using self-report methods, and I reviewed a number of studies that asked people to describe their assumptions about *if...then...* contingencies in the social world.

The critical social-cognitive mechanism is the activation of interpersonal expectancies, and reaction-time procedures have demonstrated spreading activation from the "if" to the "then" of a number of interpersonal scripts. People reporting a chronic avoidant-attachment orientation, for example, recognize the word *hurt* more quickly when given the context of trusting a romantic partner; low self-esteem individuals quickly process rejection information when given the context of failure. This approach could easily be adapted to examine the structure of interpersonal expectations hypothesized to underlie any number of individual differences, including those leading to clinical problems. Vitousek and Hollon (1990), for example, suggest that one factor in eating disorders may be a set of conditional beliefs about the outcomes associated with fatness and thinness, which could be translated into contingency statements such as "If I am fat, then others will reject me." Similarly, Arieti and Bemporad (1980) locate the interpersonal roots of depression in relational expectations about dependency and achievement, that could be expressed as "If I act independently, then my parents will be hurt," and "If I fail, then my parents will not love me." It would not be difficult to design spreading-activation tasks to assess the structure of specific interpersonal expectations that correlate with these and other individual differences.

It is precisely because of the strong links among elements of a relational schema that these structures often show a high degree of stability. Moreover, each time the structure is activated, there is the potential for new links to be formed with new memories or cues in the environment, making it more likely to be activated in a wider range of future contexts (Baldwin & Meunier, in press). Repeated activation can result also from links between *if...then...* expectancies and relevant interpersonal goals: Recent research suggests that people who are chronically anxious about and preoccupied with their relationship may ironically feel better after conflict, because it satisfies their desire for intimacy (Pietromonaco & Feldman Barrett, 1997). Combine this with the potential for self-fulfilling prophecies, as White and Shapiro (1987) and others have shown, and it is not surprising that relational schemas, including those that could be characterized as dysfunctional and distorted, are notoriously difficult to modify.

Just as a social-cognitive approach speaks to stable individual differences in behavior, it also helps explain the variability that does occur within an individual's thoughts and behaviors across contexts and relationships. For example, the nomothetic, categorical approach to attachment orientations has been critiqued for theoretical and empirical reasons (see, e.g., commentaries following Hazan & Shaver, 1994). Empirically, the test–retest stability of this measure and others like it is not particularly good, with approximately 30% of people reporting different "styles" at two different measurement occasions—even if only weeks apart (Baldwin & Fehr, 1995). Some have attributed this instability to the error introduced by the use of categorical items and have advocated continuous measures instead; Baldwin and Fehr (1995) argued, however, that although some of the instability may indeed be due to error in measuring a stable, unwavering trait, some probably reflects psychologically meaningful variability.

First, it is clear that people learn about the patterns of interaction that can be expected in their various relationships, and these relationship-specific relational schemas influence the way people anticipate and then interpret their partners' actions (Collins, 1996; Sarason, Pierce, Shearin, & Sarason, 1992). In one study of attachment, most people reported adopting a wide range of attachment orientations in their different relationships, and these orientations were correlated with their relationship-specific interpersonal expectancies regarding dependency, trust, and closeness (Baldwin et al., 1996). Thus, their interpersonal behavior would quite reasonably vary from one relationship to the next—one would not expect a person to be as trusting with a manipulative or mercurial significant other as with a reliable significant other—and this behavioral signature would follow directly from the multiple models corresponding to different interpersonal contexts.

I also reviewed a number of studies exploring phenomena of temporary accessibility whereby specific relational schemas can be activated by primes and cues in the environment. In over a dozen studies, we have shown that subtly reminding people of a certain kind of relationship—whether it be securely accepting, or critical, or avoidantly attached—can change the way they momentarily think about themselves and others. Shifts can also occur in social behavior, including choices of dating partners (Baldwin et al., 1996) or styles of interacting with a new acquaintance (Baldwin & Main, 1998). On the one hand, such temporary accessibility effects seem to argue against personality coherence, as people's perceptions and social behavior appear remarkably flexible and easily influenced by environmental factors and recent experiences. On the other hand, as our recent research into cued activation has shown, people clearly learn idiosyncratic triggers such as certain foods, contexts, or even computer-generated tones, that produce temporary accessibility effects in day-to-day life. As a result, then, even factors that apparently undermine behavioral stability are found, upon closer examination, to contribute to coherent patterns of personality functioning.

As research continues into the cognitive-affective domains that are central to people's lives, I believe it will become increasingly apparent that cognitive-affective structures representing expectancies about interpersonal events—relational schemas—are core building blocks of personality. The methods reviewed here make up a set of handy research tools for examining personality coherence and variability resulting from the representation, activation, and application of relational knowledge.

ACKNOWLEDGMENTS

Preparation of this chapter was supported by a research grant from the Social Sciences and Humanities Research Council of Canada. I thank Patricia Frazier and Evan Pritchard for their helpful comments on drafts of this chapter.

REFERENCES

Abelson, R. P. (1981). Psychological status of the script concept. *American Psychologist, 36*, 715–729.

Andersen, S. M., & Cole, S. W. (1990). "Do I know you?": The role of significant others in general social perception. *Journal of Personality and Social Psychology, 59*, 384–399.

Andersen, S. M., Glassman, N. S., Chen, S., & Cole, S. W. (1995). Transference in social perception: The role of chronic accessibility in significant-other representations. *Journal of Personality and Social Psychology, 69*, 41–57.

Andersen, S. M., Reznik, I., & Manzella, L. M. (1996). Eliciting facial affect, motivation, and expectancies in transference: Significant-other representations in social relations. *Journal of Personality and Social Psychology, 71,* 1108–1129.

Anderson, C. A., & Godfrey, S. S. (1987). Thoughts about actions: The effects of specificity and availability of imagined behavioral scripts on expectations about oneself and others. *Social Cognition, 5,* 238–258.

Arieti, S., & Bemporad, J. R. (1980). The psychological organization of depression. *American Journal of Psychiatry, 137,* 1360–1365.

Baldwin, M. W. (1992). Relational schemas and the processing of social information. *Psychological Bulletin, 112,* 461–484.

Baldwin, M. W. (1994). Primed relational schemas as a source of self-evaluative reactions. *Journal of Social and Clinical Psychology, 13,* 380–403.

Baldwin, M. W. (1997). Relational schemas as a source of if–then self-inference procedures. *Review of General Psychology, 1,* 326–335.

Baldwin, M. W., Carrell, S. E., & Lopez, D. F. (1990). Priming relationship schemas: My advisor and the Pope are watching me from the back of my mind. *Journal of Experimental Social Psychology, 26,* 435–454.

Baldwin, M. W., & Fehr, B. (1995). On the instability of attachment style ratings. *Personal Relationships, 2,* 247–261.

Baldwin, M. W., Fehr, B., Keedian, E., Seidel, M., & Thomson, D. W. (1993). An exploration of the relational schemata underlying attachment styles: Self-report and lexical decision approaches. *Personality and Social Psychology Bulletin, 19,* 746–754.

Baldwin, M. W., & Fergusson, P. (1998). [Social anxiety and interpersonal expectations]. Unpublished research data, University of Winnipeg.

Baldwin, M. W., Granzberg, A., & Pippus, L. (1997). [Cued activation of relational knowledge]. Unpublished research data, University of Winnipeg.

Baldwin, M. W., & Holmes, J. G. (1987). Salient private audiences and awareness of the self. *Journal of Personality and Social Psychology, 53,* 1087–1098.

Baldwin, M. W., & Keelan, J. P. R. (1998). *Interpersonal expectations as a function of gender and self-esteem.* Unpublished manuscript, McGill University, Montreal, Quebec.

Baldwin, M. W., Keelan, J. P. R., Fehr, B., Enns, V., & Koh-Rangarajoo, E. (1996). Social cognitive conceptualization of attachment working models: Availability and accessibility effects. *Journal of Personality and Social Psychology, 71,* 94–104.

Baldwin, M. W., & Main, K. (1998). [Social anxiety and the cued activation of relational knowledge]. Unpublished research data, University of Winnipeg.

Baldwin, M. W., & Meunier, J. (in press). Attachment orientations and the cued activation of relational schemas. *Social Cognition* [Special issue, G. Downey & H. Reis, eds.].

Baldwin, M. W., & Sinclair, L. (1996). Self-esteem and "if . . . then" contingencies of interpersonal acceptance. *Journal of Personality and Social Psychology, 71,* 1130–1141.

Bandura, A. (1986). *Social foundations of thought and action: A social cognitive theory.* Englewood Cliffs, NJ: Prentice Hall.

Barber, J. P., & DeRubeis, R. J. (1989). On second thought: Where the action is in cognitive therapy for depression. *Cognitive Therapy and Research, 13,* 441–457.

Bargh, J. A. (1992). Does subliminality matter? Awareness of the stimulus versus awareness of its influence. In R. F. Bornstein & T. S. Pittman (Eds.), *Perception without awareness* (pp. 236–255). New York: Guilford Press.

Bargh, J. A., & Pietromonaco, P. (1982). Automatic information processing and social perception: The influence of trait information presented outside of conscious awareness on impression formation. *Journal of Personality and Social Psychology, 437* 43–449.

Beck, A. T., (1967). *Depression: Clinical, experimental, and theoretical aspects.* New York: Harper & Row.

Bowlby, J. (1969). *Attachment and loss: Vol. 1. Attachment.* New York: Basic Books.

Bretherton, I. (1990). Communication patterns, internal working models, and the intergenerational transmission of attachment relationships. *Infant Mental Health Journal, 11*, 237–252.

Breuer, J., & Freud, S. (1955). Studies on hysteria. In J. Strachey (Ed. & Trans.), *The standard edition of the complete psychological works of Sigmund Freud* (Vol. 2, pp. 1–170). London: Hogarth Press. (Original work published 1895)

Cantor, N., & Kihlstrom, J. F. (1985). Social intelligence: The cognitive basis of personality. *Review of Personality and Social Psychology, 6*, 15–33.

Carlston, D. E., & Smith, E. R. (1996). Principles of mental representation. In E. T. Higgins & A. W. Kruglanski (Eds.), *Social psychology: Handbook of basic principles* (pp. 184–210). New York: Guilford Press.

Cervone, D. (1989). Effects of envisioning future activities on self-efficacy judgments and motivation: An availability heuristic interpretation. *Cognitive Therapy and Research, 13*, 247–261.

Collins, A. M., & Loftus, E. F. (1975). A spreading-activation theory of semantic processing. *Psychological Review, 82*, 407–428.

Collins, N. L. (1996). Working models of attachment: Implications for explanation, emotion, and behavior. *Journal of Personality and Social Psychology, 71*, 810–832.

Collins, N. L., & Read, S. J. (1994). Cognitive representations of attachment: The content and function of working models. In K. Bartholomew & D. Perlman (Eds.), *Advances in personal relationships* (Vol. 5, pp. 53–90). London: Jessica Kingsley.

Cooley, C. H. (1902). *Human nature and the social order.* New York: Schocken.

Davila, J., Burge, D., & Hammen, C. (1997). Why does attachment style change? *Journal of Personality and Social Psychology, 73*, 826–838.

Deci, E. L., & Ryan, R. M. (1995). Human autonomy: The basis for true self-esteem. In M. H. Kernis (Ed.), *Efficacy, agency, and self-esteem* (pp. 31–48). New York: Plenum Press.

Dovidio, J. F., Kawakami, K., Johnson, C., Johnson, B., & Howard, A. (1997). On the nature of prejudice: Automatic and controlled processes. *Journal of Experimental Social Psychology, 33*, 510–540.

Duval, S., & Wicklund, R. A. (1972). *A theory of objective self-awareness.* New York: Academic Press.

Fehr, B., Baldwin, M. W., Collins, L., Patterson, S., & Benditt, R. (in press). Anger in close relationships: An interpersonal script analysis. *Personality and Social Psychology Bulletin.*

Fiske, A. P. (1992). The four elementary forms of sociality: Framework for a unified theory of social relations. *Psychological Review, 99*, 689–723.

Frazier, P., Byer, A. L., Fischer, A. R., Wright, D. M., & DeBord, K. A. (1996). Adult attachment style and partner choice: Correlational and experimental findings. *Personal Relationships, 3*, 117–136.

Freud, S. (1958). The dynamics of transference. In J. Strachey (Ed. & Trans.), *The stan-*

dard edition of the complete psychological works of Sigmund Freud (Vol. 12, pp. 99–
    108). London: Hogarth Press. (Original work published 1912)

Gaertner, S. L., & McLaughlin, J. P. (1983). Racial stereotypes: Associations and ascrip-
    tions of positive and negative characteristics. Social Psychology Quarterly, 46, 23–
    30.

Hazan, C., & Shaver, P. R. (1987). Romantic love conceptualized as an attachment pro-
    cess. Journal of Personality and Social Psychology, 52, 511–524.

Hazan, C., & Shaver, P. R. (1994). Attachment as an organizational framework for
    research on close relationships. Psychological Inquiry, 5, 1–22.

Herr, P. (1986). Consequences of priming: Judgment and behavior. Journal of Personality
    and Social Psychology, 51, 1106–1115.

Higgins, E. T. (1996). Knowledge activation: Accessibility, applicability, and salience. In
    E. T. Higgins & A. W. Kruglanski (Eds.), Social psychology: Handbook of basic princi-
    ples (pp. 133–168). New York: Guilford Press.

Higgins, E. T., & Bargh, J. A. (1987). Social cognition and social perception. Annual
    Review of Psychology, 38, 369–425.

Higgins, E. T., Rholes, W. S., & Jones, C. R. (1977). Category accessibility and impres-
    sion formation. Journal of Experimental Social Psychology, 13, 141–154.

Higgins, E. T., Van Hook, E., & Dorfman, D. (1988). Do self-descriptive traits form a
    self-structure? Social Cognition, 6, 177–207.

Hill, C. R., & Safran, J. D. (1994). Assessing interpersonal schemas: Anticipated
    responses of significant others. Journal of Social and Clinical Psychology, 13, 366–
    379.

Holender, D. (1986). Semantic activation without conscious identification in dichotic
    listening, parafoveal vision, and visual masking: A survey and appraisal. The
    Behavioral and Brain Sciences, 9, 1–66.

Hooley, J. M., & Teasdale, J. D. (1989). Predictors of relapse in unipolar depressives:
    Expressed emotion, marital distress, and perceived criticism. Journal of Abnormal
    Psychology, 98, 229–235.

Horowitz, M. J. (1988). Introduction to psychodynamics. New York: Basic Books.

Jacoby, L. L., & Kelley, C. M. (1987). Unconscious influences of memory for a prior
    event. Personality and Social Psychology Bulletin, 13, 314–336.

Jacoby, L. L., Toth, J. P., Lindsay, D. S., & Debner, J. A. (1992). Lectures for a layperson:
    Methods for revealing unconscious processes. In R. F. Bornstein & T. S. Pittman
    (Eds). Perception without awareness (pp. 81–120). New York: Guilford Press.

James, W. (1890). The principles of psychology. Cambridge, MA: Harvard University
    Press.

Kernis, M. H., Brockner, J., & Frankel, B. S. (1989). Self-esteem and reactions to failure:
    The mediating role of overgeneralization. Journal of Personality and Social Psychol-
    ogy, 57, 707–714.

Kernis, M. H., & Waschull, S. B. (1995). The interactive roles of stability and level of self-
    esteem: Research and theory. Advances in experimental social psychology, 27, 93–141.

Krosnick, J. A., Betz, A. L., Jussim, L. J., & Lynn, A. R. (1992). Subliminal conditioning
    of attitudes. Personality and Social Psychology Bulletin, 18, 152–162.

Kuiper, N. A., & Olinger, L. J. (1986). Dysfunctional attitudes and a self-worth contin-
    gency model of depression. In P. C. Kendall (Ed.), Advances in cognitive-behavioral
    research and therapy (pp. 115–142). Orlando, FL: Academic Press.

Lewicki, P. (1985). Nonconscious biasing effects of single instances on subsequent judgments. *Journal of Personality and Social Psychology, 48,* 563–574.

Lombardi, W. J., Higgins, E. T., & Bargh, J. A. (1987). The role of consciousness in priming effects on categorization: Assimilation versus contrast as a function of awareness of the priming task. *Personality and Social Psychology Bulletin, 13,* 411–429.

Markus, H. (1977). Self-schemata and processing information about the self. *Journal of Personality and Social Psychology, 35,* 63–78.

Markus, H., & Kunda, Z. (1986). Stability and malleability of the self-concept. *Journal of Personality and Social Psychology, 51,* 858–866.

Markus, H., & Zajonc, R. B. (1985). The cognitive perspective in social psychology. In G. Lindzey & E. Aronson (Eds.), *Handbook of social psychology* (3rd ed., pp. 137–230). New York: Random House.

Meyer, D., & Schvaneveldt, R. W. (1971). Facilitation in recognizing pairs of words: Evidence of a dependence between retrieval operations. *Journal of Experimental Psychology, 90,* 227–234.

Mischel, W. (1973). Toward a cognitive social learning reconceptualization of personality. *Psychological Review, 80,* 252–283.

Mischel, W., & Shoda, Y. (1995). A cognitive-affective system theory of personality: Reconceptualizing situations, dispositions, dynamics, and invariance in personality structure. *Psychological Review, 102,* 246–268.

Mitchell, S. A. (1988). *Relational concepts in psychoanalysis.* Cambridge, MA: Harvard University Press.

Moretti, M. M., & Shaw, B. F. (1989). Automatic and dysfunctional cognitive processes in depression. In J. S. Uleman & J. A. Bargh (Eds.), *Unintended thought* (pp. 383–421). New York: Guilford Press.

Murphy, S. T., & Zajonc, R. B. (1993). Affect, cognition, and awareness: Affective priming with optimal and suboptimal stimulus exposures. *Journal of Personality and Social Psychology, 64,* 723–739.

Neuberg, S. L. (1988). Behavioral implications of information presented outside of conscious awareness: The effect of subliminal presentation of trait information on behavior in the prisoner's dilemma game. *Social Cognition, 6,* 207–230.

Newman, L. S., & Uleman, J. S. (1990). Assimilation and contrast effects in spontaneous trait inference. *Personality and Social Psychology Bulletin, 16,* 224–240.

Ogilvie, D. M., & Ashmore, R. D. (1991). Self-with-other representation as a unit of analysis in self-concept research. In R. C. Curtis (Ed.), *The relational self* (pp. 282–314). New York: Guilford Press.

Peterson, C., & Seligman, M. E. (1984). Causal explanations as a risk factor for depression: Theory and evidence. *Psychological Review, 91,* 347–374.

Pietromonaco, P. R., & Feldman Barrett, L. (1997). Working models of attachment and daily social interactions. *Journal of Personality and Social Psychology, 73,* 1409–1423.

Planalp, S. (1985). Relational schemata: A test of alternative forms of relational knowledge as guides to communication. *Human Communication Research, 12,* 3–29.

Robles, R., Smith, R., Carver, C. S., & Wellens, A. R. (1987). Influence of subliminal visual images on the experience of anxiety. *Personality and Social Psychology Bulletin, 13,* 399–410.

Rogers, C. R. (1959). Therapy, personality and interpersonal relationships. In S. Koch (Ed.), *Psychology: A study of a science* (Vol. 3, pp. 184–256). Toronto: McGraw-Hill.

Rogers, T. B. (1977). Self-reference in memory: Recognition of personality items. *Journal of Research in Personality, 11*, 295–305.

Rotter, J. B. (1954). *Social learning and clinical psychology.* Englewood Cliffs, NJ: Prentice Hall.

Safran, J. D. (1990). Towards a refinement of cognitive therapy in light of interpersonal theory: I. Theory. *Clinical Psychology Review, 10*, 87–103.

Safran, J. D., & Segal, Z. V. (1990). *Interpersonal process in cognitive therapy.* New York: Basic Books.

Sarason, B. R., Pierce, G. R., Shearin, E. N., & Sarason, I. G. (1992). Perceived social support and working models of self and actual others. *Journal of Personality and Social Psychology, 60*, 273–287.

Segal, Z. V., Hood, J. E., Shaw, B. F., & Higgins, E. T. (1988). A structural analysis of the self-schema construct in major depression. *Cognitive Therapy and Research, 12*, 471–485.

Smith, E. R. (1984). Model of social inference processes. *Psychological Review, 91*, 392–413.

Smith, E. R., & Branscombe, N. R. (1987). Procedurally mediated social inferences: The case of category accessibility effects. *Journal of Experimental Social Psychology, 23*, 361–382.

Srull, T. K., & Wyer, R. S. (1979). The role of category accessibility in the interpretation of information about persons: some determinants and implications. *Journal of Personality and Social Psychology, 37*, 1660–1662.

Stern, D. N. (1985). *The interpersonal world of the infant.* New York: Basic Books.

Strauman, T. J. (1996). Stability within the self: A longitudinal study of the structural implications of self-discrepancy theory. *Journal of Personality and Social Psychology, 71*, 1142–1153.

Tversky, A., & Kahneman, D. (1973). Availability: A heuristic for judging frequency and probability. *Cognitive Psychology, 5*, 207–232.

Vitousek, K. B., & Hollon, S. D. (1990). The investigation of schematic content and processing in eating disorders. *Cognitive Therapy and Research, 14*, 191–214.

White, G. L., & Shapiro, D. (1987). Don't I know you? Antecedents and social consequences of perceived familiarity. *Journal of Experimental Social Psychology, 23*, 75–92.

Zajonc, R. B. (1980). Feeling and thinking: Preferences need no inferences. *American Psychologist, 35*, 151–175.

6

Behavioral Expressions of a Personality System
Generation and Perception of Behavioral Signatures

YUICHI SHODA

In Akira Kurosawa's 1980 film, *Kagemusha,* when a legendary 16th-century Japanese warlord, Shingen, dies in battle, he is secretly replaced by his double in order to keep his enemies from knowing of the death and to keep his clan together. The double, trained by Shingen's advisors, begins to genuinely assume the warlord's character. The training is so complete that he not only begins to instill a sense of awe in those who come in personal contact with him but also succeeds in making enemy generals sense his presence behind his army's movements. In the eyes of others, including enemy generals, Shingen was still alive. The film raises some basic questions about personality, such as: What is it that the double acquired? What qualities underlie the continuity of a person from one day to the next, from one situation to another, or, for that matter, from the real warlord to his double? And how does continuity and stability in personality become visible in a person's behaviors?

One of the most fundamental assumptions in personality and social psychology is that each individual is characterized by a set of qualities that does not change from situation to situation and that these invariant qualities are expressed in the behaviors of the individual. Without such basic continuity, knowing the personality of an individual in one situation will not be useful in predicting or understanding the person's behavior in a different situation. The challenge, then, is to find a way to conceptualize "personality" that allows such predictions and understanding. Of course this is a question that lay persons and philosophers alike have faced throughout history, providing an integral aspect of culture and language. That can be seen, for example, by the fact that some 18,000 words describing the qualities of a person were found by Allport and Odbert (1936) when they examined the English lexicon. This tradition also became a basis of many modern "dispositional" approaches in personality that seek to characterize individuals in terms of a set of stable dispositions. The utility of these approaches may, at first, seem obvious: Why else would all these words survive so long in history if they don't somehow capture personal qualities that are invariant across situations and that determine a wide range of behaviors (e.g., Allport, 1937; Funder, 1991; Goldberg, 1993; Wiggins & Pincus, 1992)? However, although the prevalence of such trait words implies that they are useful to the users of the language, it leaves wide open the question of just how such qualities are expressed in actual behaviors. If, for example, an individual is characterized by qualities such as wisdom, empathy, bravery, moral integrity, and the belief that "honesty is the best policy," then, how do these qualities relate to observable behaviors? What are the behavioral expressions of personality?

The simplest model of behavioral expression assumes, just as intuitive psychologists do in their correspondent inference process (Jones & Davis, 1965), that, for any given behavior (e.g., friendly behavior), there is a corresponding personal quality (e.g., friendliness). This assumption is so natural that, when we discover that an otherwise reserved person once seated behind the wheel of a car can hold her own against aggressive cab drivers on the streets of New York City, or when we see the closet of an otherwise organized person in utter chaos, our first reaction is likely to be one of puzzlement. For many personality psychologists, however, when research data showed that such "anomalies" are more often the rule than the exception (e.g., Mischel, 1968; Peterson, 1968), the reaction was not benign puzzlement but, rather, a sense of paradigm crisis (e.g., Bem, 1973). It is understandable because at first glance the data may seem to challenge the very mission of the field to "embrace the problem of intra-individual consistency" (Allport, 1937, p. 23).

One purpose of this chapter is to show that the basic mission of the field can be very much alive and that the data can actually enhance it rather than invalidating it, if, and perhaps only if, we liberate ourselves from the assumption that equates personality with situation-free behavioral dispositions. Specifically, by conceptualizing the underlying personality structure from social-cognitive traditions broadly defined (e.g., Bandura, 1978, 1986; Higgins & Kruglanski, 1996; Mischel, 1973, 1990), and in particular as exemplified in a "cognitive-affective personality system (CAPS)" model (Mischel & Shoda, 1995), one can resolve this sense of paradigm crisis because an individual's stable personality is expressed as a pattern of consistency and *variation* discernible in the flow of a person's behavior. The chapter concludes by exploring the possibility that intuitive psychologists also may, at least sometimes, adopt a social-cognitive view of personality.

THE "PERSONALITY = BEHAVIORAL DISPOSITIONS" PARADIGM UNDERLIES THE PARADIGM CRISIS

The model of personality and its behavioral expressions discussed so far are represented schematically in the left panel in Figure 6.1. In this model, each person is characterized by varying amounts of dispositions toward different types of behaviors, which are reflected in the likelihood of engaging in corresponding types of behaviors (e.g., outgoing, organized, friendly). Behavior is also influenced by situations (shown by an arrow in Figure 6.1), but their influence is considered independent of personality. For example, people are usually less friendly with strangers than with acquaintances, but according to this model a "friendly" person's behavior should still be friendlier when compared to the behavior of other people, even when they are with strangers. This model predicts a consistent rank-ordering of individuals' behaviors across situations, as shown in the right panel in Figure 6.1, even though the normative level of behaviors may vary from situation to situation. Such constant rank-ordering has served as the operational definition of "cross-situational consistency," indexed by correlation coefficients, throughout the "consistency debate" (e.g., Bem & Allen, 1974; Bem & Funder, 1978; Epstein, 1979; Mischel & Peake, 1982).

Guided by this expectation, personality psychologists pursued cross-situational consistency as evidence of basic coherence in the underlying personality dispositions of individuals. To the surprise of many, however, the results in the search for this type of high cross-situational consistency were discouraging from the start (e.g., Hartshorne & May, 1928; Mischel, 1968; Mischel & Peake, 1982; Newcomb, 1929; Peterson, 1968; Vernon, 1964), and differing reactions to and interpretation of these findings led to an unfortunate division in the field between those who study personality dispositions and those who study personality functioning (Cervone, 1991; Mischel & Shoda, 1994). Typical data look more like the hypothetical ones shown in Figure 6.2, rather than those expected, shown in Figure 6.1.

It is not difficult to understand why such findings were interpreted as challenging one of the most fundamental assumptions of personality psychology. The logic that leads to this interpretation merits close scrutiny, however. It can be spelled out as the following syllogism:

1. If personality is an important determinant of a behavior, there should be cross-situational consistency in that behavior.
2. Data show that cross-situational consistency in social behavior is low.
3. Then it follows that personality is not an important determinant of behavior.

The history of the "consistency debate" thus can be seen as the uneasy tension between the data (statement 2) and the conclusion (statement 3) threat-

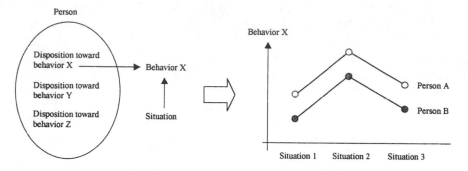

FIGURE 6.1. Behavioral disposition model of personality. In the behavioral disposition model of personality, personality is conceptualized as a set of behavioral dispositions, each of which influences the likelihood of a corresponding behavior (left panel). Situations are assumed to influence behaviors, but their effect is independent and additive. As a result, individual differences in personality, as conceptualized in this model, are expected to be in the elevation of the situation–behavior profiles, as shown in the right panel.

ening our intuitive conviction and the field's fundamental premise. Logic dictates that if statement 2 ("data show cross-situational inconsistency in behavior") is true, then statement 3 ("personality is unimportant") must follow. So the classic dilemma was posed (Bem, 1973) as to which is correct: the data, or our intuition and the premise of the field that personality plays an important role in determining behaviors? But are the data and our intuition necessarily contradictory? Examination of the syllogism above is useful in this regard. It makes clear that this reasoning depends crucially on the assump-

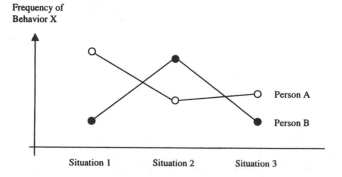

FIGURE 6.2. Typical data indicating violation of cross-situational consistency in individual differences in behavior: Person *A* displays behavior *X* more frequently than person *B* in situations 1 and 3, but in Situation 2, person *B* displays this behavior more frequently than person *A*.

tion embedded in statement 1. That assumption appears so natural that we are often not aware of making it. But what if it were not true? Then we would no longer face the dilemma of having to choose between data and intuition; the findings of cross-situational variability in behavior would no longer need to be seen as a threat to the basic premise of the field. In short, what is false may be statement 1, not statements 2 or 3 as previously assumed. Furthermore, whether statement 1 is correct or not depends entirely on how one defines and conceptualizes "personality," because different conceptions of personality imply different types of behavioral expressions, as discussed below.

Stable Situation–Behavior (*If... Then...*) Relations Characterize Individuals: Models of Stability Must Incorporate Situations

Of course, exploring alternative conceptions of personality is not warranted if the behavioral data do not show evidence of a need and a promise for an alternative. First, as mentioned above, the indication that the current model is not adequate comes from the data that show that people's behaviors often do not conform to the expectation based on the "personality=behavioral disposition" model, which assumed that behavioral expression of personality is in the overall levels of behaviors across situations. From the point of view of that model, observed cross-situational variation in behavior that deviates from the overall level was thus seen as "noise," reflecting the unreliability of the measures or unpredictable fluctuations of behavior. But they are noise only insofar as we equate personality with global behavioral dispositions. If we stop making that assumption, then it is no longer a foregone conclusion that such variations constitute noise. Perhaps there are babies in that bath water!

The indication that the effort to develop an alternative conception can be fruitful comes from the results of empirical investigations that suggest that such variability is not just random fluctuation and that the pattern of behavior variation across situations is stable and characteristic of individuals. For example, in one study conducted at a children's summer camp, behaviors of children were observed hourly, 5 hours a day, 6 days a week, for the duration of a 2-month summer program (Mischel & Shoda, 1995; Shoda, Mischel, & Wright, 1993a, 1993b, 1994). During each hour, observers systematically recorded children's behaviors when they encountered such interpersonal situations as being approached by a peer in a prosocial manner, being teased or provoked by a peer, and being warned by a counselor. Figure 6.3 shows such data for one child. Because mean levels of children's aggressive behaviors naturally varied from one situation to another (e.g., they were more aggressive when teased than when approached prosocially by a peer), the data were first standardized within each situation. The resultant Z scores, which are

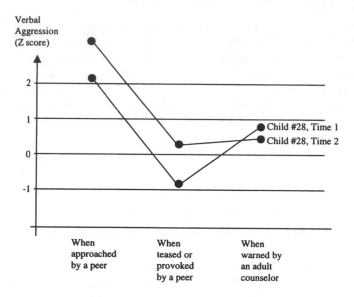

FIGURE 6.3. An illustrative, intraindividual "behavioral signature" for verbal aggression at a summer camp (based on data reported in Shoda, Mischel, & Wright, 1994). The Y axis is in Z scores, so that 0 indicates the level of verbal aggression in each situation normative for children in this sample. The two lines represent the behavioral profiles of the same individual (child 28) at two independent samples of behavior, shown as time 1 and time 2.

used in Figure 6.3, indicate how this child's behavior deviated from the normative level expected for each situation. That is, a score of 0 always indicates that the level of aggression was at the normative level for any given situation. If an individual has a Z score other than 0 in a situation, then it indicates how that person's behavior in that situation differed from the way children behaved on average in that particular situation.

Specifically, the child shown in Figure 6.3 is characterized by the markedly high level (relative to the situation norm) of verbal aggression when approached prosocially by a peer, while his levels of aggression in other situations were at about the normative level. To test if this pattern reflects chance fluctuation or if it constitutes a stable pattern that characterizes this child, data from two independent time samples were plotted. As can be seen, the pattern of behavior variation across the situations (i.e., very high verbal aggression when approached by a peer but about average level in other situations) is a recurrent pattern for this child and can be thought of as the "behavioral signature" of the child. For a significant proportion of the children who were studied, such stable intraindividual patterns of *if...then...* relations were observed (Shoda et al., 1994).

WANTED: A MODEL OF PERSONALITY THAT CAN GENERATE BEHAVIORAL SIGNATURES

The question now becomes: How might one conceptualize personality to account for this type of individual difference? The traditional conceptualization of the person as a set of dispositions toward a given type of behavior, although appealingly simple, cannot readily account for such situation–behavior relations. To do so would require a model of personality that also represents some information about situations and incorporates the situation explicitly into the representation of personality.

Personality as a Bundle of *If... Then...* Contingencies Is an Obvious Alternative, but It Is Only a First Step

One way to accomplish this is to represent each individual's personality by a set of *if...then...* contingencies that characterize that person, as shown in Figure 6.4.

While this model can accommodate behavioral variations across situations, there are some serious challenges it must still overcome. Because an individual encounters many different situations in life, the number of "ifs"

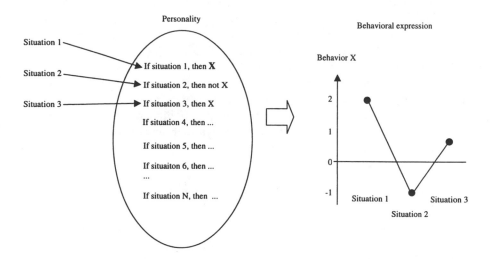

FIGURE 6.4. Personality represented as a set of separate *if...then...* situation–behavior contingencies. Behavioral expressions of individual differences are in the shape, as well as in the elevation, of the situation–behavior profile. Thus, it is capable of accounting for stable and unique patterns of intraindividual variations in behavior across situations. However, it requires representing many *if...then...* contingencies. The generality of the model crucially depends on the units chosen for the "ifs" and "thens" (see text).

that would need to be represented could be potentially large. For example, if situations like "When meeting John for breakfast," "When Alex came to see me at the office," and so on, are to be represented as separate situations, then the representation of personality would have to include a large number of *if...then...* statements. A related challenge is to find a way to generalize from the observed *if...then...* contingencies to behaviors in response to a new, yet-to-be-observed, situation. For example, based on an observation of a person's behavior when "Meeting John at the office today" how does one determine if the person will behave in a similar way when "Meeting Sam at a restaurant?" In the past, one approach to meeting this challenge has been to produce a taxonomy of situations (e.g., Schlundt & McFall, 1987) based on the premise that behaviors observed in one situation can be used to predict behaviors in other situations if the situations belong in the same taxonomic category of situations. But a relatively general category of situations, such as "Meeting someone at the office" may not be sensitive enough to the important nuances of each situation that may critically affect their psychological meaning. It is possible that "Having met Alex at the office yesterday" is psychologically very different from "Meeting John at the office today?"

In order to account for intraindividual coherence, the model must represent how the *if...then...* contingencies are related to each other. An individual may display behavior X when encountering situation 1, and behavior Y when encountering situation 2, but is there a sense that these two contingencies are related to each other, or are they two separately and independently acquired stimulus–response associations? A model of personality coherence must account for how an individual's thoughts, feelings, and behaviors are related to each other rather than being haphazard and independent psychological events. In short, one needs a model that provides a more parsimonious explanation than conceptualizing personality as a collection of separate *if...then...* reflexes in ways that achieve explanatory coherence (Thagard, 1989).

The Nature of "If," and of "Then," Is Crucial for the Usefulness of the *If...Then...* Model

In order to meet the challenges outlined above, it is not sufficient for a model of personality to just represent *if...then...* contingencies. It is a necessary condition, in that any adequate account of how a person discriminates among situations and responds in different, adaptive, ways requires at least a variant of *if...then...* contingencies represented in the personality system. But the utility of a model depends critically on the nature of the "ifs," and the nature of the "thens."

Let us consider first the challenge of generalizability. How does one generalize from one situation (e.g., meeting John for breakfast) to another situation? How does one determine what other situations are similar enough to a given situation, in which a behavior was observed, to allow generalization from it? One of the hurdles that may have prevented personality psychologists from seriously considering the possibility of incorporating situations into personality descriptions is that situations traditionally have been conceptualized in terms of what might be called "nominal" situation units. These are situations that are defined by their physical places and activities, like the school playground or the arithmetic classroom in the classic studies of the consistency of behavior across situations (e.g., Hartshorne & May, 1928; Newcomb, 1929), or specific events one encounters (e.g., "When I saw John in the coffee shop yesterday . . . "). Each nominal situation is potentially unique, and therein lies the potential limitation in generalizability.

One solution to this challenge is to characterize "nominal" units of situations in terms of their "psychologically active ingredients" of situations (Shoda et al., 1994). For example, some individuals may be particularly sensitive to what can be construed as criticism or lack of attention in the context of an intimate relationship (Downey & Feldman, 1996). Then a crucial psychological ingredient of situations for these people is the others' ambiguous behaviors that can be construed as rejecting. One would then expect that their characteristic dynamics and typical behavioral manifestations (e.g., anger and coercive, potentially abusive behaviors) will be expressed in the presence of those psychological features, regardless of the nominal setting (at home, at school, or at work). Similarly, the type of competency demanded by the situation may constitute a psychological feature (Shoda et al., 1993a). Thus, analyzing and characterizing nominal situations in terms of their functional equivalence with regard to psychological features may allow one to identify other nominal situations to which one can generalize the available observations of behavior (e.g., Bem, 1983). Note that the logic above parallels the discussion of "psychological realism" (as compared to "mundane realism") as a determinant of the external validity of a laboratory experiment (e.g., Aronson & Carlsmith, 1968).

The nature of the responses, or the "thens" represented in the *if...then...* contingencies is also crucial in meeting the challenge to address intraindividual coherence. People do not just execute one *if...then...* contingency and then move on to another. Their behavioral responses influence the situations they will encounter next (Mischel & Shoda, 1995, Figure 5). That is, the behavioral "thens" influence the situational "ifs" one faces next. But such mutual influences are not limited to externally observable "ifs" and "thens." The behavior one displays influences the thoughts and feelings activated next. And the cognitions and affects that an individual is experiencing at the time when a situation is encountered significantly influence one's encoding of the situation as well as the behavioral responses to it. Furthermore, cognitions and affects influence each other; one thought may lead to another thought and affective state as well as suppress thoughts with which it is not compatible. Thus the cognitions and affects that an individual experiences can be thought of as forming a network of *if...then...* relations *among themselves.* Such relationships can become the basis of intraindividual coherence, so that the thoughts and feelings experienced by an individual "hang together" in a pattern that is distinctive for that person.

In sum, in order to address intraindividual coherence, the conception of the "thens" must be expanded to include the cognitions and affects, or the units that make up the "internal situation" of an individual. Furthermore the "then" of one contingency may become the "if" of another, to form the basis of intraindividual dynamics and coherence. Although identification of the relevant "ifs" and "thens" is a formidable problem, recent advancements in research in a variety of areas have been providing promising leads.

PERSONALITY AS A COGNITIVE-AFFECTIVE PROCESSING SYSTEM

In fact, if one is willing to look beyond what may be considered traditional, mainstream personality psychology, finding such a model of personality that meets the challenges outlined above may not require traveling far, or inventing a whole new system of constructs. A rich set of constructs used to analyze the social-cognitive processing that underlies behaviors already exists, in essence providing a powerful potential alternative model of personality as a cognitive-affective processing system (Mischel & Shoda, 1995; see also Figure 6.5). This reflects the collective efforts of many researchers over the years not just in personality psychology but in such related areas as social and cognitive psychology as well as cultural anthropology (Higgins & Kruglanski, 1996). These constructs were not originally intended for building a model of personality; rather, they were created and have been used to understand the "why," "when," and "how" of the individual's changing experience and behavior. But that, in fact, makes it highly desirable to adopt these constructs because these are the very questions that we must address in order to understand and predict how an individual's behavior changes across situations. Furthermore, these constructs have already been shown to be useful to account for a variety of psychological phenomena. To be able to explain a new set of phenomena, namely intraindividual coherence and cross-situational variability in behavior, without inventing new constructs, is

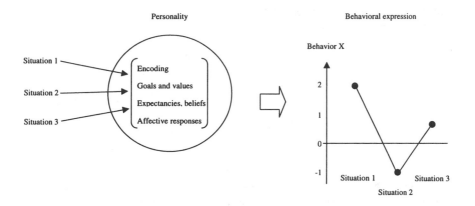

FIGURE 6.5. Personality represented as social-cognitive dispositions, consisting of accessible cognitions and affects and the stable network of relations among them that guide and constrain their activation. It accounts for stable and unique patterns of intraindividual variations in behavior across situations, without representing each *if...then...* situation–behavior contingency separately, while also making it possible to generalize to new situations (see text).

indeed desirable, because it increases the relative parsimony of the explanatory construct system as a whole.

In the social-cognitive views of personality, the central constructs include goals and motives, expectancies, and values, rather than the phenotypic characteristics of the behaviors themselves. Goals have been shown to provide useful explanatory units by a number of investigators (e.g., Alston, 1975; Gollwitzer & Bargh, 1996; Read, Jones, & Miller, 1990; Pervin, 1982). Focusing on the distinctive configuration of goals of an individual also allows one to select the features of situations that are relevant and that interact with the qualities of the person (Read & Miller, 1989). Knowing that an individual wishes to achieve a particular outcome, however, is not sufficient to understand or predict behavior. One needs to understand, for example, the individual's expectancies as well. Social behaviors critically depend on the perceived relationship between effort, on the one hand, and performance and expected consequences of behaviors on the other. And these expectancies in turn depend on the individuals' perception of the situation they are facing, which reflect the individuals' selective attention and characteristic encoding and identification of situations. Although, no doubt, there are many more than can be cited here, these social-cognitive constructs seem to provide a reasonable starting point in assessing whether a social-cognitive model of personality may satisfy the requirements for an adequate model of personality.

Social-Cognitive Variables Do Not Correspond One-to-One to Phenotypic Behavior Types

Social-cognitive constructs and global behavioral dispositions differ in one important respect. For most behavioral dispositions, there exists a direct correspondence between a disposition and the type of behaviors one expects from it (e.g., a disposition toward friendly behaviors predicts friendly behaviors, and a disposition toward aggression predisposes individuals to act aggressively). But social-cognitive variables such as goals, values, and expectancies do not necessarily have a fixed type of behavior that corresponds to them (Cervone, 1997; Cervone & Shoda, Chapter 1, this volume). A close look at the "behavioral expressions" of each type of social-cognitive variable will reveal that they are not expressed in a global tendency to engage in a given type of behavior, but rather, they are expressed in patterns of behavioral *variations* across situations, as well as "pockets" of local consistency (e.g., Wright & Mischel, 1987), as discussed below.

Goals and Values Are Reflected in How a Behavior Varies across Relevant Situations

Although most goals and values do not have general behavioral types (e.g., friendly) that correspond to them, once a situation is adequately specified, and in particular when the perceived goal- and value-relevance of various behaviors in each situation is known, it becomes possible to predict behaviors from the individual's goals and values. To the extent they are important for an individual, an individual's goals and values are expected to be visible in the "covariation" between the perceived relevance of a behavior in a given situation and the likelihood of displaying that behavior (see Figure 6.6). For example, a person who helps a homeless person on the street, but refuses to help her boss with his personal errands probably has different values from someone who has an opposite pattern, who never pays attention to homeless people but is helpful when asked for some personal favor by his boss (Shoda & Mischel, 1993). Similarly, a person who is helpful to strangers when his girlfriend is present but not when he is alone probably has different values than someone whose helping behavior depends not on the presence of an audience but on the perceived need for help. The units of "situations" can be large; for example, a person whose goal is to establish and maintain independence may be particularly motivated to immerse herself in a network of friends at college to separate from her parents, but later in life, the same goal may compel her to focus on her career even at the cost of her social life (Sanderson & Cantor, Chapter 11, this volume).

Furthermore, the behavior-generation process need not be "rational." In any given situation, a goal may activate behaviors that objectively are not

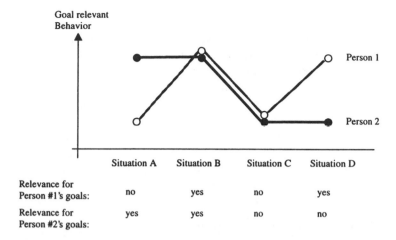

	Situation A	Situation B	Situation C	Situation D
Relevance for Person #1's goals:	no	yes	no	yes
Relevance for Person #2's goals:	yes	yes	no	no

FIGURE 6.6. Two hypothetical individuals with different goals, illustrating that different goals are manifested in different profiles of behavior variation across situations.

necessarily conducive to attaining it, but that are nonetheless associated with the goal in the actor's mind. Behavioral responses may also reflect affective states. The perception that a situation is relevant for the pursuit of a cherished goal may activate a high level of anxiety, which in turn may lead to ineffective or even self-defeating behaviors.

In sum, whether or not the process is rational or adaptive, most behavioral manifestations of goals are by definition situation-dependent, and the key aspect in the person's stream of behaviors in which goals are expressed is the *situations* in which relevant behaviors are displayed. In fact, if an individual's behavior is consistent across situations, then it would be very difficult to infer the actor's goals.

Expectancies and Beliefs Are Also Reflected in How Behavior Varies across Situations

Just as goals determine *when* and *where* a behavior is displayed, so do expectancies and beliefs. For example, if an individual has low self-efficacy beliefs about dancing, and if dancing in front of other people always activates a sense of embarrassment for her, then she may try to keep a low profile at parties where she expects peer pressure to dance. On the other hand, at parties where she doesn't expect such peer pressure, she may be much more outgoing, feeling comfortable to be at the center of attention at times. Schematically, this person's characteristic cognitive-affective information-processing pattern may be depicted as in Figure 6.7.

One would predict that her behavior across the four parties would follow a pattern such as the one shown in Figure 6.8. Note that the reason why expectancies and beliefs result in predictable patterns of cross-situational variation in behavior is because often expectancies and beliefs are about people, objects, and events in the world (e.g., "At this party people are sometimes expected to sing") constituting a part of the psychological situation for an individual. Even if it is about self (e.g., "I can't dance"), situations differ in the relevance of that aspect of self (e.g., a dance party vs. a dinner party), just as situations differ in their relevance to any given goal. Thus an expectancy, or a belief, becomes activated only in specific situations relevant for them.

Encoding Determines the Functionally Equivalent Units of Situations

Implicit in the discussions above is that the first steps in social information processing are recognizing, identifying, and interpreting a situation. In this process, of the many possible features of situations, a certain small number of them are attended and play a role in activating salient expectancies, beliefs, goals, and affects. For example, for the "dance phobic" person in the example above, the feature that distinguishes different types of parties may be the perceived likelihood of being pressured to dance. Therefore, she may pay particular attention to such aspects of situations as whether the party is attended by people who are likely to want to dance. If Figure 6.7 below describes her stable information-processing patterns, then the presence, or absence, of this feature of situations determines whether or not her characteristic patterns of

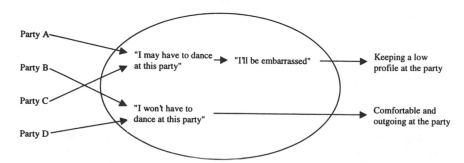

FIGURE 6.7. The processing pathways and dynamics of an illustrative case discussed in text. Parties *A* and *C* activate the cognition "I may have to dance at this party," which, in turn, activates the expectation "I'll be embarrassed," resulting in the person's keeping a low profile. Parties *B* and *D* do not activate these cognitions, and the person, feeling comfortable, behaves in an outgoing way.

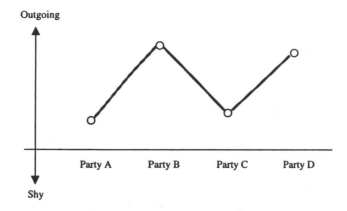

FIGURE 6.8. Behaviors expected from the hypothetical person shown in Figure 6.7.

cognitive, affective, and behavioral responses to situations with such features are activated. Thus, as shown in Figure 6.9, groups of situations (e.g., situations 1, 2, and 3 in Figure 6.9) can form a functional equivalance class, so that situations belonging to the same class activate similar encoding, resulting in similar cognitive, affective, and behavioral responses, while situations belonging to different classes will activate different cognitions, affects, and behaviors.

Furthermore, if the individual's expectancies and goals about that type of situation change (e.g., she takes a dance lesson; or she learns to overcome her fear of dancing in front of others), then the behavioral responses to *all* the situations belonging to that particular group of situations are likely to change. Thus the behavioral expression of encoding is in the grouping of situations forming the basic functional units in the cross-situational organization of behaviors—situations that for all functional purposes are the same from the individual's point of view and that elicit similar responses. To illustrate, the role of a functional equivalence class of situations in the cross-situational organization of behaviors can be analogous to that of individual pieces in a hand-held puzzle consisting of movable square tiles with patterns printed on them. The puzzle can be arranged by moving the tiles around, but that will not affect the patterns printed on each tile. Behaviors of an individual in situations belonging to the same functional equivalence unit are like the tiles, whereas the cross-situational organization of behavior is analogous to the collective pattern they form in the puzzle. When the individual's beliefs, goals, or affective states change, behaviors of that individual in those situations are expected to change as a unit (except, of course, in reality one would expect significant momentary fluctuations in behavior, so one would not see perfect units).

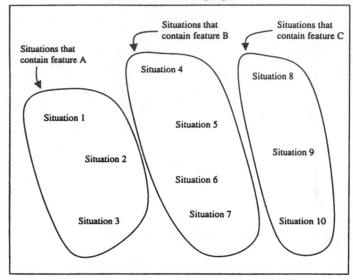

The social world according to person X

Situations that
contain feature B

Situations that
contain feature C

Situations that
contain feature A

Situation 4

Situation 8

Situation 1

Situation 5

Situation 9

Situation 2

Situation 6

Situation 3

Situation 7

Situation 10

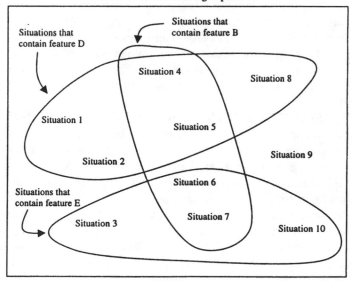

The social world according to person Y

Situations that
contain feature D

Situations that
contain feature B

Situation 4

Situation 8

Situation 1

Situation 5

Situation 2

Situation 9

Situation 6

Situations that
contain feature E

Situation 7

Situation 3

Situation 10

FIGURE 6.9. The subjective "social worlds" according to persons X and Y. For person X, situations 1, 2, and 3 form an equivalence class (because they all contain situation feature A); situations 4, 5, 6, and 7 form another equivalence class, containing feature B, and situations 8, 9, and 10 form a third equivalence class, containing feature C. Features A and C are not important for person Y, but features D and E are important. Thus, except for the equivalence class of situations containing feature B, person Y's subjective social world is organized in terms of a different set of equivalence classes of situations. Situation 9 illustrates a "loner" situation, one whose features, as seen by person Y, are not shared by other situations. The overlapping of the units illustrates that situation equivalence units need not divide up the subjective world in mutually exclusive sets as often envisioned in efforts to arrive at a "taxonomy" of situations.

Note that these functional equivalence classes, such as the one defined by the presence of "people who like to dance at parties," are in part specific to each individual. For a different person, the possibility of dancing, for example, may be completely irrelevant. Rather, it may be the presence of people who share her professional interests, that defines the functional equivalence for that person. Because the functional equivalence classes of situations are defined by the psychologically significant features they share, and because the feature that is psychologically significant depends on each individual, the result is that each individual's behavior is organized across situations with different equivalence classes of situations as basic units, in effect "carving up" the world in unique ways, as shown in Figure 6.9.

To illustrate, the left panel of Figure 6.9 shows that for person X, situations 1, 2, and 3 form an equivalence class sharing a feature ("feature A") that is psychologically significant for him. Situations 4, 5, 6, and 7 form another class sharing feature B. Situations 8, 9, and 10 contain feature C, which is another feature that is salient for him. The right panel of Figure 6.9 shows the subjective social world of person Y. For this person, the presence or absence of features D and E are salient, resulting in a very different organization of the "social world."

As discussed before, because in the present model the encoding units influence the expectancies, goals, and affects that mediate the effects of situations on the behavioral responses, for person X, one expects that his behaviors in situations 1, 2, and 3 will be similar to each other, and his behaviors in situations 4, 5, 6, and 7 form another unit. The cross-situational organization of person Y is likely to reflect the different groupings of situations shown in the right panel of Figure 6.9.

In sum, the foregoing discussion of the behavioral manifestations of representative social-cognitive variables has one clear implication for behavioral coherence: To the extent that the configuration of social-cognitive variables that characterize an individual is stable and invariant across situations, the result is a stable, distinct, and characteristic cross-situational organization of behavior (Mischel & Shoda, 1995; Shoda et al., 1994). This organization reflects the grouping of situations based on encoding units, as well as the expectancies, beliefs, goals, values, and affects activated by the encoded situation.

COGNITIVE-AFFECTIVE UNITS THEMSELVES FORM A SELF-ORGANIZING NETWORK

The foregoing discussion has focused separately on how each type of social-cognitive variable organizes and creates a coherent pattern of behavioral change and organization across situations. But are the social-cognitive variables, and the cognitions and affects they refer to, themselves organized into a coherent whole?

One key feature of the social-cognitive variables plays an important role in this respect. These variables are not just something an individual happens to "have" (Cantor, 1990), but rather they are designed to capture the dynamic variations in the salience of the cognitions, affects, and behaviors as a person interacts with the social world, and, through the interplay among the social-cognitive units, a coherent pattern is expected to emerge (Mischel & Shoda, 1995). Specifically, in order to account for such dynamic interactions, social-cognitive models of personality focus on the activation of mental representations as a key principle in the processing of social information (Higgins, 1996; Higgins & Bargh, 1987). Mental representations of the psychological meaning of situations, representations of self, others, possible future events, goals, affects, beliefs, expectations, as well as behavioral alternatives all influence each other dynamically, in response to each other and to situations (e.g., Shoda & Mischel, 1998).

Thus the multiple processes that make up each individual's social-information-processing system influence one another, imposing constraints on the configurations of cognitive and affective states that "hang together" for a given individual. If the individual components of the system, such as encoding of situations, expectancies, goals, and affects, are words in a text, then an individual is a page, or a book, of text. And not all possible combinations of words are likely, and only a few make sense. The words, or the individuals' experiences, must form a coherent whole reflecting an individual's unique personality.

One explanation of how that is possible, even without an "author" behind the scene, is that the social-cognitive processes form a self-organizing system of cognitions and affects that constrain and guide the activation, or suppression, of one another (Mischel & Shoda, 1995; Shoda & Mischel, 1998). For example, when a goal is activated, it in turn activates the cognitions and affects that are connected with it, while those that are not compatible with the goal are suppressed. Thus, when the goal of learning is highly activated, for example, an individual is likely to encode situations in terms of the opportunities for learning these situations represent, which in turn may activate expected outcomes of learning. On the other hand, when the goal of achieving favorable evaluation is activated, situations are more likely to be encoded in those terms, and the outcome expectations activated are likely to be interpersonal, rather than about learning (e.g., Grant & Dweck, Chapter 10, this volume).

A network of such units that influence and mutually constrain the activation of one another is known to have a tendency to "settle" into a configuration to form a coherent pattern that satisfies the constraints (e.g., Thagard, 1989). The process is not unlike the perceptual process that we experience when looking at a Necker cube, a line drawing of a cube that can be interpreted as seen from above or below. After a moment of confusion, one or the other view of the drawing emerges to form a coherent perception. According to one account of the process, this occurs because, initially, our interpretations of the individual parts (e.g., an edge as being in front or back) of the drawing are not coherent (e.g., Rumelhart, Smolensky, McClelland, & Hinton, 1986). That is, some parts are interpreted as if the cube is seen from above, while other parts are interpreted as if the cube is seen from below. But the interpretations of components mutually influence each other, so that when an edge is seen as being in front, then a point connected to it must be convex, and so forth. Within a second or so, our perceptual system is usually able to arrive at a configuration of interpretations of the individual parts that form a coherent whole in which the interpretation of each part is consistent with, and supports, those of others.

Similarly, units of cognitions and mental representations, such as encodings, goals, and expectancies, form a system of mutual constraints. And thus a configuration of such units that satisfies the constraints and forms a coherent whole is expected to emerge (Shoda & Mischel, 1998). The unique properties of the personality system are therefore represented in the network of relations among the cognitions and affects that guide and constrain their activation (e.g., the cognitive-affective processing system [CAPS] model; Mischel & Shoda, 1995).

Furthermore, in addition to the coherence in the cognitions and affects activated, the interrelationships that guide and constrain their activation can themselves evolve, and in doing so, they will increasingly reflect an individual's core goals and beliefs. If the formation of the network follows a process resembling a basic "learning algorithm," such as Hebb's (1949), the relationships among mental events that are activated simultaneously become strengthened. Because core beliefs and goals are likely to be activated under many circumstances throughout an individual's life, the cognitions, affects, and behaviors that are linked to them are likely to be activated simultaneously. As a result, they will be reflected in the development of an individual's distinct, coherent, network of relationships formed around the core goals and beliefs. Such formations of associations are consistent with any form of associative learning, but the focus here is on the associations among the social cognitive units and the formation of a coherent and distinctive network of associations among them, rather than the associations between external events and behavioral output.

In short, the cognitive and emotional events that social-cognitive variables refer to tend to be organized in a mutually activating network, rather than independently. People may differ stably in the network of relationships among the cognitions and affects that guide and constrain their influences on each other. Such mutual influences make social-cognitive variables self-organizing, so that from the network of mutual influences, a coherent and characteristic pattern of cognitions and affects is likely to emerge.

IS THE INTUITIVE PERCEIVER
A SOCIAL-COGNITIVE THEORIST?

Psychologists are not the only people who use the construct of "personality." In fact, most individuals in their daily interactions with others make inferences about "personalities" (e.g., Heider, 1958). And in studying this process, most research paradigms seem to start with the assumption that the "personality" that is being inferred consists of broad behavioral dispositions such as "friendly" and "aggressive." Thus the perceiver is implicitly seen as being guided by the intuitive version of the "personality = broad behavioral dispositions" model discussed earlier. Accordingly, the pattern of behaviors that was considered indicative of the "person" required consistency across situations or entities (Kelley, 1973). However, global behavioral disposition theory is not the only model of personal dispositions. With that in mind, one may then ask: Do intuitive perceivers always use a global behavioral disposition model, or might they sometimes use other models (Shoda, Mischel, & Wright, 1989)?

When Are People Likely to Be "Social-Cognitive Theorists"?

People, including scientists, prefer simple explanations, other things being equal. But of course other things are not often equal. Sometimes one has data that can't be understood by the simplest explanation, and sometimes understanding them is of crucial importance. As discussed above, cross-situational organization of behavior represents such data. When faced with observations that the behavior of a person, either someone we know, or ourselves, varies across situations in predictable ways, then we need to go beyond the simple "behavioral dispositions" explanation. For example, if a person is always very methodical in one type of situation but always quite sloppy in another, it is not adequate to describe the person merely as methodical, sloppy, or somewhere in between. One may be tempted just to ignore or dismiss such a stable pattern of cross-situational variation as a reflection of fundamental unpredictability in human behavior, but if the pattern is observed time and again, it demands explanation. That is particularly the case if we have a vested interest in the behavior of that person, such as when we are about to entrust our lives to the hands of a surgeon, who, we may discover, is due in court because of repeated speeding violations. Does she not pay attention to such matters because her priority is completely focused on patient care? Or, is she an insatiable risk seeker?

   In research on dispositional inferences, subjects are often presented with this type of information. And the expectation is that they will infer, or perhaps overinfer, a disposition that corresponds to the behavior. So in the example of a speeding surgeon above, one may infer "recklessness." Most importantly, that inference is expected to be strengthened if one learns that she speeds regardless of the situation (e.g., Kelley, 1967). On the other hand, if her speeding behavior is found to vary across situations, then intuitive observers are expected to infer dispositions to a lesser extent, or at least they should be inferring dispositions less, even though in fact they may be quite reluctant to do so. But what if one learns a bit more about the situations? What if we learned that all of her speeding tickets were issued while she was rushing to the hospital after receiving an urgent call? What if we learned that all of her parking tickets came from parking at a space reserved for the hospital executives when she couldn't find a parking spot once she reached the hospital? In that case we might be inclined to infer something about her dedication to her patients, rather than her recklessness.

How might an intuitive observer test to see which inference is correct? The answer, again, lies in obtaining relevant situational information. For example, if the surgeon's behavior is a reflection of her dedication to her patients, then one would predict that she might deviate from her otherwise cautious behavior only in situations in which doing so would benefit her patients but not in other situations. In fact if one really wanted to test the hypothesis that her behavior is driven by her dedication to her patients, one might wish to compare her behaviors in situations that differed only in the perceived benefit to the patients, while all other factors are equal. For example, one may wish to compare her behaviors when emergencies involved her patients versus other types of emergencies, such as a board meeting to discuss hospital reorganization. And if one finds that she takes risks in driving only when her patients' well-being is at stake, and not in other situations, then we will be more likely to believe that her behavior is a reflection of her dedication to her patients.

To be sure, traditional models of dispositional inferences would also predict that observers are less likely to infer that the surgeon is reckless because they would discount the original inference that she may be reckless in light of the situational information. But the traditional account would stop there and predict that observers would, or should, chalk this up to "situations," making no inferences about the person. It does not allow for the possibility that observers may be able to make a different kind of inference about the surgeon's personality—in this case her dedication to her patients. This limitation in the traditional framework for studying dispositional inferences occurs, viewed from the social-cognitive view of personality, because of the tacit assumption that personality equals behavioral dispositions, and, thus, if a behavior does not indicate a corresponding behavioral disposition, it is not personality (and if it is not personality, it is situation)! But if people behave like social-cognitive theorists, they may well infer some things about the target(s), which in the case above were the surgeon's values and goals (that she cares about her patients), as well as her expectations (that she can make a difference by rushing to the hospital). Most interestingly, from the social-cognitive view, one would predict that the more distinctively the target individual's behavior varies across situations, the more likely it is that an observer would make an inference about the individual's personality in terms of social-cognitive variables. In the example above, our likelihood of inferring the surgeon's dedication to her patients will be strengthened to the extent that she does not speed in other circumstances.

In order to test this possibility, observers were exposed to two types of targets (Lemm & Shoda, 1995). One target's behavior was consistently friendly across situations, while the other target's behavior varied across two types of situations, following a stable and distinct pattern (e.g., always friendly in an academic situation, but arrogant in a nonacademic situation). Observers recorded their impressions of the target in a free-response format, and their responses were later coded as either instances of behavioral dispositions (e.g., "friendly," "arrogant") or as instances of such social-cognitive variables as beliefs, expectations, values, and goals. As expected from classic attribution theories (e.g., Jones & Davis, 1965; Kelley, 1967), observers inferred many more behavioral dispositions when the behaviors of the target were consistent across situations, but they inferred virtually none when the behavior varied across situations. With regard to the social-cognitive variables, however, a completely opposite pattern emerged. Observers inferred significantly more social-cognitive variables when the target's behavior varied across situations, resulting in a crossover interaction between the cross-situational consistency in the target's behavior and the type of inferences (behavioral disposition vs. social-cognitive variables), as shown in Figure 6.10. Furthermore, there is also evidence that intuitive psychologists behave like social-cognitive theorists when they want to understand the target person. For example, when observers were asked to focus on what a person "is like," they tended to use behavioral dispositions in thinking about the target person. However, when they were asked to empathize with the target person, they tended to focus more on the actor's goals or the situations in which the behavior occurs (Hoffman, Mischel, & Mazze, 1981; Wegner & Giuliano, 1983). Similarly, when asked to focus on or think about *why* a target person behaved in the way she did, observers overwhelmingly tended to mention social-cognitive variables, as compared to when they were asked to think about *what kind* of person they thought the target was (Lemm & Shoda, 1995).

It has often been assumed that, when the behavior of the target varies across situations, it is undiagnostic of the target's personality. This remains true, but only as long as "personality" is conceptualized as consisting of behavioral dispositions. When one allows for the possibility that intuitive observers may act like social-cognitive theorists, permitting them to express their thoughts about the target person unconstrained by the closed-ended question that included only behavioral dispositions, then, a different picture

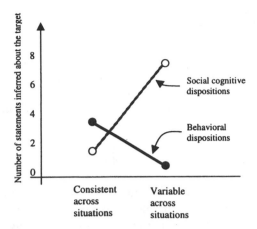

FIGURE 6.10. More social-cognitive dispositions, and fewer behavioral dispositions, were inferred when the behavior of the target person varied across situations. Adapted by permission of the authors from Lemm and Shoda (1995).

emerges. Intuitive observers do make inferences about the target person even, or especially, when the target's behavior varies across situations. But *what* they infer tends to be such social-cognitive variables as the beliefs, expectations, values, and goals of the target person (Shoda & Mischel, 1993).

LEARNING FROM THE INTUITIVE PSYCHOLOGIST

The "lay person as intuitive scientist" tradition can go both ways. In the past, when psychologists equated personality with behavioral dispositions, intuitive psychologists were also assumed to follow a similar model as they tried to gain information about others. There is no doubt that people do often operate in that way, as evidenced by many studies on dispositional inferences (e.g., Trope & Higgins, 1993) as well as the answers people gave when asked, "What kind of personality does he have?" But that view may be incomplete, as people also seem to infer other, enduring and distinctive aspects of individuals, such as their values, goals, expectations, and beliefs, that is, their social-cognitive dispositions. The "personality = behavioral dispositions" model may be parsimonious, but it also had the unfortunate consequence of treating variability of behavior across situations as "inconsistency" and as being antithetical to personality coherence, defining the task for observers and psychologists alike as one of distilling by ignoring or eliminating situational variability. In doing so, valuable data about how an individual functions, the intraindividual dynamics among cognitions, affects, and behaviors in response to changing situations, can become lost.

Thus, just as Allport and Odbert (1936) did, one might learn from the intuitive psychologists, who, when faced with the challenge of understanding distinctive variations in a person's behavior they want to understand, sometimes go beyond simple average tendencies and ask about such social-cognitive variables as the values, goals, expectations, and beliefs that underlie a person's behavior. The relevant question then becomes: In what situation did the behavior occur, and in what situation did it not? In this regard, it is interesting to note that in *Kagemusha,* one of the strategies employed by Shingen's enemy generals was to create various situations intentionally, through provocative army movements and configurations, to test if Shingen's troops' movements followed a pattern of situation–behavior contingency consistent with his personality. The film ends with the clan in ruins when one of Shingen's sons ignores the situation–behavior, *if...then...* relations that characterized his father's strategies, destroying the behavioral coherence carefully orchestrated by the advisors and the double to create the impression of Shingen's continued presence. It would be reading too much into the ending of the film if one is to see a lesson of sorts in it, but it does provide provocative questions for modern psychologists, and for intuitive observers, who are interested in understanding the functioning, and intraindividual dynamics, that characterize individuals.

REFERENCES

Allport, G. W. (1937). *Personality: A psychological interpretation.* New York: Holt, Rinehart & Winston.

Allport, G. W., & Odbert, H. S. (1936). Trait-names: A psycho-lexical study. *Psychological Monographs: General and Applied, 47,* 1–171.

Alston, W. P. (1975). Traits, consistency and conceptual alternatives for personality theory. *Journal for the Theory of Social Behavior, 5,* 17–48.

Aronson, E., & Carlsmith, J. M. (1968). Experimentation in social psychology. In G. Lindzey & E. Aronson (Eds.), *The handbook of social psychology* (Vol. 2, pp. 1–79). Reading, MA: Addison-Wesley.

Bandura, A. (1978). The self-system in reciprocal determinism. *American Psychologist, 33,* 344–358.

Bandura, A. (1986). *Social foundations of thought and action: A social cognitive theory.* Englewood Cliffs, NJ: Prentice-Hall.

Bem, D. J. (1973). Constructing cross-situational consistencies in behavior: Some thoughts on Alker's critique of Mischel. *Journal of Personality, 40,* 17–26.

Bem, D. J. (1983). Constructing a theory of the triple typology: Some (second) thoughts on nomothetic and idiographic approaches to personality. *Journal of Personality, 51,* 566–577.

Bem, D. J., & Allen, A. (1974). On predicting some of the people some of the time: The search for cross-situational consistencies in behavior. *Psychological Review, 81,* 506–20.

Bem, D. J., & Funder, D. C. (1978). Predicting mire of the people more of the time: Assessing the personality of situations. *Psychological Review, 85,* 485–501.

Cantor, N. (1990). From thought to behavior: "Having" and "doing" in the study of personality and cognition. *American Psychologist, 45,* 735–50.

Cervone, D. (1991). The two disciplines of personality psychology: Review of *Handbook of personality: Theory and research. Psychological Science, 2,* 371–377.

Cervone, D. (1997). Social-cognitive mechanisms and personality coherence: Self-knowledge, situational beliefs, and cross-situational coherence in perceived self-efficacy. *Psychological Science, 8,* 43–50.

Downey, G., & Feldman, S. (1996). Implications of rejection sensitivity for intimate relationships. *Journal of Personality and Social Psychology, 70,* 1327–1343.

Epstein, S. (1979). The stability of behavior: I. On predicting most of the people much of the time. *Journal of Personality and Social Psychology, 37,* 1097–1126.

Funder, D. C. (1991). Global traits: A neo-Allportian approach to personality. *Psychological Science, 2,* 31–9.

Goldberg, L. R. (1993). The structure of phenotypic personality traits. *American Psychologist, 48,* 26–34.

Gollwitzer, P. M., & Bargh, J. A. (Eds.). (1996). *The psychology of action: Linking cognition and motivation to behavior.* New York: Guilford Press.

Hartshorne, H., & May, M. A. (1928). *Studies in deceit: Studies in the nature of character* (Vol. 1). New York: Macmillan.

Hebb, D. O. (1949). *The organization of behavior.* New York: Wiley.

Heider, F. (1958). *The psychology of interpersonal relations.* New York: Wiley.

Higgins, E. T. (1996). Knowledge activation: Accessibility, applicability, and salience. In E. T. Higgins & A. W. Kruglanski (Eds.), *Social psychology: Handbook of basic principles* (pp. 133–168). New York: Guilford Press.

Higgins, E. T., & Bargh, J. A. (1987). Social cognition and social perception. *Annual Review of Psychology, 38,* 369–425.

Higgins, E. T., & Kruglanski, A. W. (Eds.). (1996). *Social psychology: Handbook of basic principles.* New York: Guilford Press.

Hoffman, C., Mischel, W., & Mazze, K. (1981). The role of purpose in the organization of information about behavior. Trait-based versus goal-based categories in person cognition. *Journal of Personality and Social Psychology, 40,* 211–225.

Jones, E. E., & Davis, K. E. (1965). From acts to dispositions: The attribution process in person perception. In L. Berkowitz (Ed.), *Advances in experimental social psychology* (Vol. 2, pp. 220–265). New York: Academic Press.

Kelley, H. H. (1967). Attribution theory in social psychology. In D. Levine (Ed.), *Nebraska Symposium on Motivation* (Vol. 15). Lincoln: University of Nebraska Press.

Kelley, H. H. (1973). The process of causal attribution. *American Psychologist, 28,* 107–128.

Lemm, K., & Shoda, Y. (1995, March). *Effects of cross-situational consistency in behavior in personality inferences.* Poster presented at the meeting of the Eastern Psychological Association.

Mischel, W. (1968). *Personality and assessment.* New York: Wiley. (Republished 1996 by Erlbaum: Mahwah, NJ)

Mischel, W. (1973). Toward a cognitive social learning reconceptualization of personality. *Psychological Review, 80,* 252–83.

Mischel, W. (1990). Personality dispositions revisited and revised: A view after three decades. In L. A. Pervin (Ed.), *Handbook of personality: Theory and research* (pp. 111–134). New York: Guilford Press.

Mischel, W., & Shoda, Y. (1994). Personality psychology has two goals: Must it be two fields? *Psychological Inquiry, 5,* 156–158.

Mischel, W., & Peake, P. K. (1982). Beyond *déjà vu* in the search for cross-situational consistency. *Psychological Review, 89,* 730–755.

Mischel, W., & Shoda, Y. (1995). A cognitive-affective system theory of personality: Reconceptualizing situations, dispositions, dynamics, and invariance in personality structure. *Psychological Review, 102,* 246–268.

Newcomb, T. M. (1929). *Consistency of certain extrovert–introvert behavior patterns in 51 problem boys.* New York: Columbia University, Teachers College, Bureau of Publications.

Pervin, L. A. (1982). The stasis and flow of behavior: Toward a theory of goals. In *Nebraska Symposium on Motivation* (Vol. 30, pp. 1–53). Lincoln: University of Nebraska Press.

Peterson, D. R. (1968). *The clinical study of social behavior.* New York: Appleton.

Read, S. J., Jones, D. K., & Miller, L. C. (1990). Traits as goal-based categories: The importance of goals in the coherence of dispositional categories. *Journal of Personality and Social Psychology, 58,* 1048–1061.

Read, S. J., & Miller, L. C. (1989). The importance of goals in personality: toward a coherent model of persons. In R. S. Wyer & T. K. Srull (Eds.), *Advances in social cognition* (Vol. 2, pp. 163–174). Hillsdale, NJ: Erlbaum.

Schlundt, D. G., & McFall, R. M. (1987). Classifying social situations: A comparison of five methods. *Behavioral Assessment, 9,* 21–42.

Rumelhart, D. E., Smolensky, P., McClelland, J. L., & Hinton, G. E. (1986). Schemata and sequential thought processes in PDP models. In J. L. McClelland & D. E. Rumelhart (Eds.), *Parallel distributed processing: Explorations in the microstructures of cognition — Vol. 2. Psychological and biological models* (pp. 7–57). Cambridge, MA: MIT Press/Bradford Books.

Shoda, Y., & Mischel, W. (1993). Cognitive social approach to dispositional inferences: What if the perceiver is a cognitive-social theorist? *Personality and Social Psychology Bulletin, 19,* 574–585.

Shoda, Y., & Mischel, W. (1998). Personality as a stable cognitive-affective activation network: Characteristic patterns of behavior variation emerge from a stable personality structure. In S. J. Read & L. C. Miller (Eds.), *Connectionist models of social reasoning and social behavior* (pp. 175–208). Mahwah, NJ: Erlbaum.

Shoda, Y., Mischel, W., & Wright, J. C. (1989). Intuitive interactionism in person perception: Effects of situation–behavior relations on dispositional judgments. *Journal of Personality and Social Psychology, 56,* 41–53.

Shoda, Y., Mischel, W., & Wright, J. C. (1993a). The role of situational demands and cognitive competencies in behavior organization and personality coherence. *Journal of Personality and Social Psychology, 65,* 1023–1035.

Shoda, Y., Mischel, W., & Wright, J. C. (1993b). Links between personality judgments and contextualized behavior patterns: Situation–behavior profiles of personality prototypes. *Social Cognition, 4,* 399–429.

Shoda, Y., Mischel, W., & Wright, J. C. (1994). Intra-individual stability in the organization and patterning of behavior: Incorporating psychological situations into the idiographic analysis of personality. *Journal of Personality and Social Psychology, 67,* 674–687.

Thagard, P. (1989). Explanatory coherence. *Behavioral and Brain Sciences, 12,* 435–502.

Trope, Y., & Higgins, E. T. (1993). The what, when, and how of dispositional inference: New answers and new questions [Special issue: On inferring personal dispositions from behavior]. *Personality and Social Psychology Bulletin, 19,* 493–500.

Vernon P. E. (1964). *Personality assessment: A critical survey.* New York: Wiley.

Wegner, D. M., & Giuliano, T. (1983). Social awareness in story comprehension. *Social Cognition, 2,* 1–17.

Wiggins, J. S., & Pincus, A. L. (1992). Personality: Structure and assessment. *Annual Reviews of Psychology, 43,* 473–504.

Wright, J. C., & Mischel, W. (1987). A conditional approach to dispositional constructs: The local predictability of social behavior. *Journal of Personality and Social Psychology, 53,* 1159–1177.

III

Self Processes and Personal Agency as a Basis of Personality Coherence

7

Social Cognitive Theory of Personality

ALBERT BANDURA

Many psychological theories have been proposed over the years to explain human behavior. The view of human nature embodied in such theories and the causal processes they postulate have considerable import. What theorists believe people to be determines which aspects of human functioning they explore most thoroughly and which they leave unexamined. The conception of human nature in which psychological theories are rooted is more than a theoretical issue. As knowledge gained through inquiry is applied, the conceptions guiding the social practices have even vaster implications. They affect which human potentialities are cultivated, which are underdeveloped, and whether efforts at change are directed mainly at psychosocial, biological, or sociostructural factors. This chapter addresses the personal determinants and mechanisms of human functioning from the perspective of social cognitive theory (Bandura, 1986).

The recent years have witnessed a resurgence of interest in self-referent phenomena. Self processes have come to pervade diverse domains of psychology because most external influences affect human functioning through intermediary self processes rather than directly. The self system thus lies at the very heart of causal processes. To cite but a few examples, personal factors are very much involved in regulating attentional processes, schematic processing of experiences, memory representation and reconstruction, cognitively based motivation, emotion activation, psychobiological functioning, and the efficacy with which cognitive and behavioral competencies are executed in the transactions of everyday life.

AN AGENTIC VIEW OF PERSONALITY

In the agentic sociocognitive view, people are self-organizing, proactive, and self-regulating not just reactive organisms shaped and shepherded by external events. People have the power to influence their own actions to produce certain results. The capacity to exercise control over one's thought processes, motivation, affect, and action operates through mechanisms of personal agency. These mechanisms are analyzed in some detail in the sections that follow.

Triadic Reciprocal Causation

Human behavior has often been explained in terms of one-sided determinism. In such modes of unidirectional causation, behavior is depicted as being shaped and controlled by environmental influences or driven by internal dispositions. Social cognitive theory explains psychosocial functioning in terms of triadic reciprocal causation (Bandura, 1986). The term causation is used to mean functional dependence between events. In this model of reciprocal determinism, internal personal factors in the form of cognitive, affective and biological events, behavioral patterns, and environmental events all operate as interacting determinants that influence one another bidirectionally.

In triadic causation, there is no fixed pattern for reciprocal interaction. Rather, the relative contribution of each of the constituent classes of influences depends on the activities, situational circumstances, and sociostructural constraints and opportunities. The environment is not a monolithic entity. Social cognitive theory distinguishes among three types of environmental structures (Bandura, 1997a). They include the imposed environment, selected environment, and constructed environment. Gradations of environmental changeability require the exercise of increasing levels of personal agency. In the case of the imposed environment, certain physical and sociostructural conditions are thrust upon people whether they like it or not. Although they have little control over its presence, they have leeway in how they construe it and react to it.

There is a major difference between the potential environment and the environment people actually experience. For the most part, the environment is only a potentiality with different rewarding and punishing aspects that do not come into being until the environment is selectively activated by appropriate courses of action. Which part of the potential environment becomes the actual experienced environment thus depends on how people behave. The choice of associates, activities, and milieus constitutes the selected environment. The environments that are created do not exist as a potentiality waiting to be selected and activated. Rather, people construct social environments and institutional systems through their generative efforts. The construal, selection, and construction of environments affect the reciprocal interplay among personal, behavioral, and environmental factors.

Unidirectional causality emphasizing either dispositionalism or situationalism eventually gave way to reciprocal models of causation. Nowadays almost everyone is an interactionist. The major issues in contention center on the type of interactionism espoused. At least three different interactional models have been posed, two of which subscribe to one-way causation in the link to behavior. These alternative causal structures are represented schematically in Figure 7.1. In the unidirectional model, persons and situations are treated as independent influences that combine in unspecified ways to produce behavior. The major weakness with this causal model is that personal and environmental influences do not function as independent determinants. They affect each other. People create, alter, and destroy environments. The changes they produce in environmental conditions, in turn, affect them per-

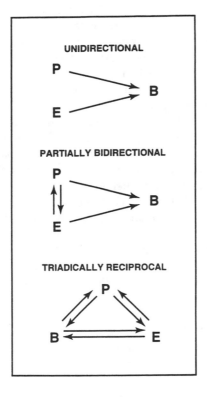

FIGURE 7.1. Schematization of the interplay of constituent determinants in alternative interactional causal models. *B* represents behavior; *P* the internal personal factors in the form of cognitive, affective, and biological events; and *E* the external environment.

sonally. The unidirectional causality with regard to behavior is another serious deficiency of this model of interactionism.

The partially bidirectional conception of interaction, which is now widely adopted in personality theory, acknowledges that persons and situations affect each other. But, this model treats influences relating to behavior as flowing in only one direction. The person–situation interchange undirectionally produces behavior, but the behavior itself does not affect the ongoing transaction between the person and the situation. A major limitation of this interactional causal model is that behavior is not procreated by an intimate interchange between a behaviorless person and the environment. Such a feat would be analogous to immaculate conception. Except through their social stimulus value, people cannot affect their environment other than through their actions. Their behavior plays a dominant role in how they influence situations which, in turn, affect their thoughts, emotional reactions and behavior. In short, behavior is an interacting determinant rather than a detached by-product of a behaviorless person–situation interchange.

As noted earlier, social cognitive theory conceptualizes the interactional causal structure as triadic reciprocal causation. It involves a dynamic interplay among personal determinants, behavior, and environmental influences. Efforts to verify every possible interactant simultaneously would produce experimental paralysis. However, because of the time lags in the operation of the triadic factors, one can gain understanding of how different segments of reciprocal causation function.

Different subspecialties of psychology center their inquiry on selected segments of triadic reciprocality. Cognitive psychologists examine the interactive relation between thought and action as their major sector of interest. This effort centers on the $P{\rightarrow}B$ segment of triadic causation. The programs of research clarify how conceptions, beliefs, self-percepts, aspirations, and intentions shape and direct behavior. What people think, believe, and feel affects how they behave. The natural and extrinsic effects of their actions ($B{\rightarrow}P$), in turn, partly influence their thought patterns and affective reactions.

Social psychologists examine mainly the segment of reciprocality between the person and the environment in the triadic system ($E{\rightarrow}P$). This line of inquiry adds to our understanding of how environmental influences in the form of social persuasion, modeling, and tuition alter cognitions and affective proclivities. The reciprocal element in the person–environment segment of causation ($P{\rightarrow}E$) is of central interest to the subspecialty of person perception. People evoke different reactions from their social environment by their physical characteristics, such as their age, size, race, sex, and physical attractiveness even before they say or do anything. They similarly activate different reactions depending on their socially conferred roles and status. The social reactions so elicited, in turn, affect the recipients' conceptions of themselves and others in ways that either strengthen or weaken the environmental bias.

Of all the different segments in the triadic causal structure, historically the reciprocal interplay between behavior and environmental events has received the greatest attention. Indeed, ethological, transactional, and behavioristic theories focus almost exclusively on this portion of reciprocity in the explanation of behavior. In the transactions of everyday life, behavior alters environmental conditions (B→E), and behavior is, in turn, altered by the very conditions it creates (E→B). The bidirectional relation between behavior and environment is not disembodied from thought, however. Consider coercive parent–child interactions. In discordant families, coercive actions by one member tend to elicit coercive counteractions from the partner in mutually escalating aggression (Patterson, 1976). But about half the time, coercion does not produce coercive counteractions. To understand fully the interactive relation between behavior and social environment, the analysis must be extended temporally and broadened to include cognitive determinants operating in the triadic interlocking system. This requires tapping into what people are thinking as they perform actions and experience their effects. Counterresponses to antecedent acts are influenced not only by their immediate effects but also by people's judgments of eventual outcomes should they stick to that course of action. Thus, aggressive children will continue or even escalate their coercive behavior, although immediately punished, when they expect persistence eventually to gain them what they seek (Bandura & Walters, 1959). But the same momentary punishment will serve as an inhibitor, rather than as an escalator, of coercion when they expect that the continuance of the aversive conduct will be ineffective. Thus, in acting on their environment, people think about where their actions are likely to lead and what they eventually produce. Forethought partly governs the form the reciprocal interplay between behavior and environment takes.

Combining knowledge of the various subsystems of causality increases understanding of the superordinate causal system. Some progress has been made in clarifying how the triadic determinants operate together and how their patterning and relative strength change in the causal structure over time. These studies involve microanalyses of triadic reciprocal causation in which people manage a dynamic computerized environment (Bandura & Jourden, 1991; Bandura & Wood, 1989). Each of the major interactants in the triadic causal structure—personal, behavioral, and environmental—functions as an important constituent in the transactional system. The personal determinant is indexed by self-beliefs of efficacy, cognized goals, quality of analytic thinking, and affective self-reactions. The options that are actually executed in the management of the organizational environment constitute the behavioral determinant. The properties of the organizational environment, the level of challenge it prescribes, and its responsiveness to behavioral interventions represent the environmental determinant. The constituent factors in the ongoing transactional system are measured repeatedly to verify the dynamics of the triadic causal system over time. The findings clarify the way in which the interlocked set of determinants operate as a whole and change in their relative contribution with experience.

Fortuitous Determinants in Causal Structures

There is an element of fortuity in people's lives. The role of fortuitous determinants in causal structures remains ever dormant in psychological theorizing even though it is often a critical factor in the paths lives take (Bandura, 1982b, 1998). People are often brought together through a fortuitous constellation of events that set in motion reciprocal interplays of influences that shape the course of their lives. Indeed, some of the most important determinants of life paths often arise through the most trivial of circumstances. In these instances, seemingly minor events have important and enduring impact on the courses that lives take.

A fortuitous event in socially mediated happenstances is defined as an unintended meeting of persons unfamiliar with each other. Although the separate chains of events in a chance encounter have their own causal determinants, their intersection occurs fortuitously rather than by design (Nagel, 1961). It is not that a fortuitous event is uncaused but, rather, there is a lot of randomness to the determining conditions of its intersections. The profusion of separate chains of events in everyday life provides numerous opportunities for such fortuitous intersects. People are often inaugurated into marital partnerships, occupational careers, or untoward life paths through circumstances. A happenstance meeting launches a new life trajectory. Had the chance encounter not occurred, the participants' lives would have taken quite different courses. The power of most fortuitous influences lies not in the properties of the events themselves but in the interactive processes they initiate.

Of the myriad fortuitous elements encountered in daily life, many of them touch people only lightly, others leave more lasting effects, and still others thrust people into new life trajectories. Psychological science cannot foretell the occurrence of fortuitous intersects, except in a very general way. Personal proclivities, the social circles in which one moves, and the kinds of people who populate those settings make some types of intersects more probable than others. However, social cognitive theory provides a conceptual scheme for predicting the nature, scope, and strength of the impact that chance encounters will have on human lives based on the reciprocal interplay of personal attributes and the characteristics of the social milieus into which one is inaugurated (Bandura, 1982b).

The personal determinants of the impact of fortuitous encounters operate by converting chance meetings into ongoing relationships. People's attributes, interests, and skills will affect whether they can gain sufficient social acceptance and satisfaction to sustain involvement with those they happened to encounter. Emotional ties also play an influential role. Interpersonal attraction seals chance encounters into lasting bonds. Values and personal standards similarly come into play. Fortuitous meetings are more apt to last if the persons involved have similar value commitments and evaluative standards than if they clash.

The social determinants of the impact of fortuitous encounters concern the holding and shaping power of the milieus into which people are fortuitously inaugurated. Individuals become attached to groups that provide valued benefits and rewards but forsake those that have little to offer. Fortuitous induction into a group also provides a new symbolic environment designed to foster affinity, solidarity, and shape ideological perspectives on life. The belief system of milieus and their reach and degree of closedness operate as other formative environmental factors. Chance encounters have the greatest potential for abruptly branching people into new trajectories of life when they induct them into a relatively closed milieu (Bromley & Shupe, 1979; Winfrey, 1979). A totalistic environment supplies a pervading new reality— new kinships, strongly held group beliefs and values, all-encompassing codes of conduct, and substantial rewarding and coercive power to alter the entire course of personal lives.

Personal Determinants versus Individual Differences

The field of personality has traditionally relied heavily on all-purpose measures of personal attributes in efforts to explain how personal factors contribute to psychosocial functioning. In this "one fits all approach," the items are decontextualized by deleting information about the situations with which people are dealing. For example, they are asked to judge their aggressiveness in an environmental void without reference to the form of aggression, who the protagonists are, their power status, the type and level of provocation, the social setting, and other conditional circumstances that can strongly influence behavioral outcomes that affect one's proneness to act aggressively. The more general the items, the more respondents have to try to guess what the unspecified situational particulars might be. The predictiveness of indefinite global measures will depend on the extent to which the visualized activities and contextual factors on which the mental averaging is performed happen to overlap with those being studied.

The everyday realities that people must manage are structured and operate conditionally. Thus, for example, behaving assertively with indifferent store clerks will bring more attentive service, whereas confrontive assertiveness toward police officers will get one roughed up or arrested. As a consequence, people will behave assertively with clerks but compliantly with police. A shapeless overall rating is ill-equipped to explain and predict the variation in assertiveness under these different circumstances. Given the highly conditional nature of human functioning, it is unrealistic to expect personality measures cast in nonconditional generalities to shed much light on the contribution of personal factors to psychosocial functioning in different task domains under diverse circumstances across all situations. Indeed, personality measures that capture the contextualized and multifaceted nature of personal causation within an agentic model have greater explanatory and predictive power and provide more effective guides for personal change than do global trait measures (Bandura, 1997a). The convenience of all-purpose global tests of personal determinants is gained at the cost of explanatory and predictive power.

A major movement in psychology is away from global structures to more domain-linked knowledge structures, self-conceptions, and competencies. Even in the field of cognitive development, the bulwark of global structuralism (Piaget, 1950) is being abandoned for more specialized cognitive competencies (Feldman, 1980; Flavell, 1978). It is ironic that, at a time when other subfields of psychology are becoming contextualized and discarding global personal structures for more particularized ones, much of the field of personality is seeking the personal causes of human behavior in omnibus conglomerate traits severed from the social realities of everyday life.

The multifaceted dynamic nature of personal causation raises the broader issue of how personal determinants are conceptualized and measured. The influence of personal factors on human functioning is often insufficiently recognized because the issue tends to be construed in static terms of individual differences rather than personal determination of action. The issue of major interest for the science of personality is not how differences between individuals on a behavioral continuum correlate with behavior, but rather how personal factors operate in causal structures in producing and regulating behavior under the highly contingent conditions of everyday life. Consider a situation in which a personal factor is essential for certain types of performances but is developed to the same high level in different individuals. The difference among individuals is negligible and would, therefore, not correlate with performance because of constricted variability. However, the personal competence is, in fact, vital for successful performance. For example, all librarians know how to read well and do not differ in this respect, but possessing the ability to read is indispensable for performing the librarianship role.

Low correlations between "individual differences" in a personal determinant and performance resulting from curtailed variability are often misinterpreted as evidence that personal factors exert little causal impact. Personal determinants operate as multifaceted dynamic factors in causal structures rather than as static entities that people possess in differing amounts. These alternative perspectives on personal causation reflect more than differences in semantic labeling. The individual differences approach is rooted in trait theory, whereas the personal determinants approach is founded on an agentic model of functional relations between dynamic personal factors that govern the quality of human adaptation and change.

Social cognitive theory does not cede the construct of "disposition" to trait theory. Dynamic dispositions must be distinguished from static trait dispositions. For example, individuals who have a resilient sense of efficacy in a given domain are disposed to behave differently in that realm of activity from those who are beset by self-doubt. Efficacy beliefs are patterned differently across individuals and spheres of activity. The issue in contention is not whether people have personal dispositions but how dispositions are conceptualized and operationalized. In social cognitive theory, an efficacious personality disposition is a dynamic, multifaceted belief system that varies across different activity domains and under different situational demands rather than being a decontextualized conglomerate. The patterned individuality of efficacy beliefs represents the unique dispositional makeup of efficaciousness for any given person. In social cognitive theory, dispositions are personal factors such as self-beliefs, aspirations, and outcome expectations that regulate behavior rather then descriptors of habitual behavior.

DISCARDING DUALISTIC CONCEPTIONS OF PERSONALITY

Theorizing in personality often contains a variety of dualities that social cognitive theory rejects. Social cognitive theory casts off mind–body dualism. Mental events are brain activities rather than immaterial entities that exist apart from brain processes. There are a number of other dualistic conceptions that are discussed briefly in the sections that follow.

Duality of Self as Agent and Object

One common dichotomy separates self into agent and object. People are said to be agents when they act on the environment but objects when they reflect and act on themselves. Social cognitive theory questions such a dualistic view of self. Proaction does not operate isolatedly from self-reaction. The dual functions of the self typically operate interactively. In their daily transactions, people formulate courses of action, anticipate their likely effects, and act on their judgments. While acting on their environment, they are also evaluating and reacting to themselves. They monitor and analyze how well their thinking and corresponding actions have served them and change their strategies accordingly. One is just as much an agent monitoring and reflecting on one's experiences and exerting self-influence as in acting on the environment. It is simply a shift in perspective of the same agent between self and environment. Even when individuals are the object of external influence, they are not just passive recipients of stimulus inputs. They act agentically on that influence in cognitive, affective, and behavioral ways that enhance, neutralize, or subvert it. Rather than splitting the self into object and agent, social cognitive theory treats this static dichotomy as a dynamic system of interlocking functions.

Social cognitive theory also rejects the fractionation of human agency into multiple selves. A theory of personality cast in terms of multiple selves plunges one into deep philosophical waters. It requires a regress of selves to a presiding overseer self that selects and manages the collection of selves to suit given purposes. Actually, there is only one self that can visualize different futures and select courses of action designed to attain desired futures and avoid aversive ones. Actions are regulated by a person not by a cluster of selves doing the choosing and guiding.

The fractionation of agency into different types of selves poses additional conceptual problems. Once one starts fractionating the self, where does one stop? For example, an athletic self can be split into an envisioned tennis self and a golfing self. These separable selves would, in turn, have their subselves. Thus, a golfing self can be subdivided into different facets of the athletic ability to include a driving self, a fairway self, a sand-trapped self, and a putting self. How does one decide where to stop fractionating selves? Here, too, there is only one self that can strive to perfect different sets of competencies required for an envisioned pursuit. Diversity of action arises not from a collection of agentive selves but from the different options considered by the one and the same agentive self. It is the person who is doing the thinking, regulating, and reflecting not a homunculus-overseeing self.

People striving to realize an envisioned future guide and motivate their efforts through a set of self-regulatory mechanisms. These are governed by appraisal of personal capabilities for different pursuits, long-range aspiration merged with working proximal subgoals that lead to its fulfillment, positive and negative outcome expectations for different life courses, the value placed on those envisioned outcomes, and the perceived environmental constraints and opportunity structures. These represent some of the influential socio-cognitive determinants of the courses that lives take. One and the same person exercises these self-influences differentially for different purposes, in different activity domains, and in different social contexts.

Duality of Structure and Process of the Self System

The affinity to global dispositional constructs has also fostered a disjoined duality of process and structure that pervades the field of personality. This dualistic view is also reflected in the dichotomization of personality theories as embodying structuralism or functionalism. Theories that specify how human agency is exercised are often mistakenly depicted as solely process theories. Trait approaches are said to be structural theories. Social cognitive theory rejects this false separateness of structural and process theories. Regulatory processes operate through guiding self structures rather than disembodied from them. Self structures do not emerge autonomously and give rise to behavior divorced from any operational processes. Developed self structures are translated into actions through regulatory functions. The experiences produced by regulatory processes operating on the environment, in turn, shape self structures. In short, both the structure of a self system and the regulatory processes must work together in human functioning.

To illustrate the interdependence of structure and process consider the self-regulation of moral conduct. Social cognitive theory provides a detailed account of how moral standards are constructed through cognitive processing of diverse sources of information conveyed by modeled moral commitments, direct instruction in moral precepts, and the evaluative reactions of others to conduct that has ethical and moral significance (Bandura, 1991a). The nature and pattern of the acquired moral standards represent an enduring cognitive structure for judging the moral status of conduct in situations containing many morally relevant decisional ingredients. One does not have a full set of moral standards on Monday, none on Tuesday, and a new set on Wednesday. The standards of conduct are enduring unless they happen to be altered by powerful experiences. Moral structure is translated into action via self-regulatory mechanisms operating through a set of agentive subfunctions. These include self-monitoring of conduct; judging the conduct in relation to one's moral standards and the circumstances under which it occurs; and applying evaluative self-sanctions depending on whether the conduct measures up to the internal standards or violates them. In short, processes do not operate in a vacuum without structural properties that provide the substance and direction for those processes. People do not run around mindlessly engaging in structure-free processing of experiences.

A social cognitive theory combining moral rule structures and self-regulative processes operating through them is no less a structural theory of personality than, for example, the psychoanalytic approach in which a superego is posited as a structural feature of personality that controls conduct. The major differences between these two theories are in globality of constructs, explicitness of acquisitional and regulative mechanisms, and explanatory and predictive power, not in whether one theory postulates a structure and the other does not (Bandura, 1973, 1991a).

Moral rule structures do not operate as invariant internal regulators of conduct. Self-regulatory mechanisms do not operate unless they are activated, and there are many processes by which self-sanctions can be disengaged from internal standards to perpetrate inhumane conduct (Bandura, 1986, 1991a). Selective activation and disengagement of internal control thus permits different types of conduct with the same moral standards. Many inhumanities are perpetrated by people who, in other aspects of their lives and other circumstances, behave in considerate, compassionate ways (Bandura, 1991a; Kelman & Hamilton, 1989; Reich, 1990; Sanford & Comstock, 1971). Consideration of the conjoint operation of moral rule structures, self-regulatory mechanisms, and contextual influences helps to explain this seeming paradox where more global structures alone do not (Gillespie, 1971). We shall return to the issue of selective self-regulation later.

The nature and regulative function of self-conceptions provides a further illustration in which relinquishment of global measures is sometimes misconstrued as abandonment of structure. Self-appraisal has traditionally been conceptualized in personality theory in terms of the self-concept (Rogers, 1959; Wylie, 1974). Such self theories are concerned, for the most part, with global self-images. A global self-conception does not do justice to the multifaceted structure of self-belief systems. They can vary substantially across different life domains and operate dynamically in concert with other psychosocial determinants. Thus, people's self-conceptions as parents may differ from their occupational self-conception and, even in the occupational realm, their self-conceptions are likely to differ for different facets of occupational competency. Composite self-images are not equal to the task of predicting with any degree of accuracy such intraindividual variability. Social cognitive theory approaches the structure of self-belief systems in more refined, domain-linked ways that have greater explanatory and predictive power (Bandura, 1986; 1997a; Pajares & Kranzler, 1995; Pajares & Miller, 1994, 1995).

A multifaceted approach does not mean that there is no structure or generality to human functioning. Given that no two situations are ever identical, life would be unbearably burdensome if one had to figure out anew how to behave in every situation one encounters. Conversely, life would be exceedingly costly and perilous if people remained blissfully inattentive to situational factors signifying appropriate courses of action and indifferent to the personal and social effects of what they do. In short, neither isolated specificity nor obtuse indiscriminativeness is adaptive (Bandura, 1986, 1997a).

Trait theorists framed the issue of human adaptiveness in terms of "consistency" with misleading connotations that perpetuated the search for behavioral fixedness. Consistency not only implies virtues of steadfastness and principled conduct, but it sets up the contrast as "inconsistency" implying instability or expediency. In fact, action devoid of discriminative forethought would produce disastrous results. Nevertheless, the inverted value implications diverted attention from analyses of the dynamic nature of human adaptation to an elusive search on how to extract consistency from variability and efforts to explain how the same global disposition can spawn highly variable conduct (Bandura, 1986).

Much ink has been spilt in fruitless debates about whether behavior is characterized by uniformity or specificity. In fact, as already noted, adaptive functioning requires both generalization and differentiation of action. Therefore, social cognitive theory addresses the determinants and mechanisms governing both generality and specificity of action rather than championing only variability. Whether people behave uniformly or variably depends heavily upon the functional equivalence of the environments. Thus, if acting intelligently in diverse settings has functional value, people will be consistently intelligent in situations that otherwise differ markedly. By contrast, if directives to subordinates improve performance but giving commands to bosses brings rebukes, people will behave authoritatively with subordinates but diplomatically with bosses. Nor is consistency across expressive modalities a blessing. If people acted on every thought that entered their minds, or if their affect ruled every action, they would get themselves into very serious trouble. Here, too, they have to regulate their actions and affective expressions discriminatively. In their conditional conception of dispositions, Mischel and Shoda (1995) document that individuals exhibit stable but discriminative patterns of social behavior. These behavioral signatures of personality are functionally related to conditional influences that facilitate or deter certain styles of behavior. The particular organization of conditional relations characterizes the uniqueness and coherence of personality for any given individual.

Behavior patterns are not necessarily locked in temporally either. Otherwise, people would not alter their behavior over the course of their development to suit their age and the changing demands of life. Changes over the life course take diverse forms across spheres of functioning rather than follow a consistent, unidirectional course (Baltes, Lindenberger, & Staudinger, in press; Bandura, 1982b). Whether social behavior is invariant or changes over time depends partly on the degree of continuity of environmental conditions over the time span that affect the functional value of different forms of behavior. However, environments are diverse rather than monolithic. In the agentic constructivist perspective of social cognitive theory, people have a hand in promoting continuities in their life. They do so by selecting environments compatible with their values, attributes, and aspirations and by constructing social environments through their actions (Bandura, 1986, 1997a; Snyder, 1981). For example, we are all acquainted with problem-prone individuals who, by their aversive conduct, breed negative social milieus wherever they go. In contrast those skilled in bringing out the best in others create beneficial social milieus. Through selection and construction of environments, personality patterns can become self-perpetuating.

Protracted disputes continue to be fought under the banners of the idiographic view that people behave idiosyncratically as though they have no processes in common, or the nomothetic view that people's behavior follows general principles that allegedly grant no individuality. These disputes often fail to distinguish between what one thinks, feels, values, and can do from the basic mechanisms by which these personal proclivities are developed and regulated. People obviously differ in their make-up because they come with different biological endowments and experience different admixtures of influences. But cultures provide numerous common direct and modeling influences that create many similar proclivities. An idiographic psychology solely of uniqueness would be a feeble scientific enterprise devoid of generalizability and operative utility. With regard to mechanisms, all people learn through modeling and the effects of their actions. Indeed, in many cultures the word for "teach" is the same as the word for "show" (Reichard,

1938). People regulate their motivation and actions anticipatorily by judgments of their capabilities, goal aspirations, outcome expectations, and perceived environmental opportunity structures and impediments (Bandura, 1986, 1997a). Thus, there is diversity in sociostructural arrangements and the forms that lives take in different social milieus but universality in the basic acquisitional and regulative mechanisms.

Continuity has meaning when applied to distinct styles of behavior. But it takes on considerable indefiniteness when judged in terms of broad categories of adaptation. One can always find linkages between early and later endeavors as, for example, between pursuit of scholarship in childhood and professional careers in adulthood. However, at this level of generality, continuity can be achieved through a variety of life paths. Personal lives, whether marked by continuities or discontinuities have their particular characters. The rapid pace of social and technological changes increasingly requires new forms of adaptation throughout the life course (Bandura, 1997a). Broad adaptational categories mask personal changes over time. As in the explanation of both generality and specificity of behavior across contextual variations, a comprehensive theory must also explain both temporal continuities and change.

The dualistic thinking is also reflected in suggestions that the processes of sociocognitive theories be combined with trait theory, such as the five-factor taxonomy, to form the comprehensive theory of personality. According to trait structuralists, factor analyses of everyday descriptors of behavior culled from dictionaries and personality questionnaires will yield the supertraits that constitute the basic structure of personality. Some of the trait theorists rallied with missionary zeal around the "Big Five" global supertraits of extraversion, agreeableness, conscientiousness, neuroticism, and openness to experience as the universal features of personality structure. McCrae and Costa (1996), the leading proponents of this approach, relied on the computer to find the supertraits in the mixture of common descriptors, and on bootstrapping to fill them out with additional variants of the descriptors. They dismiss conceptually guided approaches to personality as "armchair theories," as though theoretical propositions are never subjected to empirical verification or translated into social applications. The epistemological issue in that metaphoric armchair, which incidentally has served other scientific disciplines remarkably well, centers on whether personologists or machines do the conceptualizing. The essentially atheoretical strategy of research, the shrinking of personal characteristics to a few global traits, the empirical status of the extracted traits, and the exaggerated claims of consensuality regarding the fivefold taxonomy drew sharp critiques (Block, 1995; Carlson, 1992; Endler & Parker, 1992; Eysenck, 1991; Kroger, 1993; McAdams, 1992). Although the fivefold clustering is presented as a "model," a descriptive classification of habitual behavior is not a conceptual model, which must specify a system of postulates governing the phenomenon of interest.

Seeking the structure of personality by factor analyzing a limited collection of behavioral descriptors essentially reduces to a psychometric method in search of a theory. In an earlier expedition in the unabridged dictionary, Gordon Allport came up with thousands of trait descriptors. This vast collection required severe pruning to reduce them to a small manageable lot. The products of factor analysis are predetermined by what one puts into it. The prepruning and the methods of factor extraction used largely preordain the clusters that will be found. Adding a few more classes of trait descriptors yields more supertraits (Almagor, Tellegen, & Waller, 1995). An even more inclusive collection of descriptors with built-in assemblages of redundancies would probably yield still more clusters. Moreover, sets of descriptors of sociocognitive belief systems and other self-regulatory factors that constitute the personality structures governing human behavior would produce quite different factors than descriptors of habitual behaviors.

Not surprisingly, there are disputes among trait theorists about how many supertraits there are. Proponents of the fivefold taxonomy assert that there are five supertraits (McCrae & Costa, 1997), but others contend that there are only two (Digman, 1997), or three (Eysenck, 1991), or six (Jackson, Ashton, & Tomes, 1996), or seven (Tellegen & Waller, 1987), and still others find even more basic traits (Barrett & Kline, 1982). Variations in the claimed size of the trait collection have fueled semantic debates about what constitutes a trait, how broad it should be, and whether traits should be analyzed as untiered groupings or as tiered groupings with cardinal traits subsuming secondary ones (Guastello, 1993). This controversy is reminiscent of the debates of yesteryear about the correct number of instincts or cardinal motives.

Trait theorists disagree not only over how many supertraits there are but what factors belong in them and what they should be called (Block, 1995). To add further to classificatory fuzziness, some of the trait descriptors show up in more than one trait cluster creating significant intertrait correlations. The traits are measured by either single word descriptors or brief phrases stripped of any contextual conditions. This is a socially disembodied reclusive personality. We know that the same behavior can mean different things in different contexts. For example, the item "prefer to do things alone" is a rejective behavior in a marital relationship but self-sufficiency in a physical fitness routine. Killing is a heroic act deserving commendation on the battlefield but a homicidal act demanding imprisonment in civilian life. The behavioral descriptors that form the trait terms may, therefore, shift from one cluster to another depending on the contexts in which the behavior is performed and the purposes it is designed to serve.

The big-five adherents spend much time comparing lists of descriptors used by different trait theorists, seeking analogues of the competitors' supertraits to the fivefold clusters, and explaining misfitting ones and how they might be subsumed under the five clusters. Formal goodness-of-fit tests, however, reveal a poor fit of the empirical data to five distinct personality features (Parker, Bagby, & Summerfeldt, 1993). The substantial intercorrelations among some of the supertraits refute their distinctiveness. McCrae and his colleagues argue that the fivefold taxonomy is correct, but the statistical methods are at fault (McCrae, Zonderman, Costa, Bond, & Paunonen, 1996). The view that the supertraits are distinct yet have overlapping defining traits does not provide an adequately specified conceptual model required for definitive tests of goodness of fit. The discounting and refitting of discordant findings convey the impression that the fivefold taxonomy has become the procrustean bed of trait theorizing. Some personologists suggest that trait theorists should seek better representation of the diversity of personal characteristics by adding clusters of theoretically distinct items rather than reiterating a fivefold clustering within a stripped-down assemblage of items (Jackson, Paunonen, Fraboni, & Goffin, 1996).

Development of a comprehensive theory of personality requires an integrated conceptual scheme that classifies not only behaviors but specifies their determinants and key mechanisms through which they operate and the modes by which desired ones can be fostered and undesired ones altered. Theory guides the development of appropriate measures, specifies the conditions for empirical verification of its core propositions, and informs effective psychosocial programs of change.

The so-called supertraits are essentially clusters of habitual behaviors. People are asked to rate whether they are courteous, methodical, curious, fearful, get into arguments, and the like. It comes as no surprise, for example, that a collection of behaviors that resemble one another, such as being organized, dutiful, disciplined, and effortful form a behavioral cluster dubbed "conscientiousness." Some of the clusters cohere better than others depending on the degree of redundancy of behavioral descriptors representing them. However, descriptive behavioral clusters tell us little about the determinants and regulative structures governing the behaviors that make up a particular cluster.

In trait analyses, the behavioral descriptors tend to get reified as causes of behavior. Consider conscientiousness as an example. In measuring this factor, individuals rate such things as whether they are "a productive person who always get the job done," "work hard to accomplish my goals," and "perform the tasks assigned to me conscientiously." Conscientious behavior is said to affect how well people perform on a job. One can, of course, use past conscientious performance as a predictor of future conscientious job performance. But conscientious behavior is neither a personality structure nor is such behavior a cause of itself.

The proponents of taxonomies founded on behavioral descriptors locate the personality structure in the wrong place. As shown in Figure 7.1, the determinative personality structures are in the self system not in the behavioral expressions. To continue with the above example, the personal determinants of job performance include, among other things, people's knowledge structures, their skills, self-beliefs of efficacy to manage given activities and environmental demands, and self-regulatory capabilities operating though goals and outcome expectancies rooted in a value structure (Bandura, 1986, 1997a; Feather, 1982; Locke & Latham, 1990). These are the personality structures and processes operating within the self system that regulate level of motivation, performance attainments, and affective states.

The paucity of guiding theory in seeking the structure of personality through factor analyses of behavioral descriptors is further revealed in the ambiguity about the sources of the supertraits. They are said to be "set like plaster" by innate endowment and unspecified experiences into terminal entities by early adulthood and remain essentially unchangeable thereafter (Costa & McCrae, 1994). The apparent fixedness of personal attributes throughout adulthood most likely has more to do with the insensitivity of nonconditional global measures than with unchangeableness of personal factors over the life course. Global measures of personal attributes mask significant patterns of changes with age that domain-linked measures reveal (Brandstädter, Krampen, & Heil, 1996; Lachman, 1996; McAvay, Seeman, & Rodin, 1996). Adding conditional factors to personality assessments further increases their sensitivity to variability in the way individuals behave in different social contexts (Matsumoto, Kudoh, & Takeuchi, 1996).

Each of the supertraits is a conglomerate of facets. For example, the supertrait "openness to experience" includes such diverse activities as endorsement of daydreaming, rejection of religious authority, excitement over art and poetry, support of controversial speakers, and trying foreign foods. An individual may display high intellectual curiosity and openness to technical and commercial ideas but not care much about exotic foods or what the glitterati decree is modern art. By contrast, another individual may support diverse artistic endeavors but act like a Luddite toward technological innovations. Efforts to understand the nature, origin, and predictiveness of scientific curiosity, for example, should not clutter the personal determinant with preferences for exotic foods. It is not that a general disposition predicts behavior, but that a few of the behavioral descriptors in the conglomerate mixture may provide some overlap with the particular behavior being predicted to yield a correlate. Global conglomerates do not lend themselves to causal analyses because human experiences do not occur at the level of averaged behavioral conglomerates or life circumstances reduced to a nondescript average.

Nor are conglomerate measures equipped to explain the wide variations in behavior by the same individual in a given domain of activity under different situational circumstances. Trait theorists sought to remedy the weak predictiveness of trait indices by averaging ratings of behavior across situations and occasions, which presumably provides a truer measure of the trait

(Epstein, 1983). However, aggregation does not produce much predictive gain when actual behavior in different situations rather than self-reports of behavior is measured (Rushton, Brainerd, & Pressley, 1983). No amount of aggregation will elevate correlations between a given form of behavior under different circumstances that social sanctions have disjoined. Aggressive acts by delinquents toward parish priests and toward rival gang members will correlate poorly, however much averaging one does. In a world characterized by contingency, one can lose rather than gain predictive power by trying to predict behavior from an average value that typifies neither situation. The situational averaging solution reminds one of the nonswimmer who drowned while crossing a river that averaged only 3 feet in depth.

Other efforts to boost correlates included aggregating differing forms of conduct, such as physical aggression, verbal aggression, and antagonistic conduct into a conglomerate index. Mixing behaviors obscures the understanding of psychological functioning as does the mixing of situations. To be able to predict through aggregation that individuals will sometime, somewhere, do something within a wide assortment of acts is of no great interest. For example, people want to know whether adolescent offenders are likely to commit physical assaults, not whether sometime, somewhere, they may speak offensively or behave antagonistically, or do something else untoward.

There is little evidence that the repackaging of traits in a fivefold format has produced any better prediction of human behavior than do the traditional trait measures (Pervin, 1994), which are not much to rave about. The inflated self-congratulatory claims of breakthrough stand in stark contrast to the paucity of empirical reality tests of predictiveness. It is the replication of fivefold clustering rather than evidence of predictive power that seems to be racing the pulse of adherents to this taxonomic view of personality. It should be noted in passing that the standard correlate of omnibus trait measures is not .30, as commonly assumed. When it comes to predicting particular forms of behavior, global measures are weaker or nonsignificant predictors. Gains in social consensus among trait theorists about the number of supertraits without gains in predictive power hardly constitute an advance in the field of personality.

Job productivity is often cited as a domain in which the predictive utility of the fivefold approach has been demonstrated. In commenting on behavioral description versus prediction, Hough (1992) notes that the fivefold supertraits are not only too general and heterogeneous in facets but lack relevant factors to be useful in accounting for job performance. Innumerable studies have shown that personal goals are consistent predictors of job productivity (Locke & Latham, 1990). Barrick, Mount, and Strauss (1993) found that conscientiousness was related to actual sales productivity but neither extraversion, which presumably should make good sellers, nor any of the other supertraits had any predictive value. Even the relationship between conscientiousness and sales performance disappears when the influence of the goals employees set for themselves is removed. Given the view that personality is essentially unchangeable after early adulthood, this taxonomic approach offers little hope of self-betterment along the life course for those who happened to have gotten off to a poor start. Once cast into a nonconscientious mold by innate endowment and experience, one remains ever nonconscientious thereafter. To continue with the productivity example, goal theory offers a much more optimistic view of human changeableness with sound conceptual and empirical backing on how to instill goals and how they work. Teaching people how to regulate their motivation and activities through goal setting enables them to achieve sizable increases in productivity regardless of their age or sphere of activity (Bandura, 1991b; Locke & Latham, 1990).

The value of a psychological theory is judged not only by its explanatory and predictive power but also by its operative power to guide change in human functioning. A descriptive taxonomy of aggregated behaviors offers no guidance on how to effect personal or social change. Social cognitive theory provides a large body of particularized knowledge on how to develop the cognitive structures and enlist the processes of the self system that govern human adaptation and change (Bandura, 1986, 1997a). It lends itself readily to applications because the factors it posits are empirically anchored in indices of functioning and are amenable to change. The determinants and mechanisms through which they operate are spelled out so the theory provides explicit guidelines on how to structure conditions that foster personal and social change.

One could argue that a taxonomic scheme is not designed to be explanatory or prescriptive for change. However, trait theorists often make conflicting claims. On the one hand, their classification scheme is portrayed as simply a descriptive taxonomy. Once the major classes of behavior are firmly established, their origins and functions could be examined. On the other hand, behavioral characteristics are often reified as dynamic causal factors. This creates a serious problem of circularity: Behavior becomes the cause of behavior. Even as descriptive taxonomies, global traits cannot shed much light on the nature of personal causation because personal determinants operate conditionally at a particular contextualized level not at a socially detached conglomerate level.

Duality of Social Structure and Personal Agency

Human adaptation and change are rooted in social systems. Therefore, personal agency operates within a broad network of sociostructural influences. In these agentic transactions, people are producers as well as products of social systems. Social structures are devised to organize, guide, and regulate human affairs in given domains by authorized rules and sanctions. For the most part, social structures represent authorized social practices carried out by human beings occupying designated roles (Giddens, 1984). Within the rule structures, there is a lot of personal variation in their interpretation, enforcement, adoption, circumvention, or active opposition (Burns & Dietz, in press). It is not a dichotomy between a disembodied social structure and personal agency but a dynamic interplay between individuals and those who preside over the institutionalized operations of social systems. Social structures are created by human activity. The structural practices, in turn, impose constraints and provide resources and opportunity structures for personal development and functioning. Given this dynamic bidirectionality of influence, social cognitive theory rejects a dualism between personal agency and social structure.

Sociostructural theories and psychological theories are often regarded as rival conceptions of human behavior or as representing different levels and proximity of causation. Human behavior cannot be fully understood solely in terms of sociostructural factors or psychological factors. A full understanding requires an integrated perspective in which sociostructural influences operate through psychological mechanisms to produce behavioral effects. However, the self system is not merely a conduit for external influences. The self is socially constituted, but, by exercising self-influence, human agency operates generatively and proactively on social systems not just reactively.

In the theory of triadic reciprocal causation, sociostructural and personal determinants are treated as cofactors within a unified causal structure (Bandura, 1997a). Diverse lines of research lend support to this interdependent multicausality. For example, poverty is not a matter of multilayered or distal causation; it impinges pervasively on everyday life in a very proximal way. Elder and his colleagues show that economic hardship, by itself, has no direct influence on parents' efficacy to promote their children's development (Elder & Ardelt, 1992). Families who feel overwhelmed by the hardships experience high subjective strain, whereas those who feel they can make it through tough times experience less emotional strain. In intact households, subjective strain impairs parental efficacy by increasing marital discord. For single parents, subjective strain weakens parents' sense of efficacy both directly and by creating feelings of despondency. Thus the impact of both economic conditions and family structure operate through self processes.

Similarly, socioeconomic status does not directly affect children's academic development. Rather, it does so by influencing parents' educational aspirations for their children (Bandura, Barbaranelli, Caprara, & Pastorelli, 1996a). Parental aspirations and belief in their educational parenting efficacy, in turn, influence their children's scholastic performances by raising their educational aspirations and beliefs in their scholastic capabilities. Different facets of perceived self-efficacy operating in concert with other psychosocial factors contribute to academic achievement through different mediated paths. Multifaceted measures thus provide a refined view of causal structures that global measures of perceived efficacy cannot provide.

A similar integrated causality governs occupational trajectories of youth (Bandura, Barbaranelli, Caprara, & Pastorelli, 1999). Socioeconomic status has no direct effects on either occupational efficacy or career considerations. Rather, it has an indirect impact by influencing parents' beliefs in their efficacy to promote their children's educational development and the aspirations they hold for them. Parental efficacy and aspirations raise children's educational aspirations and their sense of academic, social, and self-regulatory efficacy. The patterning of children's perceived efficacy influences the types of occupational activities they believe they can do and, in turn, is linked to the kinds of jobs they would choose for their life's work. In other aspects of family functioning, the impact of socioeconomic status on child outcomes is entirely mediated through parents' child management practices (Baldwin, Baldwin, Sameroff, & Seifer, 1989).

Similar paths of multicausality mediated through self processes are evident in the functioning of educational systems as well as familial systems. Schools that have many poor students and those of disadvantaged minority status generally do poorly academically. However, these sociodemographic characteristics exert their impact on schools' level of achievement largely by shaping teachers' beliefs in their collective efficacy to motivate and educate their students (Bandura, 1997a). Schools that have teachers who believe strongly in their collective instructional efficacy do well academically regardless of the sociodemographic characteristics of the student bodies. In verifying the path of influence from sociostructural conditions through familial and self-regulatory processes, these types of studies clarify how personal agency operates within a broad network of sociostructural influences.

FUNDAMENTAL HUMAN CAPABILITIES

In social cognitive theory, people are neither driven by global traits nor automatically shaped and controlled by the environment. As we have already seen, they function as contributors to their own motivation, behavior, and development within a network of reciprocally interacting influences. Persons are characterized within this theoretical perspective in terms of a number of fundamental capabilities. These are reviewed in the sections that follow.

Symbolizing Capability

Social cognitive theory assigns a central role to cognitive, vicarious, self-regulatory, and self-reflective processes in human development and functioning (Bandura, 1986). The extraordinary capacity to represent events and their relationships in symbolic form provides humans with a powerful tool for comprehending their environment and for creating and managing environmental conditions that touch virtually every aspect of their lives. Symbols serve as the vehicle of thought.

Most environmental events exert their effects through cognitive processing rather than directly. Cognitive factors partly determine which environmental events are observed, what meaning is conferred on them, what emotional impact and motivating power they have, and how the information they convey is organized and preserved for future use. Through the medium of symbols, people transform transient experiences into cognitive models that serve as guides for reasoning and action. People transcend time and place in communicating with others at any distance. By symbolizing their experiences, people give structure, meaning, and continuity to their lives.

Knowledge provides the substance and thinking operations provide the tools for cognitive problem solving. Rather than solve problems solely by performing actions and suffering the consequences of missteps, people usually test possible solutions in thought. They generate alternative solutions to problems and discard or retain them based on estimated outcomes without having to go through a laborious behavioral search. The remarkable flexibility of symbolization also enables people to create novel and fanciful ideas that transcend their sensory experiences. One can easily think of cows jumping over the moon even though these feats are physically impossible. The other distinctive human capabilities are founded on this advanced capacity for symbolization. However, in keeping with the interactional perspective, social cognitive theory specifies the social origins of thought and the mechanisms through which social factors exert their influence on cognitive functioning (Bandura, 1986).

Although the capacity for symbolization vastly expands human capabilities, if put to faulty use, it can also breed personal distress. Many human dysfunctions and torments stem from problems of thought. This is because, in their thoughts, people often dwell on painful pasts and on perturbing futures of their own invention. They burden themselves with stressful arousal through anxiety-provoking rumination. They debilitate their own efforts by self-doubting and other self-defeating ideation. They constrain and impoverish their lives through phobic thinking. They drive themselves to despondency by harsh self-evaluation and dejecting modes of thinking. And they often act on misconceptions that get them into trouble. Thought can thus be a source of human failings and distress as well as a source of human accomplishments.

Vicarious Capability

A comprehensive theory of personality must explain the acquisition of competencies, attitudes, values, and emotional proclivities not just the enactments of behaviors that get dubbed as traits. There are two basic modes of learning. People learn by experiencing the effects of their actions and through the power of social modeling. Psychological theories have focused almost exclusively on learning from positive and negative response consequences. Natural endowment provides humans with enabling biological systems but few inborn skills. Skills must be developed over long periods and altered to fit changing conditions over the life course. If knowledge and skills had to be shaped laboriously by response consequences without the benefit of modeled guidance, a culture could never transmit its language, social practices, mores, and adaptive competencies. Mistakes can produce costly or even fatal consequences. The prospects of survival would, therefore, be slim indeed if one had to rely solely on trial-and-error experiences. Moreover, the constraints of time, resources, and mobility impose severe limits on the situations and activities that can be directly explored for the acquisition of new knowledge and skills. Fortunately, the tedious and hazardous trial-and-error learning can be short cut by social modeling.

Humans have evolved an advanced capacity for observational learning that enables them to expand their knowledge and competencies rapidly through the information conveyed by the rich variety of models. Virtually all behavioral, cognitive, and affective learning from direct experience can be achieved vicariously by observing people's actions and the consequences for them (Bandura, 1986; Rosenthal & Zimmerman, 1978).

Much human learning occurs either designedly or unintentionally from the models in one's immediate environment. However, a vast amount of knowledge about people, places, and styles of thinking and behaving is gained from the extensive modeling in the symbolic environment of the electronic mass media. A major significance of symbolic modeling lies in its tremendous scope and multiplicative power. Unlike learning by doing, which requires shaping the actions of each individual through repeated consequences, in observational learning, a single model can transmit new ways of thinking and behaving simultaneously to many people in widely dispersed locales. Video and computer delivery systems feeding off telecommunications satellites are now rapidly diffusing new ideas, values, and styles of conduct worldwide.

Most psychological theories were cast long before the advent of revolutionary advances in the technology of communication. As a result, they give insufficient attention to the increasingly powerful role that the symbolic environment plays in contemporary societies. For example, television has vastly expanded the range of models to which members of society are exposed day in and day out. By drawing on these modeled patterns of thought and behavior, observers transcend the bounds of their immediate environment. Because the symbolic environment occupies a major part of people's everyday lives, the study of human development and acculturation in the electronic era must be broadened to include electronic acculturation. At the societal level, symbolic modes of modeling are transforming how social systems operate and serving as a major vehicle for sociopolitical change (Bandura, 1997a; Braithwaite, 1994).

Observational learning, which can take the form of behavioral, cognitive, valuational, and affective change, is governed by four component subfunctions (Figure 7.2). "Attentional processes" determine what people observe in the profusion of modeling influences and what information they extract from what they notice. People cannot be much influenced by observed events if they do not remember them. A second major subfunction governing observational learning concerns "representational processes." Retention involves an active process of transforming and restructuring the information conveyed by modeled events into rules and conceptions for memory representation. In the third subfunction—"the behavioral production process"— symbolic conceptions are translated into appropriate courses of action. This is achieved through a conception-matching process in which behavioral enactments are restructured until they match the conception of the activity.

Behavior operates under hierarchical levels of control. Cognitive guidance is important in early and intermediate phases of competency development. Once proficient modes of behavior become routinized, they are regulated largely by lower sensory-motor systems and no longer require higher cognitive control (Carroll & Bandura, 1990). However, when routinized behavior patterns fail to produce desired results, cognitive control again comes into play in the search for better solutions. Control reverts to lower control systems after an adequate means is found and becomes the habitual way of doing things.

Partial disengagement of thought from proficient action has considerable functional value because it frees cognitive activity for matters requiring attention. If one had to think before carrying out every routine activity, it would consume most of one's attention and create a monotonously dull inner life. Efficient functioning requires a mix of routinized and mindful action. As a result of routinization, people often react with fixed ways of thinking unreflectively and with habitual ways of behaving unthinkingly. Nonconscious information processing and routinization of thought and action should be distinguished from an unconscious mind acting as a concealed agent orchestrating behavior in an unwitting host organism. To reify, from evidence of automatic and routinized responses, a subterranean agent steering perceptions and actions is to commit a serious metaphysical transgression.

The fourth subfunction in modeling concerns "motivational processes." Social cognitive theory distinguishes between acquisition and performance because people do not perform everything they learn. Performance of observationally learned behavior is influenced by three major types of incentive motivators—direct, vicarious, and self-produced. People are more likely to adopt modeled styles of behavior if they produce valued outcomes than if they have unrewarding or punishing effects. The observed cost and benefits accruing to others influence the adoption of modeled patterns in much the

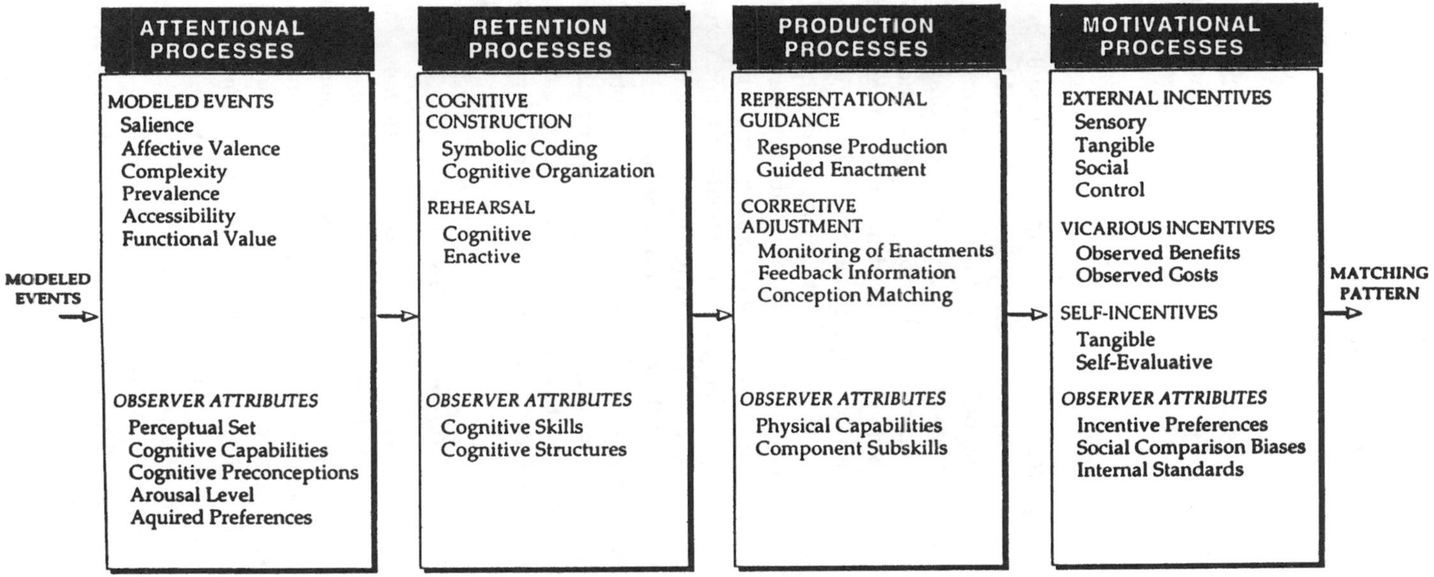

ATTENTIONAL PROCESSES

MODELED EVENTS
Salience
Affective Valence
Complexity
Prevalence
Accessibility
Functional Value

OBSERVER ATTRIBUTES
Perceptual Set
Cognitive Capabilities
Cognitive Preconceptions
Arousal Level
Aquired Preferences

RETENTION PROCESSES

COGNITIVE CONSTRUCTION
Symbolic Coding
Cognitive Organization

REHEARSAL
Cognitive
Enactive

OBSERVER ATTRIBUTES
Cognitive Skills
Cognitive Structures

PRODUCTION PROCESSES

REPRESENTATIONAL GUIDANCE
Response Production
Guided Enactment

CORRECTIVE ADJUSTMENT
Monitoring of Enactments
Feedback Information
Conception Matching

OBSERVER ATTRIBUTES
Physical Capabilities
Component Subskills

MOTIVATIONAL PROCESSES

EXTERNAL INCENTIVES
Sensory
Tangible
Social
Control

VICARIOUS INCENTIVES
Observed Benefits
Observed Costs

SELF-INCENTIVES
Tangible
Self-Evaluative

OBSERVER ATTRIBUTES
Incentive Preferences
Social Comparison Biases
Internal Standards

MODELED EVENTS →

MATCHING PATTERN →

FIGURE 7.2. Four subprocesses governing observational learning. From Bandura (1986). Copyright 1986 by Prentice-Hall. Reprinted by permission.

209

same way as do directly experienced consequences. People are motivated by the successes of others who are similar to themselves, but they are discouraged from pursuing courses of behavior that they have seen often result in aversive consequences. The evaluative reactions people generate to their own behavior also regulate which observationally learned activities they are most likely to pursue. People express what they find self-satisfying and reject what they personally disapprove.

Abstract and Creative Modeling

Modeling is not simply a process of response mimicry as commonly believed. Modeled judgments and actions may differ in specific content but embody the same rule. For example, a model may deal with moral dilemmas that differ widely in the nature of the activity but apply the same moral standard to them. Modeled activities thus convey rules for generative and innovative behavior. This higher-level learning is achieved through abstract modeling. Once observers extract the rules underlying the modeled activities, they can generate new behaviors that go beyond what they have seen or heard.

Creativeness rarely springs entirely from individual inventiveness. A lot of modeling goes on in creativity. By refining preexisting innovations, synthesizing them into new ways and adding novel elements to them, something new is created. When exposed to models of differing styles of thinking and behaving, observers vary in what they adopt from the different sources and thereby create new blends of personal characteristics that differ from the individual models (Bandura, Ross, & Ross, 1963). Modeling influences that exemplify new perspectives and innovative styles of thinking also foster creativity by weakening conventional mind sets (Belcher, 1975; Harris & Evans, 1973).

Motivational, Emotional, and Valuational Effects

In addition to cultivating new competencies, modeling influences can alter incentive motivation (Bandura, 1986). Seeing others achieve desired outcomes by their efforts can instill motivating outcome expectations in observers that they can secure similar benefits for comparable performances. These motivational effects rest on observers' judgments that they have the efficacy to produce the modeled level of attainments and that comparable accomplishments will bring them similar beneficial outcomes. By the same token, seeing others punished for engaging in certain activities can instill negative outcome expectations that serve as disincentives.

People are easily aroused by the emotional expressions of others. If the affective reactions of models only aroused observers fleetingly, it would be of limited psychological import. What gives significance to vicarious emotional influence is that observers can acquire lasting attitudes and emotional and behavioral proclivities toward persons, places, or things that have been associated with modeled emotional experiences. They learn to fear the things that frightened models, to dislike what repulsed them, and to like what gratified them (Bandura, 1992; Berger, 1962; Duncker, 1938). Fears and intractable phobias are ameliorated by modeling influences that convey information about coping strategies for exercising control over the things that are feared. The stronger the instilled sense of perceived coping efficacy, the bolder the behavior (Bandura, 1997a; Williams, 1992). Values can similarly be developed and altered vicariously by repeated exposure to modeled preferences.

During the course of their daily lives, people have direct contact with only a small sector of the physical and social environment. In their daily routines, they travel the same routes, visit the same familiar places, and see the same group of friends and associates. As a result, their conceptions of social reality are greatly influenced by symbolic representations of society, mainly by the mass media (Gerbner, 1972). To a large extent, people act on their images of reality. The more their conceptions of the world around them depend on portrayals in the media's symbolic environment, the greater is its social impact (Ball-Rokeach & DeFleur, 1976).

To sum up, modeling influences serve diverse functions—as tutors, motivators, social prompters, emotion arousers, and shapers of values and conceptions of reality. The vast body of knowledge on vicarious processes is being widely applied for personal development, therapeutic purposes, and social change (Bandura, 1986, 1997a; Bandura & Rosenthal, 1978; Rogers, Vaughan, Swalehe, Rao, & Sood, 1996; Singhal & Rogers, 1989).

Forethought Capability

Another distinctive human characteristic is the capacity for forethought. The ability to bring anticipated outcomes to bear on current activities promotes foresightful behavior. It enables people to transcend the dictates of their immediate environment and to shape and regulate the present to fit a desired future. Much human self-directedness is the product of forethought. The future time perspective manifests itself in many different ways. People set goals for themselves, anticipate the likely consequences of prospective actions, and plan courses of action likely to produce desired outcomes and avoid detrimental ones (Bandura, 1991b; Feather, 1982; Locke & Latham, 1990; Markus & Nurius, 1986; Pervin, 1989). Through the exercise of forethought, people motivate themselves and guide their actions anticipatorily. When projected over a long time course on matters of value, a forethoughtful perspective provides direction, coherence, and meaning to one's life. As people progress in their life course, they continue to plan ahead, reorder their priorities, and structure their lives accordingly.

The capacity for intentional purposive action is rooted in symbolic activity. Future events cannot, of course, be causes of current motivation and action because they have no actual existence. However, by being represented

cognitively in the present, foreseeable future events are converted into current motivators and regulators of behavior. In this form of anticipatory self-
guidance, behavior is motivated and directed by anticipated outcomes rather
than being pulled by an unrealized future state.

Outcome Expectations

People regulate their behavior partly by outcome expectations. Courses of
action that are likely to produce positive outcomes are generally adapted and
used; those that bring unrewarding or punishing outcomes are usually dis-
carded. Response consequences do not automatically shape and control
actions as claimed by radical behaviorists. Rather, people construct outcome
expectations from observed conditional relations between environmental
events and between given actions and outcomes (Bandura, 1986). In social
cognitive theory, "reinforcement" is a form of incentive motivation operating
through outcome expectations rather than an automatic strengthener of
responses.

Because outcomes exert their influence through forethought, they have
little or no motivational or behavioral impact until people discover how outcomes are linked to actions in their environment. This is no easy matter. In
everyday life, actions usually produce mixed effects: The outcomes may
occur immediately or far removed in time; the same behavior may have different effects depending on where, when, and toward whom it is performed,
and many situational factors affect behavioral outcomes. Such causal ambiguity provides a fertile ground for misjudgment. When belief about the
effects of actions differs from actuality, behavior is weakly controlled by its
actual consequences until repeated experience instills realistic beliefs. Yet it is
not always one's beliefs that change in the direction of social reality. Acting
on erroneous beliefs can alter how others behave, thus shaping the social reality in the direction of the misbeliefs (Snyder, 1980).

External consequences are not the only kind of outcomes that influence
human behavior. As noted earlier, people profit from the successes and mistakes of others as well as from their own experiences. As a general rule, they
do things they have seen succeed and avoid those they have seen fail. However, observed outcomes exert their influence through perceived similarity
that one is likely to experience similar outcomes for similar courses of action
and that one possesses the capabilities to achieve similar performances.

Observed outcomes can also affect the level of motivation by altering the
value of external outcomes through social comparison processes. People weigh
their own outcomes by those accruing to others for similar performances. For
example, the same monetary raise is likely to be viewed negatively by persons
who have seen colleagues compensated more generously, but viewed positively if colleagues have been compensated less well. The relational properties
of incentives affect not only motivation and performance but personal satisfac-

tion and discontent. Equitable outcomes foster a sense of well-being; inequitable ones breed discontent and resentment (Bandura, 1973; Martin, 1981).

Self-Regulatory Capability

People are not only knowers and performers guided by outcome expectations. They are also self-reactors with a capacity for self-direction. This capability is grounded in a self-regulatory structure. Successful development requires the substitution of internal regulation and direction for external sanctions and demands. Once the capability for self-direction is developed, self-demands and self-sanctions serve as major guides, motivators, and deterrents. In the absence of internal standards and self-sanctions, people would behave like weather vanes, constantly shifting direction to conform to whatever momentary influence happened to impinge upon them.

Subfunctions of Self-Regulation

The self-regulation of motivation, affect, and action operates through a set of psychological subfunctions (Figure 7.3). They include self-monitoring, judgmental, and self-reactive subfunctions.

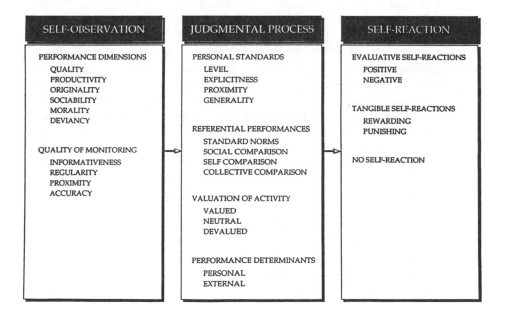

FIGURE 7.3. Structure of the system of self-regulation of motivation and action through internal standards and self-reactive influence. From Bandura (1986). Copyright 1986 by Prentice-Hall. Reprinted by permission.

People cannot influence their own motivation and actions very well if they do not pay adequate attention to their thought processes and performances, the conditions under which they occur, and to the immediate and distal effects they produce. Therefore, success in self-regulation partly depends on the fidelity, consistency, and temporal proximity of self-monitoring (Kazdin, 1974). Depending on people's values and the functional significance of different activities, they attend selectively to certain aspects of their functioning and ignore those that are of little import to them.

Observing one's pattern of behavior is the first step toward doing something to affect it, but in itself, such information provides little basis for self-directed reactions. Actions give rise to self-reactions through a judgmental function that includes several subsidiary processes. Personal standards for judging and guiding one's actions play a major role in self-motivation and in the exercise of self-directedness (Bandura, 1991b; Bandura & Cervone, 1983, 1986; Locke & Latham, 1990). Whether a given performance is regarded favorably or negatively will depend upon the personal standards against which it is evaluated. Once people commit themselves to a valued goal, they seek self-satisfaction from fulfilling it and are prompted to intensify their efforts by discontent with substandard performances. The anticipated affective self-reactions serve as incentive motivators for personal accomplishments.

For most activities, there are no absolute measures of adequacy. People must, therefore, evaluate their performances in relation to the attainments of others (Festinger, 1954; Goethals & Darley, 1977). The referential comparisons may take the form of performance attainments of others in similar situations, standard norms based on representative groups, one's own past attainments, or comparative group performance in societies organized around collectivistic principles (Bandura, 1986; Bandura & Jourden, 1991). Another factor in the judgmental component of self-regulation concerns the valuation of activities. The more relevant performances are to one's value preferences and sense of personal adequacy, the more likely self-evaluative reactions are to be elicited in that activity. Self-reactions also vary depending on how people perceive the determinants of their behavior (Weiner, 1986). They are most likely to take pride in their accomplishments when they ascribe their successes to their own abilities and efforts. They respond self-critically to faulty performances for which they hold themselves responsible but not to those they perceive as due to unusual circumstances, to insufficient capabilities, or to unrealistic demands.

Motivation based on personal standards involves a cognitive comparison process between the standards and perceived performance attainments. The motivational effects do not stem from the standards themselves but rather from several self-reactive influences. These include perceived self-efficacy to fulfill one's standards, affective self-evaluation of one's attainments, and adjustment of proximal subgoals depending on the progress one is making (Bandura 1991b; Bandura & Cervone, 1986).

Performance judgments set the occasion for self-reactive influence. Self-reactions provide the linking mechanism by which standards regulate courses of action. The self-regulatory control is achieved by creating incentives for one's own actions and by anticipative affective reactions to one's own behavior depending on how it measures up to personal standards. Thus, people pursue courses of action that give them self-satisfaction and a sense of self-worth, but they refrain from behaving in ways that result in self-censure.

Some of the self-motivating incentives may be tangible outcomes, as when people get themselves to do things they would otherwise put off or avoid altogether by making tangible rewards dependent upon performance attainments. However, people value their self-respect and the self-satisfaction derived from a job well done more highly than they do material rewards. The self-regulation of behavior by self-evaluative reactions is a uniquely human capability. Self-evaluation gives direction to behavior and creates motivators for it.

Most theories of self-regulation are founded on a negative feedback system (Carver & Scheier, 1981; Lord & Hanges, 1987; Powers, 1973). In this view, negative discrepancy between one's perceived performance and an adopted standard motivates action to reduce the disparity. However, self-regulation by negative discrepancy tells only half the story and not necessarily the more interesting half. People are proactive, aspiring organisms. Human self-motivation relies both on discrepancy production and discrepancy reduction. It requires proactive control as well as reactive control. People initially motivate themselves through proactive control by setting themselves valued performance standards that create a state of disequilibrium and then mobilizing their effort on the basis of anticipatory estimation of what it would take to reach them. Feedback control comes into play in subsequent adjustments of effort expenditure to achieve desired results. After people attain the standard they have been pursuing, those who have a strong sense of efficacy generally set a higher standard for themselves. The adoption of further challenges creates new motivating discrepancies to be mastered.

Interplay between Personal and External Outcomes

After self-regulatory capabilities are developed, behavior usually produces two sets of consequences: self-evaluative reactions and external outcomes. They may operate as complementary or opposing influences on behavior (Bandura, 1986). External outcomes are most likely to wield influence when they are compatible with self-evaluative ones. This condition exists when externally rewardable actions are a source of self-satisfaction and self-pride and when externally punishable ones bring self-censure. Behavior is also highly susceptible to external influences in the absence of countervailing internal standards. People with weak commitment to personal standards adopt a pragmatic orientation, tailoring their behavior to fit whatever the situation seems to call for (Snyder, 1987). They become adept at reading social cues and varying their self-presentation accordingly.

People commonly experience conflicts of outcomes when they are rewarded socially or materially for behavior they personally devalue. When self-devaluative consequences outweigh the force of external rewards, they have little sway. There is no more devastating consequence than self-contempt. But if the allure of rewards outweigh self-censure, the result can be cheerless compliance. However, people possess sociocognitive skills for reconciling perturbing disparities between personal standards and conduct. The mechanisms by which losses of self-respect for devalued conduct are reduced is considered shortly.

Another type of conflict of outcomes arises when individuals are punished for activities they value highly. Principled dissenters and nonconformists often find themselves in such predicaments. The relative strength of self-approval and external censure determine whether the courses of action will be pursued or abandoned. There are individuals, however, whose sense of self-worth is so strongly invested in certain convictions that they will submit to prolonged maltreatment rather than accede to what they regard as unjust or immoral. Sir Thomas More, who was beheaded for refusing to compromise his resolute convictions, is a notable example from history. It is not uncommon for people to endure hardships for unyielding adherence to ideological and moral principles.

Another common situation is one in which both the external support and reward for given activities are minimal or lacking, and individuals have to sustain their efforts largely through self-encouragement. For example, innovators persevere despite repeated failures in endeavors that provide neither rewards nor recognition for long periods, if at all during their lifetime. Innovative pursuits that clash with existing preferences bring criticism and social rejection. To persist, innovators must be sufficiently convinced of their efficacy, the worth of their pursuit to self-reward their efforts, and not be much concerned with the opinions of others (Shepherd, 1995; White, 1982).

Disengagement of Moral Self-Regulatory Agency

In development of competencies and aspirational pursuits, the self-regulatory standards selected as a mark of adequacy are progressively raised as knowledge and skills are acquired and challenges are met. In many areas of social and moral behavior, the self-regulatory standards have greater stability. People do not change from week to week what they regard as right or wrong or good or bad. Self-sanctions keep conduct in line with personal standards. However, moral standards do not function as fixed internal regulators of conduct, as implied by theories of internalization that posit global entities such as conscience and superego as constant overseers of conduct. There are many social and psychological maneuvers by which moral self-reactions can be selectively disengaged from inhumane conduct (Bandura, 1991a). Figure 7.4 shows that the disengagement may center on the conduct itself, on the sense of personal agency for the actions taken, the consequences that flow from actions, or on the victims of mistreatment.

One set of disengagement practices operates on the cognitive construal of the conduct itself. In this process of "moral justification, detrimental conduct is made personally and socially acceptable by portraying it as serving socially worthy or moral purposes. People can then act on a moral imperative. Voltaire put it well when he said, "Those who can make you believe absurdities can make you commit atrocities." Over the centuries, much destructive conduct has been perpetrated by ordinary, decent people in the name of righteous ideologies, religious principles, and nationalistic imperatives (Kelman & Hamilton, 1989; Rapoport & Alexander, 1982; Reich, 1990; Sanford & Comstock, 1971).

Language shapes thought patterns on which actions are based. Activities can take on very different appearances depending on what they are called. Not surprisingly, "sanitizing euphemistic language" is widely used to make harmful conduct respectable and to reduce personal responsibility for it (Bolinger, 1982; Lutz, 1987). How behavior is viewed is also colored by what it is compared against. The more flagrant the inhumanities against which one's destructive conduct is contracted, the more likely it will lose its repug-

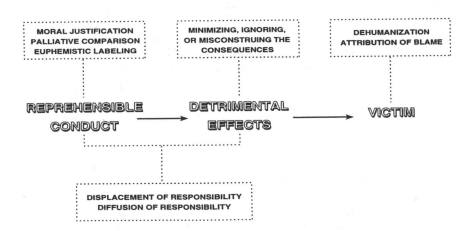

FIGURE 7.4. Mechanisms through which moral self-sanctions are selectively activated or disengaged from reprehensible conduct at different points in the self-regulatory process. From Bandura (1986). Copyright 1986 by Prentice-Hall. Reprinted by permission.

nancy or even appear benevolent. "Exonerating comparison" relies heavily on moral justification by utilitarian arguments that one's injurious actions will prevent more human suffering than they cause.

Cognitive restructuring of harmful conduct through moral justifications, sanitizing language, and exonerating comparisons is the most effective psychological mechanism for disengaging moral control. Investing harmful conduct with high moral purpose not only eliminates self-censure, but it engages self-approval in the service of destructive exploits as well. What was once morally condemnable, becomes a source of self-pride.

Moral control operates most strongly when people acknowledge that they are contributors to harmful outcomes. The second set of disengagement practices operates by obscuring or minimizing the agentive role in the harm one causes. This is achieved by "displacement and diffusion of responsibility." People will behave in ways they normally repudiate if a legitimate authority accepts responsibility for the effects of their conduct (Diener, 1977; Milgram, 1974; Zimbardo, 1995). Disclaim of personal agency removes self-condemning reactions to one's harmful conduct. As C. P. Snow insightfully observed, "More hideous crimes have been committed in the name of obedience than in the name of rebellion." The exercise of moral control is also weakened when personal agency is obscured by diffusing responsibility for detrimental behavior by group decision making, subdividing injurious activities into seemingly harmless parts, and exploiting the anonymity of collective action.

Additional ways of weakening moral control operate by "disregarding or distorting harm" caused by one's conduct (Klass, 1978). As long as the harmful effects are ignored, minimized, distorted, or disbelieved, there is little reason for self-censure to be activated. The final set of disengagement practices operates on the recipients of detrimental acts. Blaming one's adversaries or compelling circumstances can serve self-exonerative purposes. In this process, people view themselves as faultless victims driven to harmful conduct by provocation. Through "ascription of blame," injurious conduct becomes a justifiable defensive reaction to perceived provocations and mistreatments. Victims get blamed for bringing the suffering on themselves (Ferguson & Rule, 1983).

The strength of moral self-censure depends partly on how the perpetrators view the people they mistreat. To perceive another as human activates empathetic and vicarious emotional reactions through perceived similarity (Bandura, 1992). Self-censure for cruel conduct can be disengaged by "dehumanization" that strips people of human qualities. Once dehumanized, they are no longer viewed as persons with feelings, hopes, and concerns but as subhuman objects. If dispossessing one's foes of humanness does not weaken self-censure, it can be eliminated by attributing demonic or bestial qualities to them. It is easier to brutalize people when they are viewed as low animal forms (Bandura, Underwood, & Fromson, 1975; Haritos-Fatouros, 1988; Keen, 1986).

Psychological research tends to emphasize how easy it is to get good people to perform cruel deeds through dehumanization and other self-exonerative means (Milgram, 1974). What is rarely noted is the striking evidence that most people refuse to behave cruelly, even with strong authoritarian commands, toward people who are humanized (Bandura et al., 1975). The affirmation of common humanity can bring out the best in others.

Developmental research sheds some light on how the mechanisms of moral disengagement promote antisocial and destructive conduct. They weaken self-censure for harmful conduct, reduce prosocialness, and foster cognitive and emotional reactions conducive to antisocial conduct (Bandura, Barbaranelli, Caprara, & Pastorelli, 1996b). Facility in moral disengagement combined with a low sense of efficacy to resist peer pressure for transgressive activities foster heavy engagement in antisocial conduct (Kwak & Bandura, 1997).

Self-Reflective Capability

The capability to reflect upon oneself and the adequacy of one's thoughts and actions is another exclusively human attribute that figures prominently in social cognitive theory. People are not only agents of action but self-examiners of their own cognitive, affective, and behavioral functioning. Effective functioning requires reliable ways of distinguishing between accurate and faulty thinking. In verifying the adequacy of thought by self-reflective means, people generate ideas and act upon them or predict occurrences from them. They then judge from the results the accuracy and functional value of their thinking and try to improve it if necessary.

Thought Verification by Self-Reflectiveness

The process of thought verification involves comparing how well one's thoughts match some indicator of reality. There are four modes of thought verification: enactive, vicarious, persuasory, and logical. "Enactive verification" relies on the closeness of the fit between one's thoughts and the results of the actions they spawn. Good matches lend validity to the thoughts; mismatches refute them. In the vicarious mode of thought verification, seeing the effects of other people's actions provides the check on the correctness of one's own thinking. Vicarious thought verification is not simply a supplement to enactive validation. Symbolic modeling vastly expands the range of verification experiences that cannot be attained by personal action because of the constraints of time, resources, and mobility.

Some spheres of life involve highly specialized knowledge requiring dependence on experts or metaphysical ideas that are not amenable to empirical confirmation. When experiential verification is difficult or unfeasible, people evaluate the soundness of their views by checking them with what others, to whom they give credence, believe. Thoughts are also verified by inferential means. In logical verification, people can check for fallacies in their thinking by deducing from knowledge that is known and what necessarily follows from it.

Such metacognitive activities usually foster dependable thought, but they can produce faulty thought patterns as well. Forceful actions arising from erroneous beliefs often create social environments that confirm the mis-beliefs (Snyder, 1980). Verification of thought by comparison with distorted media versions of social reality can foster shared misconceptions of people, places, or things (Hawkins & Pingree, 1991; Signorielli & Morgan, 1989).

Social verification can foster bizarre views of reality if the shared beliefs of the reference group with which one affiliates are eccentric and the group is encapsulated from outside social ties and influences (Bandura, 1982a). This is most strikingly illustrated in cultist beliefs (Hall, 1987). Similarly, deductive reasoning will be flawed if the propositional knowledge on which it is based is faulty or biases intrude on reasoning processes (Falmagne, 1975).

Perceived Self-Efficacy

Among the self-referent thoughts that influence human motivation, affect, and action, none is more central or pervasive than people's judgments of the personal efficacy (Bandura, 1997a). Perceived self-efficacy is concerned with people's beliefs in their capabilities to perform in ways that give them some control over events that affect their lives. Efficacy beliefs form the foundation of human agency. Unless people believe that they can produce desired results by their actions, they have little incentive to act or to persevere in the face of difficulties.

Sources of Self-Efficacy

Self-efficacy beliefs are constructed from four principal sources of informa-tion. The most authentic and influential source is "mastery experiences." This can be achieved by tackling problems in successive attainable steps. Suc-cesses build a robust belief in one's efficacy. Failures undermine it, especially in earlier phases of self-development. Moreover, if people have only easy suc-cesses, they are readily discouraged by failure or setbacks. Development of resilient self-efficacy requires experiences in overcoming obstacles through perseverant effort.

The second way of creating and strengthening beliefs of personal effi-cacy is through "vicarious experiences." If people see others like themselves succeed by sustained effort, they come to believe that they, too, have the capacity to succeed. Conversely, observing the failures of others instills doubts about one's own ability to master similar activities. Competent mod-els also build efficacy by conveying knowledge and skills for managing envi-ronmental demands.

"Social persuasion" is the third way of strengthening people's beliefs in their efficacy. If people are persuaded that they have what it takes to succeed, they exert more effort and are more perseverant than if they harbor self-doubts and dwell on personal deficiencies when problems arise. But effective social persuaders do more than convey faith in people's capabilities. They arrange activities for others in ways that bring success and avoid placing people prematurely in situations where they are likely to fail.

People also rely on their "physical and emotional states" to judge their capabilities. They read their tension, anxiety, and depression as signs of personal deficiency. In activities that require strength and stamina, they interpret fatigue, windedness, and aches and pains as indicators of low physical efficacy. Thus, the fourth way of altering efficacy beliefs is to enhance physical status, reduce negative emotional states, and correct misinterpretations of somatic sources of information.

Cognitive Processing of Efficacy Information

Information that is relevant for judging personal efficacy is not inherently informative. It is only raw data. Experiences become informative through cognitive processing of efficacy information and self-reflective thought. The information conveyed by events must be distinguished from how that information is selected, weighted, and integrated into self-efficacy judgments. A host of factors, including personal, social, and situational ones affect how experiences are interpreted.

The cognitive processing of efficacy information involves two separate functions. The first is the types of information people attend to and use as indicators of personal efficacy. Sociocognitive theory specifies the set of efficacy indicators that are distinctive for each of the four major modalities of influence (Bandura, 1997a). For example, the judgments people make about their efficacy based on performance attainments may vary depending on their interpretive biases, the difficulty of the task, how hard they worked at it, how much help they received, the conditions under which they performed, their emotional and physical state at the time, their rate of improvement over time, and selective biases in how they monitor and recall their attainments.

The particular indicators people single out provide the information base on which the self-appraisal process operates. The second function involves the combination rules or heuristics people use to integrate efficacy information conveyed enactively, vicariously, socially, and physiologically. This involves a complex process of self-persuasion concerning one's capabilities.

Diverse Effects of Self-Efficacy

Beliefs of personal efficacy regulate human functioning through four major processes (Bandura, 1997a). They include cognitive, motivational, emotional, and choice processes. The cognitive pathway takes a variety of forms. A major function of thought is to enable people to predict events and to exercise control over those that are important to them. People of high perceived efficacy show greater cognitive resourcefulness, strategic flexibility, and effectiveness in managing their environment (Bouffard-Bouchard, Parent, & Larivée, 1991; Wood & Bandura, 1989). They also set cognized challenges for themselves and visualize success scenarios that provide positive guides for performance. Those who doubt their efficacy visualize failure scenarios that undermine performances by dwelling on things that can go wrong. In appraising situations, people who are assured in their efficacy focus on the opportunities worth pursuing rather than dwell on risks (Krueger & Dickson, 1993, 1994). They take a future time perspective in structuring their lives (Eppel, Bandura, & Zimbardo, in press).

Efficacy beliefs play a central role in the self-regulation of motivation. Most human motivation is cognitively generated. There are three forms of cognitive motivators, around which different theories have been built (Figure 7.5). These include "causal attributions," "outcome expectancies," and "cognized goals." The corresponding theories are "attribution theory," "expectancy-value theory," and "goal theory." Efficacy beliefs play a key role in each of these motivational systems.

The causal attributions people make for their performances affect their motivation (Weiner, 1986). Efficacy beliefs influence causal attributions, regardless of whether the activities involve cognitive attainments, interpersonal transactions, physical performances, or management of health habits (Bandura, 1997a). People who regard themselves as highly efficacious ascribe their failures to insufficient effort, inadequate strategies, or unfavorable circumstances. Those of low efficacy attribute their failures to low ability. The effects of causal attributions on achievement strivings are mediated almost entirely through efficacy beliefs (Relich, Debus, & Walker, 1986; Schunk & Gunn, 1986; Schunk & Rice, 1986).

We have seen in the earlier discussion of self-regulatory capabilities that

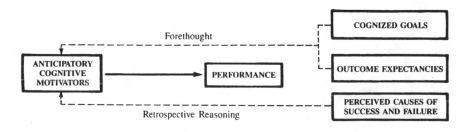

FIGURE 7.5. Schematic representation of conceptions of cognitive motivation based on cognized goals, outcome expectancies, and causal attributions.

much human motivation and behavior are regulated anticipatorily by the outcomes expected for given actions (Feather, 1982). However, there are many activities that, if done well, produce valued outcomes, but they are not pursued by people who doubt they can do what it takes to succeed. Such exclusions of large classes of options are made rapidly on efficacy grounds with little thought of costs and benefits. Rational models of decision making that exclude efficacy judgment sacrifice explanatory and predictive power (Bandura, 1997a). Moreover, making decisions in no way ensures that the needed courses of action will be executed successfully, especially in the face of difficulties. A psychology of decision making requires a psychology of action grounded in enabling and sustaining efficacy beliefs (Harré, 1983).

The capacity to exercise self-influence by personal challenge through goal setting and evaluative reaction to one's own performances provides another major cognitive mechanism of motivation and self-directedness. Efficacy beliefs play a key role in this form of cognitive motivation as well. It is partly on the basis of efficacy beliefs that people choose which goal challenges to undertake, how much effort to invest, and how long to persevere in the face of difficulties (Bandura, 1991b; Locke & Latham, 1990). When faced with obstacles, setbacks, and failures, those who doubt their abilities slacken their efforts, give up, or settle for mediocre solutions. Those who have strong belief in their capabilities redouble their efforts and figure out better ways to master the challenges. In short, people of high perceived efficacy set motivating goals for themselves, expect their efforts to produce favorable outcomes, ascribe failures to factors that are potentially controllable through ingenuity and effort, view obstacles as surmountable, and figure out ways to overcome them.

People's beliefs in their coping efficacy affect how much stress, anxiety, and depression they experience in threatening or taxing situations. There are four major ways in which efficacy beliefs regulate emotional states (Bandura, 1997a). They do so by influencing how threats are cognitively processed, by supporting coping actions that alter the threats, by exercising control over perturbing thought patterns, and by alleviating aversive affective states.

Efficacy beliefs influence how threats and taxing demands are perceived and cognitively processed. People who believe they can manage threats and adversities view them as less inimical and are not distressed by them. Those who believe they cannot control them experience high anxiety, dwell on their coping deficiencies, view many aspects of their environment as fraught with danger, magnify possible risks, and worry about perils that rarely happen. By such thinking, they distress themselves and impair their functioning (Bandura, 1997a; Sanderson, Rapee, & Barlow, 1989).

People who have a high sense of coping efficacy lower their stress and anxiety by acting in ways that transform threatening environments into benign ones. The stronger the sense of efficacy, the bolder people are in tackling the problems that breed stress and anxiety and the greater is their success in shaping the environment to their liking (Bandura, 1997a; Williams, 1992).

People have to live with a psychic environment that is largely of their own making. Many human distresses result from failures to control disturbing, ruminative thoughts. Control of one's thought processes is, therefore, a key factor in self-regulation of emotional states. The process of efficacious thought control is summed up well in the proverb: "You cannot prevent the birds of worry and care from flying over your head. But you can stop them from building a nest in your hair." What causes distress is not the sheer frequency of disturbing thoughts but the perceived helplessness to turn them off (Kent, 1987; Kent & Gibbons, 1987).

In addition, people can exercise control over their affective states by palliative means without altering the causes of their emotional arousal. They do things that bring relief from unpleasant emotional states when these arise. Belief that one can relieve unpleasant emotional states makes them less aversive (Arch, 1992a, 1992b).

Perceived inefficacy to control things one values also produces depression in varied ways. One route is through unfulfilled aspirations. People who impose on themselves standards of self-worth they judge they cannot attain drive themselves to depression (Bandura, 1991b; Kanfer & Zeiss, 1983). Depression, in turn, weakens people's beliefs in their own efficacy, creating a downward cycle (Kavanagh & Bower, 1985).

A second route to depression is through a low sense of social efficacy to develop social relationships that bring satisfaction to one's life and make chronic stressors easier to bear. A low sense of social efficacy contributes to depression both directly and by curtailing development of social supports (Holahan & Holahan, 1987a, 1987b). Perceived efficacy and social support operate bidirectionally in human adaptation and change. Supportive relationships, in turn, can enhance personal efficacy. Indeed, social support has beneficial effects only to the extent that it raises perceived coping efficacy (Cutrona & Troutman, 1986; Major, Mueller, & Hildebrandt, 1985).

The third route to depression is through thought-control efficacy. Much human depression is cognitively generated by dejecting, ruminative thought (Nolen-Hoeksema, 1991). A low sense of efficacy to control ruminative thought contributes to the occurrence, duration, and recurrence of depressive episodes (Kavanagh & Wilson, 1989).

So far, the analysis of pathways of influence has focused on how efficacy beliefs enable people to create beneficial environments and to exercise control over them. People are partly the product of their environment. By choosing their environments, they can have a hand in what they become. Beliefs of personal efficacy can, therefore, play a key role in shaping the courses lives take by influencing the types of activities and environments people choose to get into (Lent, Brown, & Hackett, 1994). In self-development through choice processes, destinies are shaped by selection of environments known to cultivate valued potentialities and lifestyles.

To sum up, people with a low sense of efficacy avoid difficult tasks, which they view as threats. They have low aspirations and weak commitment to the goals they choose to pursue. They turn inward on their self-doubts instead of thinking about how to perform successfully under pressure. When faced with difficulties, they dwell on obstacles, the negative consequences of failure, and their personal deficiencies. Failure makes them lose faith in themselves because they take it as evidence of their inherent incapability. They slacken their efforts or give up quickly in the face of obstacles. They are slow to recover their sense of efficacy after failures or setbacks and easily fall victim to stress and depression.

People with high perceived self-efficacy, by contrast, approach difficult tasks as challenges to be mastered rather than threats to be avoided. They develop interest in what they do, set challenges for themselves, and sustain strong commitments to them. They concentrate on how to perform successfully rather than on themselves and disruptive personal concerns when they encounter problems. They attribute their failures to lack of knowledge or skill, faulty strategies, or insufficient effort, all of which are remediable. They redouble their efforts in the face of obstacles and soon recover their self-assurance after setbacks. This outlook sustains motivation, reduces stress, and lowers vulnerability to depression.

Because social cognitive theory articulates the ways in which a strong sense of efficacy can be instilled and delineates the operative mechanisms, this knowledge has been extensively applied to enhance human functioning in diverse spheres of life (Bandura, 1997a, 1995; Maddux, 1995; Schwarzer, 1992). These wide-ranging applications include education, health, psychopathology, athletics, organizational innovations, and large-scale social change.

DIFFERENT FORMS OF AGENCY

The exercise of human agency can take different forms. It includes production of effects through "direct personal agency"; through "proxy agency" relying on the efforts of intermediaries; and by "collective agency," operating through shared beliefs of efficacy, pooled understandings, group aspirations, and collective action. Each of these expressions of agency is rooted in belief in the power to make things happen.

Proxy Agency

The preceding analyses addressed the direct exercise of personal agency. In many spheres of life, people do not have direct control over social conditions and institutional practices that affect their lives. Under these circumstances, they seek their well-being and security through the exercise of "proxy agency" rather than through direct control. In this socially mediated mode of agency, people try to get those who wield influence and power to act on their behalf to get what they want (Bandura, 1997a). Moreover, people often turn to proxy control in areas in which they can exert direct influence because they have not developed the means to do so, they believe others can do it better, or they do not want to saddle themselves with some of the burdensome aspects of direct control.

Personal control is neither universally desired nor universally exercised as is commonly assumed. There is an onerous side to direct personal control that can dull the appetite for it. The exercise of control requires mastery of knowledge and skills attainable only through long hours of arduous work. Moreover, maintaining proficiency under ever changing conditions of life demands continued investment of time, effort, and resources. A noted composer put it succinctly when he said, "The toughest thing about success, is that you've got to keep on being a success."

In addition to the hard work of continual self-development, in many situations the exercise of personal control carries heavy responsibilities, stressors, and risks. All too often, people surrender control to intermediaries in areas over which they can command some direct influence. They do so to free themselves of the performance demands and onerous responsibilities that personal control entails. Part of the price of proxy agency is a vulnerable security that rests on the competence, power, and favors of others.

Perceived Efficacy in Collective Agency

Conceptions of human agency have been confined to individual agency. However, people do not live their lives as isolates. They work together to produce the outcomes they desire but cannot accomplish on their own. Social cognitive theory, therefore, extends the conception of mechanisms of human agency to collective agency. People's shared beliefs in their collective power to produce desired outcomes are a crucial ingredient of collective agency. Group performance is the product of interactive and coordinative dynamics of its members. Therefore, perceived collective efficacy is not simply the sum of the efficacy beliefs of individual members. Rather, it is an emergent group-level property. A group, of course, operates through the behavior of its members. It is people acting collectively on a shared belief not a disembodied group mind that is doing the cognizing, aspiring, motivating, and regulating. Personal and collective efficacy differ in the unit of agency, but in both forms, efficacy beliefs serve similar functions and operate through similar processes. The stronger the beliefs people hold about their collective capabilities, the more they achieve (Bandura, 1993; Hodges & Carron, 1992; Little & Madigan, 1995; Prussia & Kinicki, 1996).

Some people live their lives in individualistically oriented social systems, whereas others do so in collectivistically oriented systems (Triandis, 1995). Some writers inappropriately equate self-efficacy with individualism and pit it against collectivism (Schooler, 1990). In fact, a high sense of personal efficacy contributes just as importantly to group-directedness as to self-directedness. If people are to work together successfully, the members of a group have to perform their roles with a high sense of efficacy. Personal efficacy is valued, not because of reverence for individualism, but because a strong sense of efficacy is vital for successful functioning regardless of whether it is achieved individually or by group members working together.

Cross-cultural research on organizational functioning corroborates the universal functional value of efficacy beliefs (Earley, 1993, 1994). Efficacy beliefs of personal efficacy contribute to productivity by members of collectivist cultures just as they do by those raised in individualistic cultures. But cultural context shapes how efficacy beliefs are developed, the purposes to which they are put, and the social arrangements through which they are best expressed. People from the United States, an individualistic culture, feel most efficacious and perform best under an individually oriented system. Those from collectivistic cultures, namely Hong Kong and mainland China, judge themselves most efficacious and work most productively under a group-oriented system.

Cultures are not static, uniform entities as the stereotypic portrayals would lead one to believe. Collectivistic systems, founded on Confucianism, Buddhism, or Marxism favor a communal ethic, but they differ from each other in the values, meanings, and customs they promote (Kim, Triandis, Kâgitçibasi, Choi, & Yoon, 1994). Nor are so-called individualistic cultures a uniform lot. Americans, Italians, Germans, and the British differ in their particular brands of individualism. Even within an individualistically oriented culture, such as exists in the United States, the New England brand of individualism is quite different from the Californian version, or that of the southern region of the nation.

There is substantial heterogeneity among individuals in communality within both individualistic and collectivistic cultures and even greater intra-individual variation in communality across social relationships with family members, friends, and colleagues (Matsumoto et al., 1996). There are generational and socioeconomic variations in collectivistic cultures with younger and more affluent members adopting more individualistic orientations. Moreover, people express their cultural orientations conditionally rather than invariantly depending on incentive conditions (Yamagishi, 1988). Under the sway of global markets and media forces, entrepreneurship is supplanting communality in collectivistic cultures. Conversely, some of the excesses of individualism are prompting a resurgence of efforts to restore a sense of community in individualistic cultures.

There are collectivists in individualistic cultures, and individualists in collectivistic cultures. Regardless of cultural background, people achieve the greatest personal efficacy and productivity when their personal orientation is congruent with the social system (Earley, 1994). Thus, Americans with a col-

lective orientation do better under a group-oriented system, Chinese individualists do better under an individually oriented system. The personal orientation rather than the cultural orientation is a major carrier of the effects. Both
at the societal and individual level of analysis, a strong perceived efficacy fosters high group effort and performance attainments.

Underminers of Collective Efficacy in Changing Societies

Life in the societies of today is increasingly shaped by transnational interdependencies (Keohane & Nye, 1977; Keohane, 1993). Because of extensive
global interconnectedness, what happens economically and politically in one
part of the world can affect the welfare of vast populations elsewhere. The
transnational forces, which are hard to disentangle let alone control, challenge the efficacy of governmental systems to exert a determining influence
on their own economic and national life. As the need for efficacious collective
effort grows, so does the sense of collective powerlessness. Many of the contemporary conditions of life undermine the development of collective efficacy.

Global market forces are restructuring national economies and shaping
the social life of societies. Some of the transnational market forces may erode
or undermine valued aspects of life in particular societies when these aspects
are disregarded or are considered as detractors from the level of profitability.
Social bonds and common commitments that lack marketability are especially vulnerable to erosion by global market forces. There are no handy social
mechanisms or global agencies through which people can shape and regulate
transnational practices that affect their lives. As nations wrestle with the loss
of control, the public expresses disillusionment and cynicism over whether
their leaders and institutions can work for them to improve their lives.

Under the new realities of growing transnational control, nation states
increase their controlling leverage by merging into larger regional units such
as the European Union. Other regional nation states will similarly be forced
to merge into larger blocks, otherwise they will have little bargaining power
in transnational relations. These regional marriages do not come without a
price. Paradoxically, to gain international control, nations have to negotiate
reciprocal pacts that require some loss of national autonomy and changes in
traditional ways of life (Keohane, 1993).

Modern life is increasingly regulated by complex technologies that most
people neither understand nor believe they can do much to influence. The
very technologies that people create to control their life environment can
become a constraining force that, in turn, controls how they think and
behave. The social machinery of society is no less challenging. Bureaucracies
thwart effective social action. Many of the bureaucratic practices are designed
more to benefit the people who run the social systems than to serve the public. Social change does not come easily because beneficiaries build their privi-

leges into protective institutional structures and processes. Those who exercise authority and control wield their power to maintain their advantages. Long delays between action and noticeable results discourage efforts at change. Most people relinquish control in the face of institutional and bureaucratic obstacles.

Social efforts to change lives for the better require merging diverse self-interests in support of common core values and goals. Disagreements among different constituencies create additional obstacles to successful collective action. The recent years have witnessed growing social fragmentation into separate interest groups, each exercising its own power. Pluralism is taking the form of antagonistic factionalism. In addition, mass migration of people fleeing tyranny or seeking a better life is changing cultural landscapes. Societies are thus becoming more diverse and harder to unite around a national vision and purpose.

The magnitude of human problems also undermines perceived efficacy to find effective solutions for them. Profound global changes, arising from burgeoning populations, deforestation, desertification of croplands, ozone depletion, and rapid extinction of species by razing their habitats are destroying the intertwined ecosystems that sustain life. Worldwide problems of growing magnitude instill a sense of paralysis that there is little people can do to reduce such problems. Global effects are the products of local actions. The strategy of "Think globally, act locally" is an effort to restore in people a sense of efficacy, that they can make a difference. Macrosocial applications of sociocognitive principles via the electronic media illustrate how small collective efforts can have huge impacts on such urgent global problems as the soaring population growth (Singhal & Rogers, 1989; Vaughn, Rogers, & Swalehe, 1995; Westoff & Rodriguez, 1995).

PERSONALITY AS AN INTEGRATED SELF SYSTEM

Sociocognitive theories are commonly misconstrued as atomistic without an overreaching "personality." The umbrella term "personality" represents a complex of interacting attributes, not a self-contained entity describable by a few pithy terms creating the illusion of a high-order structure. Personality is multifaceted, richly contextualized, and conditionally expressed in the diverse transactions of everyday life. The totality of an individual's cognitive, behavioral, and affective proclivities is not shrinkable to a few static descriptive categories.

Unity of Agency and Personal Identity

People express their individuality and give structure, meaning, and purpose to their lives by acting on their beliefs about themselves, their values, personal standards, aspirations, and construals of the world around them. These multiform belief systems, self structures, and self-referent processes through which one's "personality" is manifested in its totality function in concert not isolatedly. It is through coordinative and integrative activity that the diverse sources of influence produce unity of experience and action. The self embodies all of the endowments, belief systems, and distributed structures and functions through which personal agency is exercised rather than residing as a discrete entity in a particular place. In short, the self is the person—not a homunculian subpart. "Personality" is the integrated self system within which the previously identified constituents operate in complex mutual interaction in the management of diverse and changing environmental circumstances. The various constituents must be orchestrated in an integrated way because, whatever options are considered, the choices finally made and the actions taken at a given time require unity of agency. Given but a single body, one cannot perform incompatible acts simultaneously. People may, of course, exhibit contradictory behavior, but those are instances of the same being doing discordant things on different occasions not different selves doing their separate things.

Social cognitive theory and research not only examine the individual properties of these key constituents but how they contribute to personal identity and functioning within the organized multifaceted system of determinants (Bandura, 1997a). The exercise of agency through the interrelated self structures and regulatory processes shapes the kind of life people live and what they consider themselves to be. The personal identity they create for themselves derives, in large part, from how they live their life and reflect upon it. The continuity of personal identity resides more in psychological factors and the experiential continuity of the course of life followed than in physical constancy. An amnesic remains the same physically but has lost a sense of personal identity. Continuing self-identity is preserved in memories that give temporal coherence to life (McAdams, 1996), in continuance of belief and value commitments that link the present to the past and shape the course of future events, and in the connectedness of human relationships and one's life work over time.

Continuing self-identity is not solely a product of an intrapsychic autobiographical process that preserves a sense of personal continuity over time. Others perceive, socially label, and treat one as the same person over the course of life. Personal identity is partially constructed from one's social identity as reflected in how one is treated by significant others. In keeping with the model of triadic reciprocal causation, a sense of selfhood is the product of a complex interplay of social and personal construal processes. Others, of course, have only a limited sample of a given person's social life and know even much less of that individual's experiential life. Consequently, the social identity conveyed by others is more heavily dependent on the sameness of physical characteristics, social roles, and habitual behaviors that are publicly observable than on personal uniqueness and experiential factors.

Identity formation is an ongoing process not one characterized by fixedness in time. Moreover, the self view is multifaceted rather than monolithic. There are many aspects to the self. They are not equally salient, valued, or functional in different spheres of life or under different circumstances. In a dynamic, multifaceted model, continuity of personal identity requires neither high consistency among different aspects of self nor invariance across different social environments or domains of functioning. For given individuals, their personal identities are likely to be composed of unique amalgams of identities with social, political, ethnic, occupational, and familial aspects of life. Thus, for a particular individual, a strong occupational identity may coexist with a moderate ethnic identity and a weak political identity without any felt discordance. Another individual may exhibit a quite different constellation of identities, combining a strong ethnic and political identity with a weak occupational identity. Similarly, a person's self view with parents may differ significantly from the self view in relationships with peers because these social worlds tap somewhat different aspects of the self. In each case, however, it is one and the same person manifesting a multifaceted personal identity. It is the temporal stability of the patterned self view rather than high coherence of aspects that defines one's personal uniqueness and sense of continuity. Theories that construe personal identity as a fixed monolith are discordant with a vast body of evidence.

With further experiences over time, people evolve and integrate some new aspects into their self-identity. This raises the issue of how they extract continuity from variability across time, activity domains, and social contexts. To the extent that they consider mainly core aspects or focus on different aspects of themselves as relevant in different life situations, they can change in particulars but preserve a sense of continuity in their view of themselves. However, if they undergo major life changes, they consider themselves to be different persons from whom they were in the past. Taken as a whole, the findings of diverse lines of research on the various personal properties subsumed under the spacious construct of "personality" attest to the explanatory, predictive, and operative efficacy of theories that specify multiform personal structures operating conditionally through self-regulatory mechanisms within the contextual influences in which people construct and conduct their lives (Bandura, 1986, 1997a).

The Nature of Human Nature

Seen from the social cognitive perspective, human nature is characterized by a vast potentiality that can be fashioned by direct and vicarious experience into a variety of forms within biological constraints. To say that a major distinguishing mark of humans is their endowed plasticity is not to say that they have no nature or that they come structureless (Midgley, 1978). The plasticity, which is intrinsic to the nature of humans, depends upon specialized neurophysiological structures and mechanisms that have evolved over time. These advanced neural systems are specialized for detecting the causal structure of the world around one, transforming that information into abstract form and using it for adaptive purposes. This intricate, informative processing system provides the capacity for the very characteristics that are distinctly human: generative symbolization, forethought, evaluative self-regulation, reflective self-consciousness, and symbolic communication.

Although neurophysiological systems have been shaped by evolutionary pressures, people are not just reactive products of selection pressures. Through agentic action, they devise ways of adapting flexibility to remarkably diverse environments, they circumvent environmental constraints, redesign and construct environments to their liking, create styles of behavior that enable them to realize desired outcomes and pass on the effective ones to others by experiential means. Indeed, growth of knowledge has greatly enhanced human power to control, transform, and create environments of increasing complexity. We build physical technologies that drastically alter how we live our daily lives; we create mechanical devices that compensate immensely for our sensory and physical limitations; we develop medical and psychological methods that enable us to exert some measure of control over our physical and psychosocial lives; and we have developed biological technologies to change the genetic make-up of plants, and animals and we are exploring methods that could alter the genetic codes of humans. Evolution moves at a snail's pace. People have changed little genetically over the decades, but they have changed markedly through rapid cultural and technological evolution in their thinking, styles of behavior, and the roles they perform. There is much genetic homogeneity across cultures but vast diversity in belief systems and conduct. Given this variability, genetic coding that characterizes humans underscores the power of the environment.

Most patterns of human behavior are organized by individual experience and retained in neural codes rather than having been provided readymade by inborn programming. Although human behavior is fashioned largely through experience, innately determined factors enter into every form of behavior to varying degrees. Genetic factors affect behavioral potentialities, which, through their actualization, can influence the kinds of environments that are experienced and constructed. The experiences produced by agentic action shape the nature of brain development and quality of functioning. Both experientially derived factors and genetically determined ones interact, often in intricate synergistic ways, to determine behavior. The level of psychological and biological development, of course, limits what can be acquired at any given time.

Humans have an unparalleled capacity to become many things. The qualities that are cultivated and the life paths that realistically become open to them are partly determined by the nature of the societal systems to which their development is entrusted. Social systems that cultivate generalizable competencies, instill a robust sense of efficacy, create opportunity structures, provide aidful resources, and allow room for self-directedness increase the chances that people will realize what they wish to become.

ACKNOWLEDGMENTS

Preparation of this chapter and some of the cited research were supported by grants from the Grant Foundation, the Spencer Foundation, and the Johann Jacobs Foundation. Some sections of this chapter include revised, updated, and expanded material from Bandura (1986, 1997a). This chapter is a slightly abridged version of Bandura (1999). Copyright 1999 by The Guilford Press. Adapted by permission.

REFERENCES

Alland, A., Jr. (1972). *The human imperative.* New York: Columbia University.

Almagor, M., Tellegen, A., & Waller, N. G. (1995). The Big Seven model: A cross-cultural replication and further exploration of the basic dimensions of natural language trait descriptors. *Journal of Personality and Social Psychology, 69,* 300–307.

Arch, E. C. (1992a). Affective control efficacy as a factor in willingness to participate in a public performance situation. *Psychological Reports, 71,* 1247–1250.

Arch, E. C. (1992b). Sex differences in the effect of self-efficacy on willingness to participate in a performance situation. *Psychological Reports, 70,* 3–9.

Baldwin, C., Baldwin, A., Sameroff, A., & Seifer, R. (1989, April). *The role of family interaction in the prediction of adolescent competence.* Paper presented at the biennial meeting of the Society for Research in Child Development, Kansas City, MO.

Ball-Rokeach, S., & DeFleur, M. (1976). A dependency model of mass media effects. *Communication Research, 3,* 3–21.

Baltes, P. B., Lindenberger, U., & Staudinger, U. M. (in press). Life-span theory in developmental psychology. In R. M. Lerner (Ed.), *Handbook of child psychology* (5th ed.): *Vol. 1. Theoretical models of human development.* New York: Wiley.

Bandura, A. (1973). *Aggression: A social learning analysis.* Englewood Cliffs, NJ: Prentice-Hall.

Bandura, A. (1982a). Self-efficacy mechanism in human agency. *American Psychologist, 37,* 122–147.

Bandura, A. (1982b). The psychology of chance encounters and life paths. *American Psychologist, 37,* 747–755.

Bandura, A. (1986). *Social foundations of thought and action: A social cognitive theory.* Englewood Cliffs, NJ: Prentice-Hall.

Bandura, A. (1990). *Multidimensional scales of perceived academic efficacy.* Unpublished manuscript, Stanford University, Stanford, CA.

Bandura, A. (1991a). Social cognitive theory of moral thought and action. In W. M. Kurtines & J. L. Gewirtz (Eds.), *Handbook of moral behavior and development* (Vol. A, pp. 45–103). Hillsdale, NJ: Erlbaum.

Bandura, A. (1991b). Self-regulation of motivation through anticipatory and self-regulatory mechanisms. In R. A. Dienstbier (Ed.), *Nebraska Symposium on Motivation: Vol. 38. Perspectives on motivation* (pp. 69–164). Lincoln: University of Nebraska Press.

Bandura, A. (1992). Social cognitive theory and social referencing. In S. Feinman (Ed.), *Social referencing and the social construction of reality in infancy* (pp. 175–208). New York: Plenum Press.

Bandura, A. (1993). Perceived self-efficacy in cognitive development and functioning. *Educational Psychologist, 28,* 117–148.

Bandura, A. (1995). *Self-efficacy in changing societies.* New York: Cambridge University Press.

Bandura, A. (1997a). *Self-efficacy: The exercise of control.* New York: Freeman.

Bandura, A. (1997b). Self-efficacy and health behaviour. In A. Baum, S. Newman, J. Weinman, R. West, & C. McManus (Eds.), *Cambridge handbook of psychology, health and medicine* (pp. 16–162). Cambridge, England: Cambridge University Press.

Bandura, A. (1998). Exploration of fortuitous determinants of life paths. *Psychological Inquiry, 9,* 95–99.

Bandura, A. (1999). Social cognitive theory of personality. In L. A. Pervin & O. J. John (Eds.), *Handbook of personality: Theory and research* (2nd ed.). New York: Guilford Press.

Bandura, A., Barbaranelli, C., Caprara, G. V., & Pastorelli, C. (1996a). Multifaceted impact of self-efficacy beliefs on academic functioning. *Child Development, 67,* 1206–1222.

Bandura, A., Barbaranelli, C., Caprara, G. V., & Pastorelli, C. (1996b). Mechanisms of moral disengagement in the exercise of moral agency. *Journal of Personality and Social Psychology, 71,* 364–374.

Bandura, A., Barbaranelli, C., Caprara, G.V., & Pastorelli, C. (1999). *Efficacy beliefs as shapers of aspirations and occupational trajectories.* Manuscript submitted for publication.

Bandura, A., & Cervone, D. (1983). Self-evaluative and self-efficacy mechanisms governing the motivational effects of goal systems. *Journal of Personality and Social Psychology, 45,* 1017–1028.

Bandura, A., & Cervone, D. (1986). Differential engagement of self-reactive influences in cognitive motivation. *Organizational Behavior and Human Decision Processes, 38,* 92–113.

Bandura, A., & Jourden, F. J. (1991). Self-regulatory mechanisms governing the impact of social comparison on complex decision making. *Journal of Personality and Social Psychology, 60,* 941–951.

Bandura, A., & Rosenthal, T. L. (1978). Psychological modeling: Theory and practice. In S. L. Garfield & A. E. Bergin (Eds.), *Handbook of psychotherapy and behavior change* (2nd ed.). New York: Wiley.

Bandura, A., Ross, D., & Ross, S. A. (1963). A comparative test of the status envy, social power, and secondary reinforcement theories of identificatory learning. *Journal of Abnormal and Social Psychology, 67,* 527–534.

Bandura, A., Underwood, B., & Fromson, M. E. (1975). Disinhibition of aggression through diffusion of responsibility and dehumanization of victims. *Journal of Research in Personality, 9,* 253–269.

Bandura, A., & Walters, R. H. (1959). *Adolescent aggression.* New York: Ronald Press.

Bandura, A., & Wood, R. E. (1989). Effect of perceived controllability and performance standards on self-regulation of complex decision-making. *Journal of Personality and Social Psychology, 56,* 805–814.

Barrett, P., & Kline, P. (1982). An item and radial parcel factor analysis of the 16 PF questionnaire. *Personality and Individual Differences, 3,* 259–270.

Barrick, M. R., Mount, M. K., & Strauss, J. P. (1993). Conscientiousness and performance of sales representatives: Test of the mediating effects of goal setting. *Journal of Applied Psychology, 76,* 715–722.

Belcher, T. L. (1975). Modeling original divergent responses: An initial investigation. *Journal of Educational Psychology, 67,* 351–358.

Berger, S. M. (1962). Conditioning through vicarious instigation. *Psychological Review, 69,* 450–466.

Block, J. (1995). A contrarian view of the five-factor approach to personality description. *Psychological Bulletin, 117,* 187–215.

Bolinger, D. (1982). *Language: The loaded weapon.* London: Longman.

Bouffard-Bouchard, T., Parent, S., & Larivée, S. (1991). Influence of self-efficacy on self-regulation and performance among junior and senior high-school age students. *International Journal of Behavioral Development, 14,* 153–164.

Braithwaite, J. (1994). A sociology of modeling and the politics of empowerment. *British Journal of Sociology, 45,* 445–479.

Brandstädter, J., Krampen, G., & Heil, F. E. (1996). Personal control and emotional evaluation of development in partnership relations during adulthood. In M. M. Baltes & P. B. Baltes (Eds.), *The psychology of control and aging* (pp. 265–296). Hillsdale, NJ: Erlbaum.

Bromley, D. G., & Shupe, A. D. (1979). *"Moonies" in America: Cult, church, and crusade.* Beverly Hills: Sage.

Burns, T. R., & Dietz, T. (in press). Human agency and evolutionary processes: Institutional dynamics and social revolution. In B. Wittrock (Ed.), *Agency in social theory.* Thousand Oaks, CA: Sage.

Carlson, R. (1992). Shrinking personality: One cheer for the Big Five. *Contemporary Psychology, 37,* 644–645.

Carroll, W. R., & Bandura, A., (1990). Representational guidance of action production in observational learning: A causal analysis. *Journal of Motor Behavior, 22,* 85–97.

Carver, C. S., & Scheier, M. F. (1981). *Attention and self-regulation: A control-theory approach to human behavior.* New York: Springer-Verlag.

Costa, P. T., Jr., & McCrae, R. R. (1994). "Set like plaster?" Evidence for the stability of adult personality. In T. Heatherton & J. Weinberger (Eds.), *Can personality change?* (pp. 21–40). Washington, DC: American Psychological Association.

Cutrona, C. E., & Troutman, B. R. (1986). Social support, infant temperament, and parenting self-efficacy: A mediational model of postpartum depression. *Child Development, 57,* 1507–1518.

Diener, E. (1977). Deindividuation: Causes and consequences. *Social Behavior and Personality, 5,* 143–156.

Digman, J. M. (1997). Higher-order factors of the Big Five. *Journal of Personality and Social Psychology, 73,* 1246–1256.

Duncker, K. (1938). Experimental modification of children's food preferences through social suggestion. *Journal of Abnormal Social Psychology, 33,* 489–507.

Earley, P. C. (1993). East meets West meets Mideast: Further explorations of collectivistic and individualistic work groups. *Academy of Management Journal, 36,* 319–348.

Earley, P. C. (1994). Self or group? Cultural effects of training on self-efficacy and performance. *Administrative Science Quarterly, 39,* 89–117.

Elder, G. H., & Ardelt, M. (1992, March 18–20). *Families adapting to economic pressure: Some consequences for parents and adolescents.* Paper presented at the meeting of the Society for Research on Adolescence, Washington, DC.

Endler, N. S., & Parker, J. D. A. (1992). Interactionism revisited: Reflections on the continuing crisis in the personality area. *European Journal of Personality, 6,* 177–198.

Eppel, E. S., Bandura, A., & Zimbardo, P. G. (in press). Escaping homelessness: Influence of self-efficacy and time perspective on coping with homelessness. *Journal of Applied Social Psychology.*

Epstein, S. (1983). The stability of behavior across time and situations. In R. Zucker, J. Aronoff, & A. I. Rabin (Eds.), *Personality and the prediction of behavior* (pp. 209–268). San Diego, CA: Academic Press.

Eysenck, H. J. (1991). Dimensions of personality: 16, 5 or 3?—Criteria for a taxonomic paradigm. *Personality and Individual Differences, 12,* 773–790.

Falmagne, R. J. (1975). *Reasoning: Representation and process in children and adults.* Hillsdale, NJ: Erlbaum.

Feather, N. T. (Ed.). (1982). *Expectations and actions: Expectancy-value models in psychology.* Hillsdale, NJ: Erlbaum.

Feldman, D. H. (1980). *Beyond universals in cognitive development.* Norwood, NJ: Ablex.

Ferguson, T. J., & Rule, B. G. (1983). An attributional perspective on anger and aggression. In R. G. Geen & E. I. Donnerstein (Eds.), *Aggression: Theoretical and empirical* (Vol. 1, pp. 41–74). New York: Academic Press.

Festinger, L. (1954). A theory of social comparison processes. *Human Relations, 7,* 117–140.

Flavell, J. H. (1978). Developmental stage: Explanans or explanadum? *Behavioral and Brain Sciences, 2,* 187–188.

Gerbner, G. (1972). Communication and social environment. *Scientific American, 227,* 153–160.

Giddens, A. (1984). *The constitution of society: Outline of the theory of structuration.* Cambridge: Polity Press.

Gillespie, W. H. (1971). Aggression and instinct theory. *International Journal of Psycho-Analysis, 52,* 155–160.

Goethals, G. R., & Darley, J. M. (1977). Social comparison theory: Attributional approach. In J. M. Suls & R. L. Miller (Eds.), *Social comparison processes: Theoretical and empirical perspectives* (pp. 259–278). Washington, DC: Hemisphere.

Gould, S. J. (1987). *An urchin in the storm.* New York: Norton.

Guastello, S. J. (1993). A two-(and-a-half)-tiered trait taxonomy. *American Psychology, 48,* 1298–1299.

Hall, J. R. (1987). *Gone from the promised land: Jonestown in American cultural history.* New Brunswick, NJ: Transaction Books.

Haritos-Fatouros, M. (1988). The official torturer: A learning model for obedience to the authority of violence. *Journal of Applied Social Psychology, 18,* 1107–1120.

Harré, R (1983). *Personal being: A theory for individual psychology.* Oxford, England: Blackwell.

Harré, R., & Gillet, G. (1994). *The discursive mind.* Thousand Oaks, CA: Sage.

Harris, M. B., & Evans, R. C. (1973). Models and creativity. *Psychological Reports, 33,* 763–769.

Hawkins, R. P., & Pingree, S. (1991). Divergent psychological processes in constructing social reality form mass media content. In N. Signorielli & M. Morgan (Eds.), *Cultivation analysis: New directions in media effects research* (Vol. 108, pp. 35–50). Beverly Hills, CA: Sage.

Hodges, L., & Carron, A. V. (1992). Collective efficacy and group performance. *International Journal of Sport Psychology, 23,* 48–59.

Holahan, C. K., & Holahan, C. J. (1987a). Self-efficacy, social support, and depression in aging: A longitudinal analysis. *Journal of Gerontology, 42,* 65–68.

Holahan, C. K., & Holahan, C. J. (1987b). Life stress, hassles, and self-efficacy in aging: A replication and extension. *Journal of Applied Social Psychology, 17,* 574–592.

Hough, L. M. (1992). The "Big Five" personality variables—Construct confusion: Description versus prediction. *Human Performance, 5,* 139–155.

Jackson, D. N., Ashton, M. C., & Tomes, J. L. (1996). The six-factor model of personality: Facets from the Big Five. *Personality and Individual Differences, 21,* 391–402.

Jackson, D. N., Paunonen, S. V., Fraboni, M., & Goffin, R. D. (1996). A five-factor versus six-factor model of personality structure. *Personality and Individual Differences, 20,* 33–46.

Kanfer, R., & Zeiss, A. M. (1983). Depression, interpersonal standard-setting, and judgments of self-efficacy. *Journal of Abnormal Psychology, 92,* 319–329.

Kavanagh, D. J., & Bower, G. H. (1985). Mood and self-efficacy: Impact of joy and sadness on perceived capabilities. *Cognitive Therapy and Research, 9,* 507–525.

Kavanagh, D. J., & Wilson, P. H. (1989). Prediction of outcome with a group version of cognitive therapy for depression. *Behaviour Research and Therapy, 27,* 333–347.

Kazdin, A. E. (1974). Comparative effects of some variations of covert modeling. *Journal of Behavior Therapy and Experimental Psychiatry, 5,* 225–232.

Keen, S. (1986). *Faces of the enemy.* San Francisco: Harper & Row.

Kelman, H. C., & Hamilton, V. L. (1989). *Crimes of obedience: Toward a social psychology of authority and responsibility.* New Haven, CT: Yale University Press.

Kent, G. (1987). Self-efficacious control over reported physiological, cognitive and behavioural symptoms of dental anxiety. *Behaviour Research and Therapy, 25,* 341–347.

Kent, G., & Gibbons, R. (1987). Self-efficacy and the control of anxious cognitions. *Journal of Behavior Therapy and Experimental Psychiatry, 18,* 33–40.

Keohane, R. O. (1993). Sovereignty, interdependence and international institutions. In L. Miller & M. Smith (Eds.), *Ideas and ideals: Essays on politics in honor of Stanley Hoffman* (91–107). Boulder, CO: Westview Press.

Keohane, R. O., & Nye, J. S. (1977). *Power and interdependence: World politics in transition.* Boston: Little, Brown.

Kim, U., Triandis, H. D., Kâgitçibasi, C., Choi, S., & Yoon, G. (1994). *Individualism and collectivism: Theory, method, and applications.* Thousand Oaks, CA: Sage.

Klass, E. T. (1978). Psychological effects of immoral actions: The experimental evidence. *Psychological Bulletin, 85,* 756–771.

Kroger, R. O. (1993). Reification, "faking," and the Big Five. *American Psychology, 48,* 1297–1298.

Krueger, N. F., Jr., & Dickson, P. R. (1993). Self-efficacy and perceptions of opportunities and threats. *Psychological Reports, 72,* 1235–1240.

Krueger, N., Jr., & Dickson, P. R. (1994). How believing in ourselves increases risk taking: Perceived self-efficacy and opportunity recognition. *Decision Sciences, 25,* 385–400.

Kwak, K., & Bandura, A. (1997). *Role of perceived self-efficacy and moral disengagement in antisocial conduct.* Unpublished manuscript, Osan College, Seoul, Korea.

Lachman, M. E. (1986). Personal control in later life: Stability, change, and cognitive correlates. In M. M. Baltes & P. B. Baltes (Eds.), *The psychology of control and aging* (pp. 207–236). Hillsdale, NJ: Erlbaum.

Lent, R. W., Brown, S. D., & Hackett, G. (1994). Toward a unifying social cognitive theory of career and academic interest, choice, and performance. *Journal of Vocational Behavior, 45,* 79–122.

Little, B. L., & Madigan, R. M. (1994, August). *Motivation in work teams: A test of the construct of collective efficacy.* Paper presented at the annual meeting of the Academy of Management, Houston, TX.

Locke, E. A., & Latham, G. P. (1990). *A theory of goal setting and task performance.* Englewood Cliffs, NJ: Prentice-Hall.

Lord, R. G., & Hanges, P. J. (1987). A control system model of organizational motivation: Theoretical development and applied implications. *Behavioral Science, 32,* 161–178.

Lutz, W. D. (1987). Language, appearance, and reality: Doublespeak in 1984. In P. C. Boardman (Ed.), *The legacy of language—A tribute to Charlton Laird* (pp. 103–119). Reno: University of Nevada Press.

Maddux, J. E. (Ed.). (1995). *Self-efficacy, adaptation, and adjustment: Theory, research and application.* New York: Plenum Press.

Major, B., Mueller, P., & Hildebrandt, K. (1985). Attributions, expectations, and coping with abortion. *Journal of Personality and Social Psychology, 48,* 585–599.

Markus, H., & Nurius, P. (1986). Possible selves. *American Psychologist, 41,* 954–969.

Martin, J. (1981). Relative deprivation: A theory of distributive injustice for an era of shrinking resources. In B. Staw & L. Cummings (Eds.), *Research in organizational behavior* (Vol. 3, pp. 53–107). Greenwich, CT: JAI Press.

Matsumoto, D., Kudoh, T., & Takeuchi, S. (1996). Changing patterns of individualism and collectivism in the United States and Japan. *Culture and Psychology, 2,* 77–107.

McAdams, D. P. (1992). The five-factor model in personality: A critical appraisal. *Journal of Personality, 60,* 329–361.

McAdams, D. P. (1996). Personality, modernity, and the storied self: A contemporary framework for studying persons. *Psychological Inquiry, 7,* 295–321.

McAvay, G. J., Seeman, T. E., & Rodin, J. (1996). A longitudinal study of change in domain-specific self-efficacy among older adults. *Journal of Gerontology: Psychological Sciences, 51B,* 243–253.

McCrae, R. R., & Costa, P. T. (1996). Toward a new generation of personality theories: Theoretical contexts for the five-factor model. In J. S. Wiggins (Ed.), *The five-factor model of personality: Theoretical perspectives* (pp. 51–87). New York: Guilford Press.

McCrae, R. R., & Costa, P. T. (1997). Personality trait structure as a human universal. *American Psychologist, 52,* 509–516.

McCrae, R. R., Zonderman, A. B., Costa, P. T., Bond, M. H., & Paunonen, S. V. (1996). Evaluating replicability of factors in the Revised NEO Personality Inventory:

Confirmatory factor analysis versus procrustes rotation. *Personality and Social Psychology, 70,* 552–566

Midgley, M. (1978). *Beast and man: The roots of human nature.* Ithaca, NY: Cornell University Press.

Milgram, S. (1974). *Obedience to authority: An experimental view.* New York: Harper & Row.

Mischel, W., & Shoda, Y. (1995). A cognitive-affective system theory of personality: Reconceptualizing situations, dispositions, dynamics, and invariance in personality structure. *Psychological Review, 102,* 246–268.

Moerk, E. L. (1995). Acquisition and transmission of pacifist mentalities in Sweden. *Peace and Conflict: Journal of Peace Psychology, 1,* 291–307.

Nagel, E. (1961). *The structure of science.* New York: Harcourt, Brace, & World.

Nolen-Hoeksema, S. (1991). Responses to depression and their effects on the duration of depressive episodes. *Journal of Abnormal Psychology, 100,* 569–582.

Pajares, F., & Kranzler, J. (1995). Self-efficacy beliefs and general mental ability in mathematical problem-solving. *Contemporary Educational Psychology, 20,* 426–443.

Pajares, F., & Miller, M. D. (1994). Role of self-efficacy and self-concept beliefs in mathematical problem solving: A path analysis. *Journal of Educational Psychology, 86,* 193–203.

Pajares, F., & Miller, M. D. (1995). Mathematics self-efficacy and mathematics performances: The need for specificity of assessment. *Journal of Counseling Psychology, 42,* 190–198.

Parker, J. D. A., Bagby, R. M., & Summerfeldt, L. J. (1993). Confirmatory factor analysis of the Revised NEO Personality Inventory. *Personality and Individual Differences, 15,* 463–466.

Patterson, G. R. (1976). The aggressive child: Victim and architect of a coercive system. In E. J. Mash, L. A. Hamerlynck, & L. C. Handy (Eds.), *Behavior modification and families* (pp. 267–316). New York: Brunner/Mazel.

Pervin, L. A. (1989). *Goal concepts in personality and social psychology.* Hillsdale, NJ: Erlbaum.

Pervin, L. A. (1994). A critical analysis of current trait theory. *Psychological Inquiry, 5,* 103–113.

Piaget, J. (1950). *The psychology of intelligence.* New York: International Universities Press.

Powers, W. T. (1973). *Behavior: The control of perception.* Chicago: Aldine.

Prussia, G. E., & Kinicki, A. J. (1996). A motivational investigation of group effectiveness using social cognitive theory. *Journal of Applied Psychology, 81,* 187–199.

Rapoport, D. C., & Alexander, Y. (Eds.). (1982). *The morality of terrorism: Religious and secular justification.* Elmsford, NY: Pergamon Press.

Reich, W. (Ed.). (1990). *Origins of terrorism: Psychologies, ideologies, theologies, states of mind.* Cambridge, England: Cambridge University Press.

Reichard, G. A. (1938). Social life. In F. Boas (Ed.), *General anthropology* (pp. 409–486). Boston: Heath.

Relich, J. D., Debus, R. L., & Walker, R. (1986). The mediating role of attribution and self-efficacy variables for treatment effects on achievement outcomes. *Contemporary Educational Psychology, 11,* 195–216.

Rogers, C. R. (1959). A theory of therapy, personality, and interpersonal relationships, as developed in the client-centered framework. In S. Koch (Ed.), *Psychology: A study of a science: Vol. III. Formulations of the person and the social context* (pp. 184–256). New York: McGraw-Hill.

Rogers, E. J., Vaughan, P. W., Swalehe, R. M. A., Rao, N., & Sood, S. (1996). *Effects of an entertainment–education radio soap opera on family planning and HIV/AIDS prevention behavior in Tanzania.* Unpublished manuscript, Department of Communication and Journalism, University of New Mexico, Albuquerque.

Rottschaefer, W. A. (1991, February). Some philosophical implications of Bandura's social cognitive theory of human agency. *The American Psychologist, 46,* 153–155.

Rosenthal, T. L., & Zimmerman, B. J. (1978). *Social learning and cognition.* New York: Academic Press.

Rushton, J. P., Brainerd, C. J., & Pressley, M. (1983). Behavioral development and construct validity: The principle of aggregation. *Psychological Bulletin, 94,* 39–53.

Sanday, P. R. (1981). The socio-cultural context of rape: A cross-cultural study. *The Journal of Social Issues, 37,* 5–27.

Sanderson, W. C., Rapee, R. M., & Barlow, D. H. (1989). The influence of an illusion of control on panic attacks induced via inhalation of 5.5% carbon dioxide-enriched air. *Archives of General Psychiatry, 46,* 157–162.

Sanford, N., & Comstock, C. (1971). *Sanctions for evil.* San Francisco: Jossey-Bass.

Schooler, C. (1990). Individualism and the historical and social-structural determinants of people's concerns over self-directedness and efficacy. In J. Rodin, C. Schooler, & K. W. Schaie (Eds.), *Self-directedness: Cause and effects throughout the life course* (pp.19–58). Hillsdale, NJ: Erlbaum.

Schunk, D. H., & Gunn, T. P. (1986). Self-efficacy and skill development: Influence of task strategies and attributions. *Journal of Educational Research, 79,* 238–244.

Schunk, D. H., & Rice, J. M. (1986). Extended attributional feedback: Sequence effects during remedial reading instruction. *Journal of Early Adolescence, 6,* 55–66.

Schwarzer, R. (1992). Self-efficacy in the adoption and maintenance of health behaviors: Theoretical approaches and a new model. In R. Schwarzer (Ed.), *Self-efficacy: Thought control of action* (pp. 217–243). Washington, DC: Hemisphere.

Shepherd, G. (Ed.). (1995). *Rejected: Leading economists ponder the publication process.* Sun Lakes, AZ: Thomas Horton.

Signorielli, N., & Morgan, M. (Eds.). (1989). *Cultivation analysis: New directions in media effects research.* Newbury Park, CA: Sage.

Singhal, A., & Rogers, E. M. (1989). Pro-social television for development in India. In R. E. Rice & C. K. Atkin (Eds.), *Public communication campaigns* (2nd ed., pp. 331–350). Newbury Park, CA: Sage.

Snyder, M. (1980). Seek, and ye shall find: Testing hypotheses about other people. In E. T. Higgins, C. P. Herman, & M. P. Zanna (Eds.), *Social cognition: The Ontario Symposium on Personality and Social Psychology* (Vol. 1, pp. 105–130). Hillsdale, NJ: Erlbaum.

Snyder, M. (1981). On the self-perpetuating nature of social stereotypes. In D. L. Hamilton (Ed.), *Cognitive processes in stereotyping and intergroup behavior* (pp. 182–212). Hillsdale, NJ: Erlbaum.

Snyder, M. (1987). *Public appearances/private realities: The psychology of self-monitoring.* New York: Freeman.

Tellegen, A., & Waller, N. G. (1987, August). *Re-examining basic dimensions of natural language trait descriptors.* Paper presented at the 95th Annual Convention of the American Psychological Association, New York.

Triandis, H. C. (1995). *Individualism and collectivism.* Boulder, CO: Westview Press.

Vaughan, P. W., Rogers, E. M., & Swalehe, R. M. A. (1995). *The effects of "Twende Na Wakati," an entertainment-education radio soap opera for family planning and HIV/ AIDS prevention in Tanzania.* Unpublished manuscript, University of New Mexico, Albuquerque.

Weiner, B. (1986). *An attributional theory of motivation and emotion.* New York: Springer-Verlag.

Westoff, C. F., & Rodriguez, G. (1995). The mass media and family planning in Kenya. *International Family Planning Perspectives, 21,* 26–31.

White, J. (1982). *Rejection.* Reading, MA: Addison-Wesley.

Williams, S. L. (1992). Perceived self-efficacy and phobic disability. In R. Schwarzer (Ed.), *Self-efficacy: Thought control of action* (pp. 149–176). Washington, DC: Hemisphere.

Winfrey, C. (1979, February 25). Why 900 died in Guyana. *The New York Times Magazine,* p. 39.

Wood, R. E., & Bandura, A. (1989). Social cognitive theory of organizational management. *Academy of Management Review, 14,* 361–384.

Wylie, R. C. (1974). *The self-concept: A review of methodological considerations and measuring instruments* (Rev. ed.). Lincoln: University of Nebraska Press.

Yamagishi, T. (1988). The provision of a sanctioning system in the United States and Japan. *Social Psychology Quarterly, 51,* 265–271.

Zimbardo, P. G. (1995). The psychology of evil: A situationist perspective on recruiting good people to engage in anti-social acts. *Japanese Journal of Research in Social Psychology, 11,* 125–133.

8

Yin and *Yang* of the Japanese Self
The Cultural Psychology of Personality Coherence

SHINOBU KITAYAMA
HAZEL ROSE MARKUS

Yuko Arimori won a bronze medal in the women's marathon in the 1996 Olympic Games in Atlanta. Right after the race, as she was surrounded by reporters from Japan, she said that she wanted to "give a praise" to "the self who persevered and hung on until the end" (*ganbaru* in Japanese). This episode moved many Japanese—those who watched the scene on the TV and those who learned about it the next day, when her comments appeared on the front pages of major newspapers and on the nationally broadcast news shows. Overnight, the runner became a sort of national hero.

From a Western perspective, one can imagine that the runner was simply proud of herself. Or, if she cried as she made her comments, it was probably because she was upset with herself for failing to win the gold and perhaps was indulging in self-pity. Yet, from a Japanese perspective, close scrutiny reveals otherwise. The linguistic expression "giving a praise to someone" (*homete-ageru*), which is quite colloquial in Japanese, carries several distinct connotations. To begin with, the expression is used only when the giver of the praise is more resourceful, stronger, or higher in status or power (even if only temporarily and transiently) than the receiver. Thus, for example, a mother may often "give a praise" to her child, but the child never "gives a praise" to the mother (unless a joke or pun is intended by the child). Likewise, a teacher can "give a praise" to a pupil, but not vice versa. Hence, the very linguistic structure used by the runner entails the involvement of two separate subjects who differ in status or power. Furthermore, because of this implied difference in status and power, the act of praising in this context necessarily involves caring emotions (e.g., sympathy) that are extended by the more resourceful giver to the lesser receiver.

Is it unusual for someone to extend sympathy to someone else who happens to be herself? How can it be that two selves differing in status or power reside within the same person? From a Western perspective, the duality of self implied in this instance could seem a case of split personality. Aside from this unusual construal of the self and selves, the athlete would appear to be quite self-indulgent, childish, or immature. Given these "deficiencies in personality," it is all the more paradoxical that the reactions to the athlete's remarks by most Japanese were almost all unequivocally positive. For many Japanese, the episode was both morally compelling and emotionally moving. As interpreted and understood this way, then, the runner's episode raises several fundamental questions that pertain to the topic of this volume: What do we mean by the "unity" and "coherence" of personality? How do cultures vary in the meanings of personality coherence? And what consequences does this variation entail?

We suggest that embodied in the runner's episode is a central cultural narrative in Japan—one that portrays a "good [i.e., coherent and integral] person" as someone who persists with strict and critical attitudes toward the self, and yet who is fragile, warm-hearted, and even sympathetic to the self. The tough mind and the warm heart supplement each other; neither is sufficient by itself; each can only be sustained in balance by the antagonistic force exerted by the other; and each can be highlighted, augmented, and held in relief only in the other's presence. Thus the runner's toughness, which indicated her resolute commitment to her role identity as an athlete, simultaneously made her fragility and warmness all the more meaningful. Her tears were not just the tears of any person on the street; rather, they carried the weight of days, months, and years of hard training and difficult time. They came from a person who had knowingly engaged in such difficulties, persisted, hung on till the end, and eventually overcome them. Conversely, her warm-heartedness transformed, in a quite extraordinary fashion, a tough person into someone rather ordinary who was capable of everyday feelings and emotions and who was willing to share these feelings with others and to be receptive and appreciative of their caring acts; she was thus fully deserving of whole-hearted sympathy.

Moreover, these two selves inhabited the same physical body in balance, despite the fact that they might seem incompatible with each other. Altogether, the runner's response indicated her exemplary moral character. The ability to switch between one's perspectives or one's modes of engaging in the world—from an athlete on a national team to a child of a family, or from a strong public figure to a vulnerable private figure—is required in a cultural world that highlights the inevitable multiplicity of one's relationship and in which selves are defined in reference to such relationships.

This Japanese cultural narrative brings us right into the heart of the claim we make in this chapter: namely, that even though seemingly contradictory when analyzed in isolation, two aspects of the Japanese self—toughness and warm-heartedness—cohere together once they are combined, as *yin* and *yang*, to produce a person of integrity and coherence. Chinese philosophical thinking holds that reality is a process; it is active and changeable (Tu, 1994). Objects and concepts, including persons, are typically understood as fluid; they are not defined by essences or attributes or properties. Often a concept or an aspect of reality involves the idea that any given whole—say, the whole of a person—is more than the sum of its parts. And the parts of a given whole may often contradict or oppose one another. Existence requires actively maintaining a harmony or a balance among these parts; it requires the integration of the *yin* and the *yang* that make up the way, as described in the *I-Ching* (*The Book of Changes*). These Chinese understandings and a network of everyday practices associated with them are pervasive in everyday experience throughout Asia. Within such a framework, personality is found not in the defining traits, but in the dialectic, or the process of relation or balance, among the parts. Accordingly, the toughness of Yuko Arimori can only be understood against a background of warm-heartedness, and her warm-heartedness can only be understood against a background of toughness.

TWO VIEWS OF COHERENCE: BALANCE OR CONSISTENCY

In what follows, we distinguish between two perspectives on personality coherence. One perspective is illustrated by the example above. One needs both *yin* and *yang* to assure the coherence of personality, because the sense of personal coherence and integrity is produced by the dynamic equilibrium or balance between forces that are opposed, incompatible, and inconsistent with each other. This view of personality coherence as the balance of *yin* and *yang* in a person can be contrasted with an alternative view, which regards personality coherence as consistency among elements of a person, such as traits and behaviors.

Both views are social constructions, enabled simultaneously by psychological, interpersonal, collective, and cultural processes. An exploration of personality coherence in any cultural context requires a systematic knowledge of what it means to be a person and how behavior is understood to be produced and maintained in this context (Markus & Kitayama, 1998). Cultural groups in every historical period are associated with characteristic patterns of sociocultural participation—that is, with characteristic ways of being a person in the world. Hence, personality coherence is not a property inherent in a person; rather, it is produced and sustained by an array of sociocultural practices and meanings. Nevertheless, the social and collective processes underlying personality coherence are more obviously highlighted with the balance view, since personality coherence in this view is established out of the configuration of various facets of the self that are contingent on relatively specific social relationships and contexts. By contrast, the notion of consistency within a bounded person lends itself to a rather decontextualized view of personhood. Both psychological and cultural processes that are rooted in the consistency view of personality coherence conspire to leave the psychological or the unitary agentivity of the self in the foreground of the conscious experience. Simultaneously, they tend to hide the very social surrounding that affords this experience in a background.

The idea of transsituational consistency in behavior has been often invoked as the key criterion of personality coherence (Pervin, 1990). Indeed, even when the notion of balance is used, it is taken to be synonymous with consistency (Heider, 1958). Nevertheless, cross-cultural research in recent years (Heine & Lehman, 1997; Markus & Kitayama, 1991) has indicated that people in many cultures often disagree with Leon Festinger (1957) and many of his followers in North American social psychology, who have claimed that consistency among one's personal attributes centrally defines one's integrity. It is possible that the balance view of personality is more pervasive, better accepted and appreciated, and more highly valued in cultures outside North America.

The current analysis is informed by the recently emerging discipline of cultural psychology (Bruner, 1990, 1996; Cole, 1996; Fiske, Kitayama, Markus, & Nisbett, 1998; Greenfield, 1997; Kitayama, 1998; Kitayama & Markus, 1994; Markus, Kitayama, & Heiman, 1996; Shweder et al., 1998; Shweder & Sullivan, 1993). Cultural psychology begins with the premise that all human experience, by its very nature, is social and situated. A person comes into being only when engaged in culture-specific systems of meanings and practices that afford this personhood. Even a bounded, independent person becomes conceivable, let alone actually possible, only within a social context that affords this form of personhood. Likewise, even when one is alone, isolated from the rest of the world, it is this outer world that makes the isolation both possible and often intolerably miserable. Human psychological functions, structures, and processes are interdependent with, closely attuned to, invited by, and afforded by the attendant pattern of cultural practices and public meanings.

Cultural psychology takes very seriously the idea that there are multiple worlds of practices and meanings (Shweder, 1991). These worlds can be equally viable and comprehensible, and to that extent can be equally rational, but they can be very different in their potential to invite and sustain various psychological processes and structures. Hence events that are seemingly identical (say, parties or sports events) may differ greatly in the meanings they entail when situated in different cultural contexts. For example, a base-ball game can be a sheer competition, as in the United States, where the stron-ger team tries to beat the weaker by the widest possible margin. But in Japan, the best game is construed to be the one where neither team obviously excels the other and one team wins by just a face-savingly small amount (Whiting, 1990). Living in different cultural worlds amounts to developing correspond-ingly divergent minds and hearts. From this perspective, personality coher-ence, like many other psychological constructs and processes (e.g., self, honor, conflict, love, and rationality), cannot be understood outside the rele-vant social and cultural context. Personality coherence does refer to a certain quality of the person him- or herself. Yet what it is and how it is accom-plished are inevitably socioculturally mediated. On the basis of this premise of cultural psychology, we argue that both the meaning of personality coher-ence and the specific psychological and interpersonal processes involved in it may be highly contingent on the relevant cultural contexts.

As we search for patterns in individual behavior, it is important to point out that the balance view and the consistency view of personality coherence are linked to two very different sets of understandings about the nature, source, and purpose of behavior. The balance view of personality coherence is rooted in Eastern philosophical traditions, which emphasize overcoming the idea of the self as a separate, enduring entity. The notion of a stable self is believed to be erroneous, and the pursuit of egoistic goals is assumed to be the source of suffering (Paranjpe, 1988). Suffering is identified with a desire for esteem, recognition, or security (Crook & Rabgyas, 1988). A focus on the self as a permanent entity works against the appreciation of interdependence and the nonparticularity of things.

In contrast, the consistency perspective on coherence is rooted in West-ern philosophical traditions, which have repeatedly made the case for the "natural" self-interest or selfishness of the individual. And the scientific study of personality in the West has not been value-free, but has tacitly incor-porated this individualistic ontology into its theories and models. This is hardly surprising, because the model of the person as an autonomous, inde-pendent free entity is the model of most of the Western social sciences (including psychology, sociology, and economics), and of most of biology as well (Lillard, 1998). As Wallach and Wallach (1983) have noted, Western psy-chology has sanctioned self-determination, self-interest, and selfishness through its promotion of a particular set of models of human nature. Modern European and North American personality theory is anchored in a philo-sophical legacy that includes Hobbes in the 17th century, Bentham in the 19th, and Dawkins in the late 20th (Schwartz, 1986). Moreover, this model of the person has been objectified and made real through the practices and insti-tutions that have been structured according to these understandings. Both of these perspectives on human behavior are powerful and viably animate their respective worlds; the point is not to argue for one or the other. Instead, our goal is to underscore how cultural frameworks structure both everyday and scientific understandings of personality.

This chapter consists of four major sections. Following this introductory section, the second section begins by describing a cultural-psychological perspective on personality coherence. A theoretical framework is presented to account for the collective construction of person and personality, with a particular emphasis on the construction of the two alternative views of personality coherence: consistency and balance. In the third section we discuss in detail the ways in which the balance view of personality coherence is reflected in practices and public meanings of contemporary Japanese culture and Japanese selves. In particular, we explore what personality coherence is like when it is defined in terms of the balance of ostensibly competing or even contradictory elements. In the fourth section of this chapter, we illustrate our theoretical analysis by focusing on one domain that is central in the construction of personality—namely, self-evaluation. Specifically, pertinent psychological evidence is reviewed to show that most of the time, self-critical perceptions predominate in the Japanese phenomenology of the self and yet they are in balance with—and, in fact, even prerequisites for—an implicit glow of warm feelings toward the self. We conclude by suggesting that the question of personality coherence can only be addressed by taking into detailed account the nature of the cultural context in which this person is constructed.

A CULTURAL-PSYCHOLOGICAL VIEW OF PERSONALITY COHERENCE

Some Historical Background

Dispositional Views of Personality

For the most part, personality psychology has been deeply wedded to an individualistic model of the person, in which a separate, bounded individual is seen as the primary fact (Pervin, 1994; Markus & Kitayama, 1998). The assumption is that there in fact exist some stable internal qualities of the person, "dispositions" or "traits," which manifest themselves across different situations (Goldberg, 1993; McCrae & Costa, 1997). This "presocial" individual is assumed to be characterized in terms of attributes (such as the Big Five trait features) that are internal and perhaps even inherent in this person. Furthermore, these internal attributes or dispositions are considered to guide, direct, and organize the person's overt behavior, the person's inner experience (both thinking and feeling), and the coherence of these. Personality coherence is, then, synonymous with personal consistency. Indeed, if personality is an entity that is autonomous, bounded, and independent, what else can its coherence be, other than a matter of stability and consistency in the arrangement of cognitions, emotions, motivations, and behaviors bounded within the person? Personality coherence is thus a stable, trait-like structure of each individual's cognitive, emotional, motivational, and behavioral functions. If Mary is in fact a sociable person, then she is likely to be more or less sociable across different situations.

Empirically, cross-situational consistency of behaviors has long been known to be quite weak, no stronger than $r = .20$ (Mischel, 1973). Likewise, many psychologists eager to demonstrate any degree of attitude–behavior consistency have been repeatedly discouraged by the correlations of a similar magnitude. These findings notwithstanding, the belief in personal consistency as the criterial feature of personality has persisted (Funder & Ozer, 1997). Some have argued that the failure to recover the expected cross-situational consistency of behavior is due to the unreliability of behavioral measures, and therefore that the best remedy is to make the measures more reliable by collapsing data across a wide range of observations (e.g., Epstein, 1979). Others have suggested that behavioral stability applies only to those people for whom stability in that particular domain personally matters, and thus who believe themselves to be consistent in that domain (Bem & Allen, 1974). In essence, one may hope to find personal consistency if one looks at it at the right place with the right methods.

Social-Cognitive Views of Personality

A number of opinions dissenting from this standard view can be discerned in the literature. The dissenting views have been championed by personality researchers with social-cognitive orientations, who have assumed that personality systems are best understood, described, and analyzed not in terms of static dispositions that are ascribed to each person, but in terms of goals, values, strategies, affective responses, expectations, and beliefs that constitute a person as a whole (Cantor, 1994; Cantor & Kihlstrom, 1987; Dodge, 1993; Dweck & Leggett, 1988; Higgins, Chapter 3, this volume; Kelly, 1955; Markus, 1977; Mischel, 1973, 1990; Mischel & Shoda, 1995). In this conceptualization, the cross-situational consistency of behavior is weak because the researchers have sought an entity—consistent disposition—that may in fact be nonexistent. Personality coherence is not a matter of consistency of each individual's traits across situations. Instead, it is assumed to manifest itself at the level of goals, values, strategies, affects, and beliefs that characterize each person. Because these "lower-level" constructs of personality are likely to be highly contingent on specific features of different situations one is likely to encounter in daily life, the often negligible trait-level consistency of the person should not come as any surprise. Instead, stability and consistency may be observed in the ways in which each individual engages in different types of social situations (Mischel & Shoda, 1995).

The social-cognitive theories reconceptualize personality coherence in terms of the consistency of behaviors in specific social situations. How certain types of social situations are construed and made meaningful can vary considerably across individuals. For example, a meeting with a counselor at a summer camp can be a threat for some children, but it can be an opportunity to be a "good child" for others. Hence different individuals respond differently to the "same" situation in accordance with the idiosyncratic meanings they assign to it. Furthermore, the same person may respond to similar situations differently, depending on his or her idiosyncratic constructs of the situation, demonstrating no explicit consistency in behavioral tendency. Yet the relationship between situational construals (e.g., a "threat" situation) and behavioral tendencies (e.g., aggression) may still be stable; if so, it may provide a solid basis for perceived consistency of personality, and thus its coherence for actors and observers alike. Mischel and Shoda (1995) provide evidence for this possibility in North America by demonstrating that the judgment of behavioral consistency of the self is highly correlated with the extent to which behavioral tendencies are reliably associated with different types of situations. On the basis of this evidence, these researchers have argued that behavioral consistency can be analyzed meaningfully in terms of the association of behaviors and attendant social situations in which they take place.

The social-cognitive camp of personality research has come a long way toward a more contextualized view of personality, in which types of psychological systems are afforded and enabled by social situations, which by themselves are constructed by individuals who differ in their psychological systems (Cantor, 1994; Mischel & Shoda, 1995). The social context is assumed to be a constitutive element of the person. To understand the person, it is important to examine the nature of the social situations, the everyday practices, the lay knowledge, and the common narratives that together define the sociocultural context in which the person participates. These elements are required to fashion or to realize experience; they are not a cultural or social overlay that is applied after basic behavior has occurred. There is, then, a very close affinity between the social-cognitive approach to personality and cultural psychology. Yet, given the very wide-angle perspective afforded by the study of personality across diverse cultures, cultural psychologists are in a position to argue even more radically than theorists of the social-cognitive approach for the socially and collectively constructed nature of personhood, self, or personality, and thus for the socially constructed nature of its coherence.

Cultural Psychology: Mutual Constitution of Culture and Personality

The last decade has seen an explosive surge of findings and theories that have alerted researchers in many behavioral and social science disciplines to the cultural boundedness of some of the fundamental assumptions and phenomena of the respective fields. In our home turf of social, personality, and developmental psychology, for example, a great many "anomalies" have been discovered in cultures outside North America. For example, verbs are acquired before nouns by infants in Mandarin China (Tardif, 1996); Japanese self-criticize without any trace of depression (Kitayama, Markus, Matsumoto, & Norasakkunkit, 1997); Chinese are often persuaded quite effectively by arguments that defy the fundamental premise of logical consistency (such as "losing is winning"; Peng, 1997); the fundamental attribution error fails to occur in India (Miller, 1984), China (Morris & Peng, 1994), and Japan (Kitayama & Masuda, 1997); and the Japanese do not seem to engage in dissonance reduction (Heine & Lehman, 1997). The initial discoveries of such anomalies have prompted many theorists to raise questions about some of the assumptions hidden in the historical development of the field itself, not the least important of which is the assumption of a "bounded, independent person" as the "natural" unit of analysis in social, personality, and developmental psychology (e.g., Cole, 1996; Geertz, 1973; Gergen, 1973; Markus & Kitayama, 1991, 1994; Miller, 1994; Sampson, 1977, 1988; Shweder & Bourne, 1984; Shweder & Sullivan, 1993; Triandis, 1989, 1995).

In sociology and anthropology, some theorists who have become impatient with more traditional, mostly static analyses of social structures, rituals, and kinship typologies have begun to theorize about the ways in which human agency, subjectivity, and personal experience may be understood as active elements of the social structure itself (e.g., Berger & Luckmann, 1967; Bourdieu, 1976; Giddens, 1984; Kleinman, 1989; Lutz, 1988; Myers, 1991; Schutz & Luckmann, 1974; White, 1994). Likewise, in linguistics, instead of the syntactic analysis of language that has dominated the field since Chomsky, many theorists have begun to focus more closely on the pragmatic use of language, the discourse practices, and the narratives that give shape to personal experience, to social relationships, and thus eventually to social structures (e.g., Lakoff & Johnson, 1980; Ochs, 1988; Wierzbicka, 1994). All these new developments in the divergent disciplines have converged to the cultural-psychological agenda of illuminating how cultural practices and meanings and human agency composed of psychological processes and structures mutually constitute, reinforce, and sustain one another. Thus the present attempt to formulate the contextual and culturally constructed nature of personality can be placed squarely within the wider movement that is now beginning in the behavioral and social science disciplines under the banner of cultural psychology.

The cultural-psychological perspective is illustrated in Figure 8.1. On the left-hand side are listed various collective and social practices and meanings that as a whole constitute a given cultural group. On the right-hand side are found a number of psychological processes and structures. The practices and meanings of culture, and the psychological processes and structures of each member of the culture, are *mutually constitutive.*

This mutually constitutive relation is formed between culture and the person through development. Everyone is born into a culture consisting of a set of practices and meanings, which have been laid out by generations of

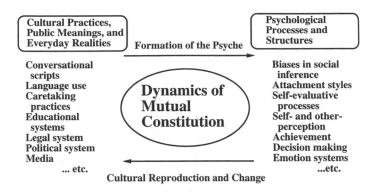

FIGURE 8.1. Theoretical framework of cultural psychology: Mutual constitution of culture and the psyche.

people who have created, carried, maintained, and altered them. To engage in culturally patterned relationships and practices and to become mature, well-functioning adults in the society, new members of the culture must come to coordinate their responses to their particular social milieu. That is, people must come to think, feel, and act with reference to local practices, relationships, institutions, and artifacts; to do so, they must use the local cultural models, which consequently become an integral part of their psychological systems. Each person actively seeks to behave adaptively in the attendant cultural context, and in the process different persons develop their own unique sets of response tendencies, cognitive orientations, emotional preparedness, and structures of goals and values.

The practices and meanings of a culture can function as tools (Bateson, 1972; Cole, 1996; Vygotsky, 1978), resources (Geertz, 1973), and capital for everyone and anyone who participates in it. Like a sailor who uses a map to navigate a ship, or like a mathematician who uses Greek symbols to perfect a proof of a new theory, we all use a number of cultural artifacts to live our everyday lives including "things" like tables, chairs, and money; "images" such as happiness or the future; "ideas" such as liberty and duty; and "scripted routines" such as saying hello and good-bye, eating a working lunch, or taking a break. Unlike many of the earlier analyses drawing on the culture-as-a-toolkit metaphor, however, our suggestion is that cultural tools are not just to be used by a person; they also create, alter, and eventually fully constitute this person him- or herself. Like using any tools and resources, actively using cultural practices and meanings not only requires but also gradually gives rise to certain styles of responding to and acting with them (Kitayama, Markus, et al., 1997; Markus, Mullally, & Kitayama, 1997). Put another way, cultural practices and meanings invite a particular mode of responding and living—the mode that is attuned to and coordinated with the specific characteristics of the practices or meanings at issue. It is the active engagement in the pattern of social life that exerts formative influences on psychological processes.

Notably, different individuals have different biological propensities, potentials, and temperamental inclinations. Furthermore, humans as a species have important biological propensities that have made cultural adaptation possible (Brown, 1991; Durham, 1991; Fiske et al., 1998). Yet virtually none of these biological propensities is likely to determine in full the nature of the cognitive, emotional, and motivational organizations a person develops in the course of becoming a mature adult. The psychological structures and processes are one's characteristic ways of "handling" and "living with" an assortment of cultural affordances. Thus the ways in which any given biological propensities are appropriated in use for this or that psychological structure (e.g., how cardiovascular systems are involved in coping with stress); the meanings that are assigned to such propensities (e.g., a facial musculature pattern as "spontaneous expression of emotion" or as "social mask"); and which temperamental inclinations (e.g., "extraversion" as marked by contraction of zygomatic muscles in infants) are valued, fostered, and reinforced, or despised, inhibited, and suspended—all of these are closely intertwined with the attendant cultural pattern.

In sum, cultural psychology rests on the notion of the mutual constitution of culture and the person. Personality as a system of many psychological tendencies, processes, and structures, including cognitions, emotions, and motivations, is established through the coordination and attunement of individual responses to cultural practices and meanings. Personality is a result of the routinization of response patterns that are coordinated with the gestalt of cultural practices and meanings. Furthermore, once these psychological systems operate naturally and spontaneously, they are bound to reproduce the initial pattern of cultural practices and meanings. Thus, as Shweder (1990) puts it, culture and the psyche make each other up. And the goal of cultural psychology is to delineate the dynamics involved in this mutually constitutive relationship between the two.

European-American notions of personality are afforded by and maintained by a great many cultural meanings, including the idea that difference among people is obvious and good; the belief that a person can be separated from society or the social situation; and the assumption that social behavior is rooted in, and largely determined by, one's underlying traits. These notions of personality are also fostered by a host of routine practices, such as employment ads, personal ads, the self-administered personality tests that appear regularly in lifestyle magazines, and diverse counseling and therapy methods—all of which encourage the view that people have different trait-like qualities, and that these attributes will be important in employment, marriage, and life in general. As soon as these specific meanings and practices are spelled out, it is evident that many of them are quite specific to European-

American cultural contexts and are not shared across divergent cultural contexts. In many Asian cultural contexts, for example, one's uniqueness or positive difference from others is not emphasized or rewarded, and one's internal dispositions are not accorded the same importance in understanding social behavior, whether it is getting married or holding a job. Efforts to delineate the cultural models and practices that undergird psychology's current theories of personality are important in their own right, but perhaps more importantly, they also show that a comprehensive understanding of coherence in individual behavior will require knowledge of other cultural models of the person and social behavior.

The cultural-psychological perspective, then, allows us to broaden the currently narrow focus on the bounded individual, and thus to reconceptualize personality from a more encompassing, dynamic point of view—a viewpoint that regards a human as a social being, and his or her personality and human agency as collectively afforded and maintained. From the cultural-psychological perspective, coherence in personality can only be meaningfully analyzed when we understand in detail the precise ways in which personality is culturally contextualized, socially situated, and thus collectively constructed.

Specifically, we suggest that a judgment about the coherence or integrity of a person depends on the stability of the person's embeddedness in the psychocultural complexes held in place in a given cultural context. Behaving in accordance with the generic blueprint laid out by tacit assumptions, meanings, and practices of a given cultural community should amount to being coherent both in one's own eyes and in those of others in the same cultural community. Hence, to ask a question about personality coherence is to pose a question about the specific model of the person through which the behavior is made meaningful by both the actor and observers. What are the root models of the person in a culture? How are various aspects of the culture constructed, maintained, and held in place by and through these models? And what types of behaviors, thoughts, feelings, and motivations are construed to be attuned and coordinated with such cultural patterns? Furthermore, to the extent that perceived coherence is one active element in the making of the self, the appropriation of others, and the forming of social relationships, we may also ask questions about how personality coherence, constructed as such in the culture, may mediate these social psychological processes.

Independent and Interdependent Models of the Self

The possibility that the person or the self may be constructed very differently across cultures is one of the major themes of the cultural psychology (e.g., Markus & Kitayama, 1991; Shweder & Sullivan, 1993; Triandis, 1995). Elsewhere (Markus & Kitayama, 1991), we have proposed that in European American cultures the self is construed to be an *independent*, autonomous entity, but in East Asian cultures, it is construed to be an *interdependent,* mutually connected entity. The independent model of the person incorporates the following ideas: (1) A person is an autonomous entity defined by a distinctive set of attributes, qualities, or processes; (2) this configuration of internal attributes or processes determines or causes behavior; (3) individual behavior will vary, because people vary in their configuration of internal attributes and processes, and this distinctiveness is good; and (4) people should express their attributes and processes in behavior, so there should be consistency in behavior across situations and stability over time, and this consistency and stability are good.

The interdependent model of the person incorporates a different set of ideas: (1) A person is part of an encompassing set of social relationships; (2) behavior is a consequence of being responsive to the others with whom one is interdependent, and the origins of behavior are in relationships; and (3) the precise nature of a given social situation often varies, so individual behavior will be variable from one situation to another and from one time to another. This sensitivity to social context and consequent variability are good. (For an in-depth look at these divergent models of the person, see Fiske et al., 1998, and Markus & Kitayama, 1998.)

The theoretical analysis rooted in the distinction between these two models of the self has proved to be quite powerful in integrating cross-cultural differences in cognition, emotion, and motivation (see, e.g., Fiske et al., 1998, and Markus et al., 1996, for reviews). From this observation, it may seem quite sensible to assume that people in different cultural contexts tend to internalize and thus to believe the cultures' respective models of the self, and that by virtue of this internalizing of cultural models, psychological systems show cross-culturally divergent characteristics.

Several notable attempts to measure self-construals at the individual level, and then to relate the individual differences in self-construal to differences in psychological functions in other domains (e.g., Kiuchi, 1995; Kwan, Bond, & Singelis, 1997; Okazaki, 1997; Singelis, 1994; Takata & Matsumoto, 1995), are all grounded in the assumption that cultural views of the self have to be internalized and individually, cognitively, or affectively represented in order for them to have any significant influences on psychological processes. The same assumption can be found in analyses on influences of lay theories in social thinking and social behavior (e.g., Dweck, 1993). The same type of theorizing used to be common in the "personality and culture" school that flourished in the 1950s. As some theorists have pointed out (Miller, 1994), cultural influences were often conceptualized as unidirectional transmission of culture-level information to the person. In this view, the person is a culture made small and compact, and perhaps partial, so as to be fitted into a single body. The isomorphic relation posited between culture and the person in this perspective may turn out to be too limiting, however.

We regard a culture as a pattern of practices and meanings that dynamically change over time, and that more often than not are kept tacit, embodied in routinized behaviors, rather than being stored in people's brains as "instructions" for behaviors. Participating in a culture is like receiving an invitation to do certain things. Cultural participation is inherently active, because cultural invites (as well as coerces) and affords (as well as constrains) active and creative human actions, thoughts, feelings, and motivations. Culture may thus be better conceptualized as a structure or a frame within which one seeks an adaptation by actively thinking, feeling, and acting, rather than as an entity that is to be learned or understood. The cultural psychology holds that the construction of the person is mediated not only by "enbrained" information or knowledge about *what* is right and wrong or *what* to do and believe, but also, more significantly, by practices and meanings that are historically constructed and embodied in *how* people in the community think, feel, and act. Hence a much greater emphasis must be given to the social and collective processes by which cultural views of the self are transformed into culturally divergent systems of psychological processes and structures.

Theoretical Framework: The Collective Construction of the Person

In accordance with this line of analysis, we have proposed a collective-constructionist theory of the self, which assumes that cultural models' influences on psychological functions are significantly mediated by the ways in which social situations are collectively constructed (Kitayama, Markus, & Lieberman, 1995; Kitayama, Markus, et al., 1997; Markus & Kitayama, 1994; Markus, Mullally, & Kitayama, 1997). The theory helps us conceptualize the dynamic relationship between processes at macrosocietal, historical, and collective levels, and those at microsocial, contemporaneous, and personal or interpersonal levels. The theoretical framework is schematically illustrated in Figure 8.2.

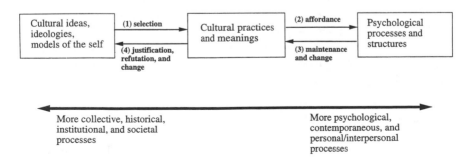

FIGURE 8.2. The collective-constructionist theoretical framework.

Historical Selection of Cultural Practices

The theory begins with the assumption that the models of the self as independent or as interdependent are reflected in philosophical and ontological ideas and ideologies constructed and preserved in the respective cultural contexts. In conjunction with other processes at the historical, societal, and collective levels, including ecological, economic, and political processes, these philosophical and ontological assumptions of culture have given rise over many generations to a set of social situations, daily practices, and public meanings associated with them.

Some practices may be explicitly designed in the society with the guidance of its predominant ideology. For example, a relatively well-articulated rule regarding the subtle gradient of the "depth" of bowing in modern Japan was probably introduced into the society to promote the social hierarchy based on Confucian ideology. It is also possible that some preexisting practices are reinterpreted to foster a new model of the self. For example, mundane practices derived from a Protestant ethical code of asceticism during the era of the Reformation might have been gradually appropriated to form the core of the contemporary model of the "economic man," as we shall see in more detail shortly. And of course, once distinct mentalities are fostered by an assortment of practices rooted in a particular view of the self, many other practices that are produced by or introduced to the culture are motivated by such mentalities; as a consequence, they should tend to be congruous with and thus to provide de-facto proof for the validity of that very model of the self. For example, psychological orientations toward self-control (supposedly derived in part from the belief in asceticism) in contemporary North American society may have contributed to a number of health practices (e.g., daily jogging and swimming) that require these very mental orientations, thereby affirming the supposition about the necessity of self-control.

It is very difficult to be exact about the etiology of practices of any contemporary cultures. The social history of mundane cultural practices is one area that has yet to be fully developed (Stearns & Stearns, 1986). Yet, at the most general level, it is safe to assume that as a consequence of selective accumulation of practices and meanings, each culture has its own unique semiotic world—a world that has the potential to evoke certain meanings, interpretations, and patterns of thoughts, emotions, desires, and actions. Such potential inherent in cultural practices may be called the "cultural affordances" (cf. Gibson, 1966).

Cultural Affordances

Cultural affordances can take a variety of forms. To illustrate, let us consider a cultural script of "friendly [i.e., tactful], adversarial [i.e., self-assertive], and egalitarian [i.e., democratic] discussion," which is quite common in North

American graduate education. Participating in conversations grounded in this script will encourage the development of mental preparedness to identify, express, and justify one's own opinions and judgments. Pertinent information is likely to be organized so as to facilitate this communicative (as opposed to receptive) mode of thinking (cf. Zajonc, 1960), resulting in a variety of cognitive and judgmental biases (Lord, Ross, & Lepper, 1979). Furthermore, restraint of anger and other fierce emotions, which can often accompany interpersonal disagreement and dispute, is both a prerequisite for and a consequence of repeatedly participating in such discussions (see Stearns & Stearns, 1986, for an excellent social-historical analysis of anger and its restraint in the contemporary United States). Thus, this particular cultural practice of a "friendly, adversarial, and egalitarian discussion" may be said to carry an affordance for the mental qualities of expressive rationalism and emotional restraint (especially restraint of anger). Or consider the domestic practice of "who sleeps by whom" (Shweder, Jensen, & Goldstein, 1995). Cultural groups vary considerably in preferred sleeping arrangements, and sleeping patterns are likely to reflect and often reinforce (and thus afford) certain mythologies about family and social relationships. For example, the typical North American pattern of a husband and wife, but nobody else, sharing the same bedroom lends itself to a culturally sanctioned image of the "sacred couple" and to associated cultural discourses about romantic love. Similarly, ads that appear on TV and popular magazines are explicitly designed (with a certain degree of success) to maximize their potential to evoke certain thoughts, emotions, and motivations.

In short, as an amalgam of practices, associated meanings, and social situations, each cultural world is likely to afford, solicit, or invite various psychological processes and structures that resonate with the elements of the culture. It is a challenging task of cultural psychology to articulate this construction of psychological processes and structures. The construction is collective, not only because it is mediated by the selecting and pruning of cultural practices over the course of the history of a given cultural group (arrow 1 of Figure 8.2), but also because it is an integral part of how the psychological processes of each individual operate in attunement with those of others within shared social space defined largely by conventionalized cultural practices and meanings (arrow 2 of Figure 8.2).

Maintenance and Change of Culture

It is important to emphasize that once established, the psychological processes and structures become instrumental in reproducing and reconstituting the cultural practices, meanings, and social situations from which they have been originally derived. Furthermore, insofar as such psychological processes are likely to become functionally autonomous (at least in part) of the surrounding cultural practices from which they have been derived, they should become capable of operating without much support from the cultural context. Hence individuals are able to and often do initiate changes in the immediate social realities (arrow 3 of Figure 8.2). Finally, the ever-fluctuating set of cultural practices and meanings is often used either to justify or to refute underlying ideologies, core cultural ideas, and associated models of the self. Hence these cultural representations are also likely to change. Yet, for the most part, the change may well be gradual and partial. For one thing, core cultural representations are only infrequently contested as focal issues of public debate. For another, they may still be consistent with a large number of other existing cultural practices and meanings (see arrow 4 of Figure 8.2).

The implication of the theoretical framework depicted in Figure 8.2 is that the two models of the person we have proposed (Markus & Kitayama, 1991) are historically constructed and have given rise to an array of cultural practices and meanings that as a whole constitute each concrete individual. There then results an integration of psychological processes and structures with cultural practices and meanings within a systemic whole, which has been variously characterized by Kroeber (1917) as "superorganic," by Whiting and Child (1953) as "custom-complex," and by Bruner (1990, 1996) as "narrative." More recently, we (Markus, Mullally, & Kitayama, 1997) have focused specifically on the aspects of this psychocultural complex that pertain to the self and called these "selfways." Despite differences in the conceptual emphasis given to, and the spatiotemporal scope of the phenomena to be covered by, each concept, all these efforts are directed toward characterizing a system in which culture and the person make each other up.

The Protestant Heritage of the Modern West

The notion that each individual person is a collective and historical product is certainly not a new idea. One could easily find similar ideas in the writings of the founding fathers of modern social psychology, such as Asch (1952), Bartlett (1932), Lewin (1935), and Vygotsky (1978) (see Fiske et al., 1998, and Markus et al., 1996, for reviews). These ideas are currently being rediscovered and elaborated by a number of socioculturally oriented psychologists (e.g., Cole, 1996; Saito, 1996; Wertsch, 1991; see Berline, 1992, and Jahoda, 1992, for the broader historical roots of sociocultural theories in the West). Instead of tracing the intellectual history of modern sociocultural psychology, however, we would like to focus only on one prominent sociologist who accomplished an excellent cultural and historical analysis of modern capitalistic mentalities at the turn of the 20th century.

In his celebrated treatise, *The Protestant Ethic and the Spirit of Capitalism,* Max Weber (1930/1992) identified rationalism and asceticism as the core elements of the mentality required in modern capitalistic culture. This mentality, he further argued, can be traced back to the Protestant model of an elect individual who engages continuously and ascetically in a "calling" to increase the glory of God. Importantly, Weber clearly recognized that this connection between the Protestant model of the person and the ascetic and rational character of each concrete individual of the contemporary industrial world is collectively and historically mediated. He thus noted:

> When asceticism was carried out of monastic cells into everyday life, and began to dominate worldly morality, it did its part in building the tremendous cosmos of the modern economic order. This order is now bound to the technical and economic conditions . . . which to-day determine the lives of all the individuals . . . with irresistible force. (p. 181)

As a consequence, the capitalistic culture thus constructed needs no support from the very model of the person that originally encouraged and constituted the culture. This cultural world has become self-maintaining, functionally detached from its historical precursor, by virtue of its capability to reproduce the mentality that is attuned to it in each of the concrete individuals who participate in it. Thus Weber continued:

> To-day the spirit of religious asceticism—whether finally, who knows?—has escaped from the cage. . . . The rosy blush of its laughing heir, the Enlightenment, seems also to be irretrievably fading, and the idea of duty in one's calling prowls about in our lives like the ghost of dead religious beliefs. . . . The individual generally abandons the attempt to justify it at all. . . . The pursuit of wealth, stripped of its religious and ethical meaning, tends to become associated with purely mundane passions, which often actually give it the character of sport. . . . Of the last stage of this cultural development, it might well be truly said: "Specialists without spirit, sensualists without heart; this nullity imagines that it has attained a level of civilization never before achieved." (p. 182)

Weber's analysis is quite compatible with our framework. As summarized in Figure 8.3, the Protestant model of the elect contributed over the his-

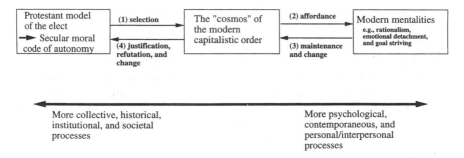

FIGURE 8.3. The Protestant heritage of "modern mentalities" as suggested by Max Weber (1930/1992).

tory of the modern West to the establishment of the "cosmos of the modern economic order" and an assortment of associated cultural practices. This "cage" does two things simultaneously. On the one hand, it defines the mundane social realities that influence, "with irresistible force," everyone who participates in it, hence affording and encouraging a particular mode of thought (rationalism), feeling (interpersonal detachment), and motivation (devotion to one's life task) (Giorgi & Marsh, 1990). On the other hand, it has also helped replace the Protestant ethic with a more secular moral code of independence and autonomy, and with a wider range of discourses in terms of freedom, individual rights, and self-expression (Taylor, 1989).

This analysis helps explain why there exists an uncanny resemblance between many theories and focal issues of contemporary psychology and the Protestant model of the person. These theories and issues include a cost–benefit analysis of rational decision making and its subjective-utility variant in the attitude literature (e.g., Ajzen, 1996; cf. rationalism); the fundamental attribution error, or a tendency to presuppose a hidden, fixed disposition in social perception (e.g., Gilbert & Malone, 1995; Ross, 1977; cf. predestination); a life task analysis of social-cognitive theory of personality (e.g., Cantor, 1994; cf. calling); delay of gratification (e.g., Mischel, Shoda, & Rodriguez, 1989; cf. asceticism); and many more. Thus, the fact that the Protestant ethic in its narrow, religious sense "has escaped from the cage" should not obscure two equally important possibilities. The first concerns the likelihood that the mentalities of contemporary European-Americans have been shaped or at least encouraged by the social realities promoted by the set of originally religious ideas. Second, we should also be aware that psychological theories themselves may be influenced by these ideas quite indirectly, by virtue of the fact that the concepts, images, examples, and forms of argumentation used in the theories are all derived from a subset of the meanings that have been accumulated in the European-American cultural group. Hence there exists at a very rough level an isomorphic relationship between the mentalities of people in this cultural world and the theories advanced in this world to account for these mentalities. This, of course, is to say that the theories are valid in respect to the mentalities to be explained. Yet their validity is assured, at least in part, by the historical fact that both the phenomena to be explained and the theories to explain them are grounded in the same root model of the person, here carefully traced by Weber to a Protestant cultural heritage.

Having examined Weber in some detail, we should hasten to add that the Protestant model of the person is only one (albeit an important and powerful one) of many variants of what we have called the independent view of the self. Another variant—related but distinct, and in any case quite important in its own right in respect to the "modern economic order"—consists of the core ideas in the discipline of economics, which have served not only as a description of but as a prescription for this order from the days of Adam Smith onward. These ideas include the actions of a free market made up of individual players, social contracts, and rational profit making. It is within the independent view of the self, with all such variants encompassed in it, that the notion of personality coherence as consistency and the assorted mental processes and tendencies that support this notion have historically been constructed (cf. Baumeister, 1987; Gergen, 1973; Jahoda, 1986; Pepitone, 1976).

Personality Coherence in the West and the East: Consistency and Balance

The Consistency View of Personality Coherence

In the history of the modern West, ideas such as the natural rights and free will of each individual, true, authentic self, or each market consisting of free members who choose to enter it via mutual consent and contract, have played a dominant role in forming many aspects of cultural practices, everyday discourses, and institutions (e.g., Bellah, Madsen, Sullivan, Swindler, & Tipson, 1985; Farr, 1991). These ideas are all variants or derivatives of the model of the self as independent. According to the independent model of the person, behavior is considered an expression of one's internal attributes or dispositions.

Evidence suggests that in Western cultures, attitudes are typically more powerful predictors of behavior than social norms (Triandis, 1995). Furthermore, although personal consistency cannot be always attained because various social forces (some very subtle) are likely to influence the course of any action, psychological processes are likely to be established in such a way that seemingly inconsistent behaviors are readily reconstrued to restore perceived consistency through constant updating of the pertinent dispositions (say, attitudes) in accordance with the behaviors, via the mechanisms of self-perception and self-justification (Bem, 1967; Festinger, 1957). As may be expected, individuals are most strongly motivated to engage in an action that is perceived to be initiated by their own choice and free will (Deci & Ryan, 1987, 1995). Likewise, a procedure to remind people of their behavioral intentions has proved to be very effective in producing actions that are congruous with the intentions (Gollwitzer, 1993). Although diverse and obviously different in detail, all these processes are consequences of having repeatedly participated in a cultural world framed in terms of the independent view of the self; furthermore, they serve as prerequisites for becoming more effective members of this cultural group.

These actor characteristics are supplemented by characteristics of observers, inasmuch as behaviors construed in that way by actors are likely to be observed and interpreted by others with similar interpretive schemes; this is called by Ross and Nisbett (1991) "lay dispositionism" (see also Gilbert & Malone, 1995; Jones, 1979). Thus, in European-American cultural contexts,

laypeople often interpret others' behaviors in terms of underlying dispositions even when there exist obvious situational constraints on the behaviors.
In a classic experiment, Jones and Harris (1967) had subjects read an essay
allegedly written by another student and estimate the true attitude of the
essay writer. When subjects were told that the writer had freely chosen the
essay position, they inferred that his true attitude corresponded to the essay
position. Interestingly, even when subjects were told that the writer had been
forced to take that position by a coach in a debate club, his true attitude was
inferred to correspond to the essay position. If a behavior is caused by situation, it should not indicate anything informative about the actor him- or herself. Thus the tendency to ignore or fail to take full account of situational-
force information in person perception is often considered to be an error; it
violates a normative inferential standard (Ross, 1977).

Importantly, however, when this inferential bias takes place in actual
social situations, it may more often than not correspond to the subjective
experience of the actor, who engages in self-perception and self-justification
(whereby dispositions are updated or even created from scratch in accordance with the actions that are subtly induced by situational factors). Not
surprisingly, when one simultaneously examines the perceptions of an actor
by observers and the self-perceptions of the actor him- or herself, the two
tend to coincide (e.g., Bem, 1967; Ross, Lepper, & Hubbard, 1975). Hence the
meaning of the act as an expression of the actor's disposition tends to be
shared by the actor him- or herself and the observers, even when the act can
be shown to have been caused by subtly manipulated situational factors. In
short, consistency-restoring operations can be found in both self-perception
and other-perception—and, from the perspective of mutual constitution, this
convergence of the two may turn out to be crucial in socially constructing the
independent, bounded notion of the self.

What emerges in the social field of actors and observers is that actor
characteristics tend to resonate with or be attuned to observer characteristics.
An automatic and obligatory reference to attitude in guiding one's own
actions (Fazio & Zanna, 1981), for example, may immediately be met with an
equally spontaneous bias on the part of the observers to infer the actor's corresponding dispositions (Newman & Uleman, 1989; Winter & Uleman, 1984).
The actor's propensity to refer to his or her internal attributes in accounting
for his or her own act (Bem, 1967; Festinger, 1957) is likely to satisfy the
observers' cognitive need or desire to see the actor's dispositions underneath
it (Jones, 1979; Ross, 1977). This interpersonal resonance structure enables the
actor to further confirm, by virtue of the act's having elicited supporting
responses from observers, the meaning of the act as guided by his or her own
internal attributes; simultaneously, it enables the observers to be assured of
the character of the actor.

Furthermore, somewhat paradoxically, once the psychological structure
has been established so that consistency-restoring operations of self-

perception or behavioral justification are well automatized and habitualized (and thus are in fine attunement with the strong normative demands for consistency), these operations will become part of the background. The socially afforded nature of the perceived consistency between disposition and behavior will be left unnoticed. Instead, the self is placed in the foreground; it is perceived to be an entity that is separate from and, in fact, in charge of the social surrounding (Bandura, 1982; Heckhausen & Schultz, 1995). In other words, the very subjective experience of being independent, agentic, self-efficacious, and bounded is likely to be enhanced by an immersion into a sociocultural context that affords such experience (Kitayama, Matsumoto, Takagi, & Markus, 1997; Weisz, Rothbaum, & Blackburn, 1984). And this experience makes it difficult to acknowledge its own culturally afforded nature.

The resulting experience of the self is schematically illustrated in Figure 8.4A. The self is perceived to be composed of a set of attributes internal to it, such as motives, desires, attitudes, traits, and needs. These internal attributes or dispositions are further perceived to be bounded within the self and to organize one's behaviors and interactions with people in the surrounding social contexts. Managing to maintain this structure in one's perceptions of the self and its relationship with the social world amounts to establishing coherence in one's personality. It is important that this phenomenology is part and parcel of the cultural system rooted in the corresponding view of the person as independent. As such, it is anything but natural; it is entirely contingent on the particular arrangement of culture.

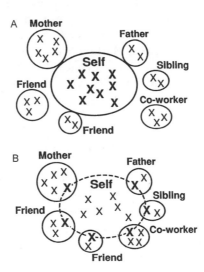

FIGURE 8.4. (A) Independent view of self. (B) Interdependent view. From Markus and Kitayama (1991). Copyright 1991 by the American Psychological Association. Reprinted by permission.

The Balance View of Personality Coherence

By contrast, in the history of East Asian cultures, the world views expressed in Buddhist teachings, Taoist writings, and Confucian ideologies, among others, have exerted considerable influence on the composition of daily practices, discourses, and social institutions (Ames, Dissanayake, & Kasulis, 1994). These world views are variants of the model of the self as interdependent. The collective-constructionist theory implies that social situations available in East Asian cultural contexts, when taken as a whole, should exhibit certain characteristics that promote the view of the self as interdependent. Hence, once individuals are socialized in this cultural context, they are likely to develop various psychological processes that are attuned to such social situations.

Within the interdependent model, a person is defined primarily in reference to his or her relationship with a pertinent social unit—or, more specifically, the extent to which he or she adjusts and fits into standards of excellence or ideal images appropriate in this relationship. Hence there exists a strong demand for attunement of the self with the social surrounding. Actions are construed, guided, and generated by psychological processes that incorporate expectations, norms, and rules of the social surrounding (Markus & Cross, 1990). Thus, for example, one may actively search for and identify what significant others in the context expect of the self and what they may need or want. The person is then inclined to use these situational anchors in organizing his or her own thoughts, feelings, and actions. The emerging experience of the self is characterized by its embeddedness in the context. One's agency is identified and made meaningful in reference to the encompassing social context. It is this "self in a specific social context" that predominates in subjective experience (see Markus & Kitayama, 1998, for a review of evidence). And when this type of construal is attained, individuals experience themselves to have been symbolically completed and to have become "fully human" (Lebra, 1976).

One piece of evidence consistent with the current analysis comes from research on behavioral regulation. Triandis (1995) summarizes evidence that in Asia social norms are bound to be relatively more important than attitudes in predicting behavior (see also Suh, Diener, Oishi, & Triandis, 1998). Although a fine attunement between the self and the social surrounding is not always attainable, psychological processes are likely to be established in such a way that actions that are seemingly unrelated or even incongruous with situational expectations are readily reinterpreted to maintain the sense of the self as fully embedded and encompassed in the context. It is not uncommon in Japan for acts that seem from a North American perspective to be intrinsically appealing (e.g., going to an amusement park with the family over a weekend) to be framed in terms of an idiom of social duty and obligation. For example, one might hear a Japanese parent say, "I really don't like to go, but kids are kids, and I have to go along with them." Yet this very posture of unwillingness to go to the amusement park with one's children may signify the importance of the self as a responsible parent who is needed and sought after by the children.

From the Western perspective, in which the disposition is the core of the person, responsibilities to others are often cast in terms of individual preferences or desires. Doing something because of obligations to others or because of their needs or requirements, even when these others are members of one's immediate family, can be seen as passive or dependent and as sacrificing one's autonomy and control. For example, when North Americans are thanked for doing things for others, it is not uncommon to hear them say, "Oh, I like to do these kinds of things; it was fun," or "It was my pleasure." Revealing that one was merely responding to social pressure or to the appeals of others can indicate weakness and a lack of clear ego boundaries. Overcommitted people, for example, are often advised to "just say no," as if the state of being multiply obligated were the result of a sickness or a pathological inability to resist the illegitimate entreaties of others. Moreover, allowing others to entrap one is not only bad for the actor; it is also bad for the others, because it can foster dependence in these persons rather than self-reliance.

Yet, given an interdependent, balance-based view of the person, it is one's very social embeddedness—one's willingness to incur social obligation—that gives meaning to existence. Being "part of it" with multiple ties and social entailments is the basis of being a person. Indeed, individuals are most strongly motivated to engage in an intrinsically appealing action when they perceive the action to have been requested or expected of them by significant others (Sethi & Lepper, 1997). Such an expectation highlights one's embeddedness in a social relationship, providing a much needed frame in which to locate and securely anchor the self. Given the interdependent, balance-based view of the self, social relationships provide the very means of deriving full meaning from one's being.

The psychological processes that constantly update one's own beliefs and attitudes so as to maintain the perceived embeddedness of the self are fostered by strong normative expectations held by others who believe in the lay theories of the person as fully interdependent and socially enabled. For example, in Japanese cultural contexts, individuals are often asked to state social roles and positions, as well as their relationships with some common acquaintances (e.g., "What is your relationship with Mrs. X?"). Such a question is predicated on the belief in the socially embedded nature of the person. Moreover, responding to it encourages the development of the psychological structure that immediately satisfies this demand for social responsiveness. See Markus, Mullally, and Kitayama (1997) for a summary of many practices grounded in a view of the self as interdependent (see also Barnlund, 1989; Clancy, 1986; Hendry, 1993). Once these psychological structures have been established so that they are in fine attunement with the strong normative demands, the demands will be perceived to be part and parcel of the self. The social responsiveness becomes so automatized and habitualized that the situational anchors to which the person responds are often experienced as being part of the self in that situation. The socially afforded nature of the self will be highlighted, and attributes internal to the self in general are bound to become part of the background.

The self constructed in this way tends to be multicomponential and multiperspectival. Because there are many possible social contexts for any single person, each individual is likely to develop multiple representations of selves in social relationships. It is explicitly recognized that the self in one context and the self in another context may show very different characteristics. For example, the self may be very tough-minded and strict in one set of situations, but it may be quite warm-hearted and sympathetic in another. The resulting experience of the self is schematically illustrated in Figure 8.4B. The self is perceived to be part of multiple social units. One switches between these social units in accordance with the nature of the social situations one happens to be in.

Recently, Hermans (1996) has suggested that the self may be seen as a collection of voices positioned differently in a social space (see Bachnik & Quinn, 1994, for a similar approach as applied to Japan). For example, a teenage boy may say to himself that he wants to go downtown with his friends for a late-night movie. But immediately afterward, he may take his mother's position to say to himself that it might not be a very prudent idea, which then changes his initial desire into a more compromised plan—say, playing Nintendo at home with friends. In this example, the self is constituted by a dialogue between the "I" and "mother," and through this dialogue the entire constellation of the self can unfold. The notion that very different configurations of the self can emerge, depending on the exact position or perspective one takes in seeing, interpreting, and construing things in the world, is quite consistent with the balance view of personality. Within the balance-based mode of construction of the self, however, the notion that the self can take very different forms according to its exact positioning in the social space is explicitly acknowledged and inscribed in various cultural practices, conventions, and lay theories. For example, a switching of one's perspectives on him- or herself, called *kejime*, is one element that is highly emphasized in Japanese socialization practices (Bachnik, 1992a).

Within this construction, internal attributes of the self that are relatively stable (i.e., dispositions), although acknowledged, are perceived to be among the multiple facets of the self that are contrasted against, yet in fine balance with, the selves in specific contexts. The dispositions, then, may not have any more privileged roles in guiding one's actions than do more situation-specific representations. Furthermore, what is good from one perspective may be very bad from another. From an independent perspective, it may seem possible and even desirable to increase positive evaluations in as many situations and contexts as possible. But from the interdependent perspective, this is not so: The act of maximizing the positivity of the self, by itself, may be seen as negative once a perspective is taken wherein, say, vanity is despised and jealousy is to be avoided. Resulting from this realization is not a tendency to overemphasize one perspective in lieu of others, but a tendency to keep a balance across the divergent perspectives associated with one's own social relationships (Kitayama & Markus, in press). Coherence of personality constructed in this way is likely to be assessed not in terms of consistency of various elements within any single perspective, but in terms of balance or harmony among the divergent perspectives. And the maintenance of balance across divergent perspectives symbolically affirms the sense of the self as socially embedded, engaged, responsive, and eventually responsible.

THE JAPANESE CULTURAL CONSTRUCTIONS OF THE SELF

The balance view of personality is quite widespread throughout East Asia, yet one can find considerable regional variations around this central theme. In this section we focus specifically on Japanese elaborations of the idea—how they have arisen in the history of Japan, and how they have shaped the cultural practices of contemporary Japan and the attendant mentality of the contemporary Japanese people. The intent is not to emphasize the uniqueness of Japanese culture; we believe that contemporary Japan can best be seen as one offshoot or variant of a larger trend in civilization that has unfolded in South and East Asia in the last several thousand years. The notion of balance, for example, has been extensively elaborated in traditional Chinese medicine as the fundamental principle of physical and mental health (Ohnuki-Tierney, 1984; Wang, 1998). Nevertheless, each specific region in Asia today, as in other areas of the world, shows a remarkably distinct constellation of cultural practices that are both influenced by major historical and ideological events of the larger area *and* grounded in idiosyncratic regionalities; Japan is no exception.

Multiperspectival selves in Japan correspond to the arrangement of the social world as historically constructed in this cultural context. Depending on the types of social relations available in his or her life (e.g., home, school, work, bar, party, etc.), each individual may configure his or her own unique organization of selves. Nevertheless, along with these different content domains of life, we can discern a duality that cuts across them—namely, the division between two very generic frames of an individual's life: *official* and *personal*. As pointed out by a number of observers of Japanese social life (Bachnik, 1992a, 1992b, 1994; Benedict, 1946; Doi, 1986; Kelly, n.d.; Kitayama & Karasawa, 1995; Lebra, 1976; Roland, 1988; Rosenberger, 1992; Smith, 1983), nowhere can the multiplicity of the Japanese self be seen more vividly than in this duality. Our argument in this section is summarized in Figure 8.5. This is an initial, admittedly crude attempt to define the two frames for organizing

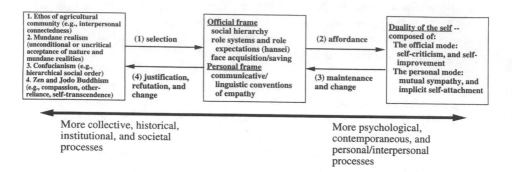

FIGURE 8.5. The collective construction of Japanese selves: Cultural models of the self, cultural practices, and psychological tendencies and structures.

the social world in contemporary Japanese culture, and then to relate the set of practices associated with each of the frames to the following: first, to ideas and models of the self historically developed in India, China, other regions of Asia, and Micronesia, and incorporated into Japanese culture; and second, to psychological structures and processes involved in the construction of selves in contemporary Japanese culture.

The Official Frame

The official frame involves one's activities in relatively formal and official social relations. The guiding principles here are mostly cognitive and rule-based. A hierarchical structure is assumed for society and cosmos. Rules are drawn for the structure of the hierarchical order; prescriptions are made for appropriate conducts for different roles. Typical contemporary examples include business, work, and other social organizations.

One major historical source for this frame is Confucianism, which is predicated on the vertical order of society. In modern Japan, role prescriptions, role expectations, and social rules based on the idealized image of social hierarchy are often justified in terms of loyalty, duty, devotion, and filial piety—all aspects of Confucian teaching (Benedict, 1946; DeVos, 1973, 1985; Kondo, 1990; Nakane, 1970). Although some recent observers have noted a gradual decline in the rigidity of the vertical societal structure with the advent of, for example, supposedly more individualistically oriented youth, feminism, and failures of more traditionally organized corporate businesses in international competition (e.g., Kashiwagi, 1997), the change appears to be slow, even if it should continue to unfold in the same direction in the future.

A related idea, which has ancient roots in Confucianism, Taoism, and

Zen Buddhism, among others, concerns an emphasis on an immersion or identification with a heavenly "path," which in turn allows one to transcend the worldly self. Originally conceived and conceptualized in Chinese thought, the path is considered to be an absolute standard or universal truth of the cosmos (Tu, 1994). But since its incorporation into Japanese thought around the 6th or 7th century A.D., the idea has undergone a considerable transformation. That is, the path has been secularized and made plural to signify idealized ways of doing things in every matter of daily concern.

Nakamura (1989) suggests that the Japanese have shown a strong tendency to provide secular, worldly interpretations for various ideas of Indian or Chinese origin, and that this tendency is due in part to a Japanese indigenous mythology and ontology that the ultimate truth lies not in any unworldly domain of "pure reason," but in worldly realities taken as such. What "really" exists is not any abstract principle or logic, but the flow of mundane daily life activities, as well as "natural" emotions and desires immersed in those activities. This ontology has resulted in the near-absence of critical thought, let alone any indigenous systems of abstract logic or thought, throughout the history of Japan. It has also promoted the secularization of the idea of the cosmic path.

Thus, in contemporary Japan various arts in high culture are considered to represent different paths, such as the "path of tea" (*Sa-dou*, the art of tea) or "the path of the sword" (*Ken-dou*, Japanese fencing). More generally, from this notion of path has evolved an idea that there are ideal, socially shared forms (e.g., ideal forms for pitchers in baseball, for quarterbacks in football, and for those performing every single move in the traditional arts of *Sa-dou* and *Ken-dou*), as well as ideal images for every matter of concern in the secular world (e.g., images for "good child," "good parent," "good superior," etc.; White & LeVine, 1986).

Furthermore, as Plath (1980) has shown, there exists in contemporary Japan a strong, albeit rather tacit, emphasis on finding one's own "path" through a long-term engagement with the social surrounding and his or her cohort. Thus the path is considered to be fully embedded in the mundane social order, and thus to be discovered gradually, incrementally, and effortfully through devoted engagement in the social matrix of everyday life. In its emphasis on the socially embedded nature of the path, this Japanese notion of "engagement" is markedly distinct from, say, the Protestant idea of "life task" or "calling."

Within the official frame, social relations are defined in terms of roles, status, wealth, educational rank, and other relatively impersonal markers of a person's place in the cultural world, and one's merit is assessed by success and failure in attaining them. Both to acquire and defend one's honor (one's "face" conceived of as his or her place in the symbolic system of social hierarchy) and to avoid shame (a "loss of face") become important concerns

(Edwards, 1997; Kuwayama, 1992; see Ho, 1976, for a Chinese perspective on honor and face). The emphasis on hierarchical formality and structure was developed by the Samurai ruling class of feudal Japan (Nitobe, 1905/1969). During the early period of feudal Japan, when regional wars were routine, honor acquisition played a significant role for Samurai warriors; but through-out the subsequent peaceful era of 250 or so years in the Tokugawa regime, honor acquisition may have been replaced by shame avoidance as a domi-nant constitutive principle of the Samurai culture, which inevitably and strongly influenced the culture of merchants that had become a major eco-nomic and thus political force of the time. The landscape of contemporary Japanese culture has been strongly influenced by this historical transforma-tion (Benedict, 1946; Edwards, 1997).

The self is an element in this social space; as such, its worth depends on its place (e.g., status and role) in the space, and thus the central criterion for judging the self is its standing in the space—how well it fares in it. Evaluation of the self as good or bad, superior or inferior, and worthy or unworthy pre-figures the experience of the self. For the marathon runner, to win a race is to locate the self high up in the official social space. For many "salary men," moving up the ladder of the social hierarchy carries the same meaning. Given this construction of the official social world, the self is always compared with a socially defined ideal image for the self in a particular social position, and it becomes possible to improve within the space by eliminating any personal shortcomings that are identified in the comparison. This representation of the self in the official frame provides a dominant system for participating in vari-ous public social units (e.g., classroom and workplace), and thus governs one's subjective experience in these relatively public social situations.

The Personal Frame

The personal frame involves one's activities in relatively informal and more personal social relations. The guiding principles here are mostly affective and other-oriented. Benevolent human emotions of empathy, sympathy, and com-passion are emphasized. A complete reliance or dependence on the mercy of others, and an immersion of the individual self in such benevolent others, are held to be both feasible and desirable (cf. Doi, 1971; Yamaguchi, 1994). Typical contemporary examples of aspects of life that fall within the personal frame include family relations (especially the mother–child relationship), close friendships, and other more informal interpersonal relations.

Sympathetic, affectionate, interpersonal discourses are embedded in a variety of linguistic conventions and mundane daily routines. For example, when the day's work is over at an office, a boss may say to his or her subordi-nates in a warm tone of voice, "*Gokurousama*," which literally means "Mr./ Ms. Hardship." Or at one of the training gyms now quite common in bigger cities in Japan, one will find young clerks at the front desk saying in a very friendly and casual fashion to clients who have just finished their day's exercise, "*Otukaresama!*," the literal translation of which is "Mr./Ms. Tired!" In these cultural and linguistic conventions, people treat others as individuals who have gone through some hardship and thus have been plagued with fatigue, so as to extend warm feelings of sympathy to them.

Such conventions of sympathy are even embedded in the grammar of the Japanese language. One case in point relates to words used in self-reference. Thus, when a person refers to him- or herself while speaking with someone of lower status or age, the person has to take the perspective of the other person and call the self from that perspective. For example, when referring to herself in front of her own baby, a mother has to call herself "the mother" (e.g., "The mother really loves you"). Likewise, elementary school teachers refer to themselves as "the teacher" in front of their pupils (e.g., "The teacher is very happy!"). This perspective reversal is no longer permitted once the partner of the conversation is too old or mature to be regarded as needy, weak, or powerless. Thus school teachers will refer to themselves by using the first-person pronoun, "I," in talking with their colleagues. Likewise, college professors will not take their undergraduates' perspective when they refer to themselves in classes. Again, an emphasis on sympathy can be discerned in this complex use of personal pronouns in Japanese.

An empathetic stance toward others appears to be part and parcel of the Japanese mode of thought in both social and nonsocial situations. Thus, when asked to explain another person's morally questionable behavior, Japanese respondents often take the protagonist's perspective and consider what he or she must have thought and felt in the situation; as a consequence, their judgments tend to be quite lenient (Azuma, 1994; Yeh, 1995). Indeed, the propensity to look into what and how someone feels, rather than only examining what he or she has said in words, may be highly automatized. Kitayama and Ishii (1998) showed that when asked to judge, as quickly as possible, the emotional meaning of a spoken word as good or bad, Japanese respondents failed to ignore the attendant vocal intonation of emotion. Thus it took them longer to make the judgment if the attendant tone of voice was incongruous with the emotional meaning of the focal word than if it was congruous with the latter. Under comparable conditions, however, U.S. respondents did not show any such difficulty. The time required in the word meaning judgment was nearly identical, regardless of the tone of the voice with which the target word was spoken.

Several major historical antecedents can be suggested for the personal frame. Nakamura (1989) argues that the indigenous ethos that had existed in Japan before Buddhism and Confucianism were imported from the Asian continent (during the 6th–7th centuries A.D.) was characterized by an acceptance and appreciation of worldly realities "as they are," which in turn bred a relatively unconditional acceptance of natural, free, affirmative affection for both nature and other people ("mundane realism" in Figure 8.5). This ethos of ancient Japan influenced how foreign ideas were accepted.

For example, when Buddhism was imported from the Asian continent, the ideas of compassion and sympathy had an especially strong appeal to the preexisting Japanese ethos, and thus they were selectively incorporated in lieu of other ideas, such as impurity of the secular world (which contradicted the ancient ethos of mundane realism). Hence, the most influential of various Buddhist teachings was that of *Jodo* ("Pure land"). The teaching, as extensively developed after the introduction of the original Chinese ideas by two Japanese monks of the 12th and 13th centuries (Honen and Shinran), emphasizes the powerlessness of the self, the absolute compassion and benevolence of a motherly Buddha, and hence the necessity of repeated prayers using the Buddha's name for benevolence, which is considered to be the only means for salvation. The ethos of empathy and reliance on others might have had a considerable fit to the mentalities of farmers who formed a cohesive, stable, and relatively small rural community, and urgently needed to cooperate in their daily production and life ("ethos of agricultural community" in Figure 8.5).

As developed and conceptualized in Japan, Buddha's benevolence and compassion are indeed quite extraordinary. Thus, for example, Shinran, the monk who founded the Real-Jodo sect in the 13th century (which now attracts the largest number of followers among the contemporary Buddhist sects in Japan), is said to have argued that criminals are those who have the most legitimate right to or opportunity for salvation. Buddha helps those who do *not* help themselves, because these individuals have the most urgent need for salvation. Those who have already helped themselves need not be helped! This mentality, which is diametrically opposed to the Judeo-Christian, especially Protestant ethic of independence and autonomy (God helps those who *do* help themselves), can be found in Japanese classrooms. In general, teachers spend much more time in instructing and helping students who are falling behind, and parents of both these children and other, higher-achieving ones find no reason to complain. This is in stark contrast to North American classrooms, where the gifted are considered to have a legitimate right to receive more advanced instruction (cf. Stevenson & Stigler, 1992).

Although occasionally adopted as official ideologies of the governing class, the ideals of Buddhism and especially of its Jodo variants, such as compassion, benevolence, sympathy, and other-reliance, have had only limited influences on the larger societal order. Yet these ideas have had a major effect on social relations in more personal and informal domains of life. Unlike the official frame, which is defined in terms of formal rules and role structures, the personal frame is defined by implicit assumptions of affectionate, sympathetic, or empathetic bonds and ties; thus, in this frame, status differences and merits in the official domain are to be suppressed as much as possible. The self is perceived to be an element in the more informal or personal social space. As a consequence, the central criterion for judging the self is whether it is being accepted, *as it is*, by significant others in the relationship. Evaluation of the self as good or bad becomes irrelevant. Good selves may be accepted because they are respected, but bad selves may also receive an even greater amount of acceptance because they need to be cared for. And it is in these circumstances that Japanese individuals are most likely to experience unqualified good feelings of happiness, relaxation, and calm (Kitayama, Markus, & Kurokawa, 1998).

For the marathon runner described at the beginning of this chapter, her family members and friends may have provided "spiritual support." And the runner may have believed that these "real" friends would accept her, regardless of the outcome of the race. Likewise, "salary men" may have some informal network of friends and family members that gives them the sense that they are accepted, regardless of their status in the workplace. This representation of the self in the personal frame subsides into the back of the conscious experience in many more formal or official social situations, but it does exist and becomes active once one retreats from the official social setting into a more personal setting.

Coexistence of the Two Frames

Socialization

One can easily discern the assumptions about the duality of the social world in the socialization practices of contemporary Japanese culture. It has been observed that Japanese parents and grandparents indulge their children till they reach school age (Azuma, 1994; Befu, 1986; Johnson, 1993). Dependence on parents that would appear excessive by Western standards is not only tolerated, but also encouraged to an important degree. A child's misbehaviors are often tolerated, with the assumption that only through such misbehaviors does the child become capable of appreciating the benevolence of others and the significance of sympathy. The same applies to preschools. As compared to U.S. and Chinese preschools, Japanese preschools often appear chaotic. For example, teachers rarely intervene to resolve problems caused by mischievous children (Tobin, Wu, & Davidson, 1989). To an important extent, preschool may be considered to be an extension of the personal space that is identified at this stage mostly with home and family. Yet, when elementary school begins at about age 6, the social world that surrounds the child changes dramatically. Parents become more strict and put high demands on the child to be a "good child" (Azuma, 1994; White & LeVine, 1986). Schools too are structured as official social organizations, where roles (e.g., those of teacher and student) are clearly differentiated and the relations among them are explicitly stipulated.

From our theoretical perspective, what is happening here is the sequential introduction of the two frames. A child is first immersed in the personal, affectionate, sympathetic world, followed at about age 6 by participation in the official, rule-based, role-governed system. This does not mean, however, that the child's life during the period of formal schooling, is demarcated sharply into two well-defined spheres of school and home. On the contrary, once a child has reached school age, parents generally become more strict and oriented toward discipline and appropriateness of the child's behavior in different occasions at home, while maintaining the sympathetic, affective bond that was established earlier. Likewise, sympathy and affectionate interpersonal relations are much emphasized in school education as well through a variety of daily activities: group learning, where students assigned to small groups are encouraged to help one another in learning; a lunchtime program, where meals are provided by the school and students take turns serving each other; and a group cleaning time, when all students work together to clean their classrooms. Indeed, these activities that demand intricate interpersonal coordination seem to presuppose earlier training, conducted at home, to nurture sympathy and other-reliance. Thus, intermixed both at home and in school are both the ethos of the official frame, where adherence to social rules and duties are emphasized, and the ethos of the personal frame, where sympathetic attitudes toward one another and cooperation and mutual support are nurtured. The goal is to help children acquire the social competence to switch back and forth between the two frames flexibly in a socially appropriate fashion (Bachnik, 1992a).

Public versus Private Spheres of Life?

The contrast between the official and the personal frames for Japanese must be distinguished from the contrast between the public and the private spheres for European-Americans (cf. Stearns & Stearns, 1986). Unlike the public–private distinction, which in the West is relatively well demarcated in terms of time and space between, say, public work during the day and private life afterward, the official–personal contrast in Japan is grounded in the organizing themes of any given relationship at any given moment in time. Thus any given social relationship can be colored by both of these two frames. In fact, considerable evidence exists in leadership research in Japan that a mixture of these two organizational principles is the single most important quality of a good leader (Misumi, 1985; see also Rohlen, 1989). Unlike North American findings that the effectiveness of any leadership style is fully contingent on various features associated with task, situation, and followers, a large number of Japanese studies unequivocally suggest that an effective leader is almost always someone who is both strict and warm-hearted, and who can go back and forth between the two frames smoothly and naturally. One can easily discern a strong emphasis on a balance of competing requirements, rather than on a single-minded consistency.

Public versus Private Forms of Self-Consciousness?

Another distinction that bears some similarity to the personal versus official frames identified for Japanese constructions of the self concerns the notions of private versus public self-consciousness (Feningstein, Scheier, & Buss, 1979; Scheier & Carver, 1983). "Private self-consciousness" refers to a reflection on the self as an object of conscious awareness from one's own private vantage point, whereas "public self-consciousness" refers to a reflection on the self from the vantage point of other individuals in the general public.

Extrapolating from this distinction, one could easily suppose that the two Japanese frames map precisely into private versus public self-consciousness. Thus it might be supposed that in the personal frame one is acting as a private person defined in terms of beliefs, desires, or wishes that are internal to oneself, whereas in the official frame one is acting as a public figure in accordance with role expectations, socially sanctioned rules, and other types of knowledge that are external to the self.

Many attempts at such mapping can be found in the literature. For example, Greenwald and Pratkanis (1984) and, more recently, a number of social identity theorists (e.g., Turner, Oakes, Haslam, & McGarty, 1994; see Deaux, 1996, for a review) have suggested a model of the self that is composed of three layers: the private, the social, and the collective. Triandis (1989) has also focused on the distinction between private attributes of the self and public attributes of the self, and has suggested that individualists are defined primarily in terms of private attributes and collectivists in terms of public attributes (Trafimow, Triandis, & Goto, 1991). And it may be conceded that private, solitary thoughts are more common at home, which is the typical social site that invites the personal frame, and that public, role-based considerations are more common at work, which is the typical social site that highlights the official frame. Moreover, historically speaking, discourses, idioms, and practices encompassed in the official frame may have been originally invented or incorporated from the Asian continent and elaborated as the ethical code of public sharers of life, whereas those of the personal frame may have been grounded more in private spheres of life (Nakamura, 1989). Nevertheless, the equation of the personal frame with private self-consciousness (or private self) and the official frame with public self-consciousness (or public self) cannot be pushed too far.

The two frames identified for Japanese constructions of the self are sets of discourses, practices, and meanings that can be used to configure meanings for the self in relation to others in virtually every domain of life. Hence, for example, within the personal frame a person is likely to define his or her relationships with others in terms of mutual sympathy and compassion. Although any formal, societal roles are rarely implicated in this frame, both "private" features of the self and more "public" features of the self may occur to the person. For example, the person may say to him- or herself during a social interaction, "I feel very relaxed." This appraisal pertains to the self's inner experience and thus can count as an aspect of private self-consciousness, but the person may also wonder whether his or her partner in the social interaction may have recognized the sympathetic remark he has subtly conveyed. Here the target person is considering another's appraisal of his or her own behavior, and thus this may be regarded as an aspect of public self-consciousness. Likewise, both "private" and "public" self-relevant thoughts may be easily identified within an official frame. Thus a person operating in an official frame may be keenly aware of expectations held by others in respect to the public role he or she plays in the setting (public self-consciousness). Yet the person may also focus on his or her ability to play the role, critically appraising what he or she can could do in the situation (private self-consciousness).

The private and public forms of self-consciousness refer to the characteristics of thoughts or feelings. By contrast, the personal and official frames pertain to culturally sanctioned positions or perspectives from which all such thoughts and feelings are generated. Whichever position one happens to take to reflect on one's own self and social relationships, both private thoughts and public concerns are likely to enter one's conscious experience. It is more reasonable to assume, then, that various forms of thought and emotion—either nonsocial or social, private or public, and solitary or embedded—are all implicated in both the personal and the official frames. What varies between the two frames is the manner in which these forms of thought and feeling are configured. Thus, in the personal frame the key organizing themes are affectionate interpersonal engagement, sympathy, and other-reliance, whereas in the official frame they are role commitment, self-criticism, and self-improvement.

Frame Switching

Switching back and forth between the two frames is very common in everyday Japanese life. Although an analogous shifting or switching of frames is pervasive in any social interaction (Goffman, 1959, 1967; Hermans, 1996; Sakita, 1998), rarely has this switching been culturally elaborated and authorized as extensively in European-American cultural contexts as in Japanese contexts. For example, a boss at an office of a Japanese firm may be extremely friendly during a brief tea break, but the very next moment, when the work begins, the frame may be switched.

Such switching can also happen within a single person. Thus any single act based on one frame can be reflected on and evaluated from the perspective associated with the alternative frame. For example, the Japanese runner described at the beginning of this chapter, Yuko Arimori, may have competed in the race with a representation of herself as a marathon runner (i.e., the official frame). Once the race was finished, however, she may immediately have switched the perspective so as to reflect on the race and her effort within a framework associated with a different representation of, say, herself as a child, woman, or girlfriend (i.e., the personal frame). Obviously, the meaning and attendant evaluation of the self can vary, often dramatically, from one context to another. Hence the harsh attitude the runner took toward herself during the race was replaced by warm feelings directed toward herself right after the race. In such an instance, there then result *yin* and a *yang*. A *yin* from one perspective may be a *yang* from another. The same action may take very different meanings, depending on the perspectives from which one looks at it and evaluates it. As noted above, the self grounded in the interdependent view is thus bound to be multiperspectival and multivocal.

The duality of Japanese patterns of social behavior and self-perceptions has been noted repeatedly in the anthropological and sociological literatures on Japan. It is most colorfully suggested by the title of the classic volume by Ruth Benedict (1946), *The Chrysanthemum and the Sword.* Beneduct observed the curious coexistence of tender-heartedness and tough-mindedness in Japanese mentalities and culture. Lebra (1976) also noted the social relativism of Japanese moral judgments, where standards employed in moral discourses vary with and depend significantly on the attendant social relationships; the frequent result is an acute conflict between the morality of interpersonal obligation grounded in role relationships (*giri*) and that motivated by sympathetic interpersonal ties (*ninjo*). Likewise, Azuma (1994) pointed out that when value judgments are examined with a semantic differential method, Japanese data often show two distinct dimensions of "goodness," which correspond to "beauty" and to "rightfulness." Thus, for example, extramarital relationships may be judged to be good in the sense of "beautiful" and simultaneously bad in the sense of "wrong." This sort of moral dilemma, defining a central theme of many tragedies in Japanese fiction and drama, and explicitly captured in the term "beauty of betraying the virtue" (*haitoku-no-bi*), produces a state of nostalgic wishfulness that is often either augmented or counterbalanced by the coexisting anxiety (Buruma, 1984; Morris, 1975). It is also interesting to note in passing that statements by a number of Japanologists after World War II have themselves been characterized by a systematic shift of perspectives from one pessimistic, self-derogatory extreme (which was typical shortly after the war) to the other, optimistic, often grandiose extreme (which was more common during the period of the rapid economic growth of the 1970s and 1980s) (Aoki, 1990).

PSYCHOLOGICAL EVIDENCE FOR JAPANESE CONSTRUCTIONS OF THE SELF

So far, we have extensively discussed the possibility that Japanese selves are multifaceted and yet coherent. We have specifically focused on the duality defined by the two frames, personal and official. In this section we review some initial psychological evidence for this duality.

Duality and Consistency in Self-Perception

In our recent work, we have focused on an aspect of the duality that permeates the Japanese constructions of the self. Our own and others' studies of the self in Japan have suggested that Japanese self-perceptions are indeed quite context-specific and often dualistic, in that what is true to the self in one frame may be perceived to be otherwise once the frame is switched (Cousins, 1989). One study (Markus, Kitayama, Mullally, Masuda, & Fryberg, 1997) compared Japanese and U.S. students' self-descriptions in two conditions that corresponded to the two frames, official and personal. In one condition corresponding to the personal frame, participants were asked to describe themselves by responding "yes" or "no" to a series of attributes. In a second condition, corresponding to the official frame, respondents were asked to describe themselves as others expected them to be. The attributes were selected from previous studies in which U.S. and Japanese students were asked to characterize themselves. Table 8.1 shows the 10 most frequently endorsed attributes for the Japanese students and the U.S. students in both the personal-frame condition and the official-frame condition. Self-descriptions that overlap in the two conditions are indicated by asterisks in the table. As can be seen, the Japanese respondents had 20% overlap in the content of their frequent self-descriptions in the two conditions, whereas the Americans had more than 50% overlap. In the personal frame, the Japanese described themselves the way they might be in very informal interpersonal relations: "relaxed," "laid-back," "calm," "undisciplined," and "free-spirited." These findings suggest that in Japan, self in the personal frame feels accepted and cared for, and is the recipient of empathy—the very comfortable and positively regarded state of "ordinary."

The U.S. students included very positive descriptions among their most frequent descriptors, as well as many terms that would seem to require validation by others—"cooperative," "responsible," "hard-working," and "reliable." The Japanese students endorsed these terms with only moderate frequency. Some of the descriptors most frequently endorsed by the U.S. students (especially "ambitious," "special," and "respectful") were endorsed with relatively low frequency (48%, 55% and 14%, respectively) by the Japanese in the personal frame. Comparing the responses in the two frames suggests that in the United States, the personal aspects of the self are closely attuned to, synchronized with, or functionally coordinated with the social surroundings, but that in Japan the personal aspects of the self are relatively detached from, or insulated from, the social or official surroundings. This suggests an awareness among the Japanese that a person who is engaged with others and behaving as required or expected is a different self than one

TABLE 8.1. The 10 Most Frequently Endorsed Attributes for Japanese Students and U.S. Students in the Personal-Frame Condition and the Official-Frame Condition

U.S. students		Japanese students	
Attribute	% of responses	Attribute	% of responses
The personal frame condition			
Responsible*	100	Happy	94
Respectful*	100	Fun-loving*	94
Persistent	100	Relaxed	92
Cooperative*	98	Direct	92
Special	96	Assertive	90
Happy	95	Laid-back	86
Unique	95	Calm*	86
Reflective	95	Free-spirited	86
Fun-loving	93	Undisciplined	84
Sympathetic*	93	Ordinary	84
Hard-working*	93	Ambitious	93
Reliable*	93	Independent	93
The official-frame condition			
Respectful*	100	Sympathetic	100
Responsible*	100	Responsible	100
Self-confident	100	Reliable	100
Reliable*	100	Attentive	100
Hard-working*	100	Fun-loving*	100
Independent	100	Cooperative	98
Cooperative*	100	Calm*	98
Sympathetic*	100	Persistent	98
Attentive	100	Attractive	98
Balanced	100	Spontaneous	98
Ambitious	100		
Relaxed	100		
Direct	100		

Note. Asterisks indicate self-descriptions that overlap in the two conditions. The data are from Markus, Kitayama, Mullally, Masuda, and Fryberg (1997).

not so engaged or committed; it also indicates that for the Japanese, the difference between the official and the personal constructions of the self are experience-near. In contrast, the U.S. students showed significantly fewer differences in how they described themselves in the personal-frame and official-frame conditions. This suggests that people in the United States understand themselves as consistent and stable selves who are for the most part as others expect them to be, or, alternatively, that Americans believe others should not expect them to be any way except the way they are.

Critical Self-Perceptions in Japan

The dualistic nature of Japanese constructions of the self is further illuminated by recent empirical work on two self-relevant response tendencies of

Japanese (Kitayama, 1998). Self-criticism and self-attachment appear to Westerners to be unlikely bedfellows. By contrast, Japanese individuals do show markedly critical self-perceptions; at the same time, however, these individuals can also be shown to be positively attached to themselves once implicit measures of self-attachment are employed. These two tendencies are both reliable and robust. The coexistence of self-criticism and self-attachment illustrates how personality coherence can be achieved not in terms of personal consistency, but in terms of the balance of *yin* and *yang*. Although seemingly contradictory, a closer scrutiny of the phenomena may reveal that they are integrated within a coherent system of personality.

Self-Criticism as Collectively Afforded

Considerable evidence has been accumulated by now that Japanese often respond quite critically to themselves (Kitayama, Takagi, & Matsumoto, 1995; Heine, Lehman, Markus, & Kitayama, 1998). In a recent study, we (Kitayama, Markus, et al., 1997) prepared 400 social situations involving either a success or a failure, described in sentences, which were randomly sampled from a larger set of situations that had been generated by Japanese undergraduates and those generated by their U.S. counterparts. Both Japanese and U.S. undergraduates were asked to read each of these situations and to judge whether and to what extent their own self-esteem would increase or decrease in each situation if they were in it. The U.S. group responded with a strong self-enhancing tendency; that is, they judged that their self-esteem would increase more in the success situations than it would decrease in the failure situations. By contrast, the Japanese group showed a marked tendency toward self-criticism; that is, they judged that their self-esteem would decrease more in the failure situations than it would increase in the success situations.

Furthermore, we had another group of both Japanese and U.S. undergraduates judge how a typical undergraduate would respond to each of the 400 situations. The pattern of the self-esteem change estimated for the typical undergraduate was nearly identical to the pattern observed for the self, indicating that these judgments were not mediated by any tactical self-presentations. The hypothesis that Japanese are often genuinely self-critical has been supported by other studies that manipulate anonymity of responses in self-evaluation. When estimating their own performance in an ability task, Japanese respondents have been shown to be quite self-critical—underestimating their own performance relative to others' performance, even when the anonymity of responses was fully assured (Karasawa, 1998; Kitayama, 1997; Muramoto, 1998; Takata, 1987). A similar self-critical pattern has been found in Japanese respondents' causal attribution of their own success and failure (Kitayama, Takagi, & Matsumoto, 1995). Finally, Japanese respondents can be self-critical even when they are evaluating not themselves, but groups to which they belong (Heine & Lehman, 1997; Kitayama, Palm, Masuda,

Karasawa, & Carroll, 1996, but also see Muramoto & Yamaguchi, 1997, for a possible exception).

The critical perceptions and appraisals of the self prevalent in Japan are not only psychological, but also collective and socially shared, in that they are afforded, encouraged, and invited by the very ways in which common social situations in this cultural context are constructed. Half of the situations used in the aforementioned study (Kitayama, Markus, et al., 1997) had been sampled from the Japanese cultural context, and the remaining half from the U.S. cultural context. In addition to the self-critical appraisal in Japan and the self-enhancing appraisal in the United States described above, we found that the situations sampled from Japan and those sampled from the United States had unique influences on these appraisals. Thus the U.S. success situations were judged by both Japanese and U.S. respondents to increase their self-esteem more than the U.S. failure situations were judged to decrease it. Hence the U.S. self-enhancement was produced in part because the social situations that were common in this cultural context encouraged or invited this tendency. Conversely, the Japanese failure situations were judged by both Japanese and U.S. respondents to decrease their self-esteem more than the Japanese success situations were judged to increase it. Hence self-criticism in Japan was a response tendency that was resonant with and in fact invited by the very social situations prevalent in this cultural context. Together, U.S. respondents were most self-enhancing when responding to U.S. situations, and the Japanese respondents were most self-critical when responding to Japanese situations.

The Kitayama, Markus, et al. (1997) study is an experimental analogue of an exposure to a different cultural context. It suggests that self-critical response tendencies of Japanese are afforded by the practices and meanings of the Japanese cultural contexts. Likewise, the self-enhancing response tendencies of North Americans are afforded by those of the North American cultural contexts. Can the same point be made with a broader brush, such that long-term acculturation to one or the other cultural context fosters the respective response tendencies? Two recent studies allow us to answer this question both conclusively and affirmatively.

In one study, Heine and Lehman (1998) conducted a meta-analysis of existent studies on self-esteem in both European-descent Canadians and Asians, including Japanese (the total $n > 4,000$). The self-esteem scores of these respondents increased steadily as a function of their exposure to North American culture. Thus the scores were lowest (1) for those Japanese who never had any exposure to North American culture, but they increased steadily in the following order: (2) for those who had spent time in a Western country, (3) for recent Asian immigrants to Canada, (4) for Asians who had immigrated to Canada several years ago, (5) for second-generation Asian-descent Canadians, (6) for third-generation Asian-descent Canadians, and finally (7) for European-descent Canadians. Importantly, the last two groups were no different in their levels of self-esteem; therefore, the sizable ethnic difference observed in a cross-cultural comparison was accounted for in full by the exposure to divergent cultural contexts. Thus, once Japanese individuals are exposed to a North American cultural context, they are much less likely to show such tendencies.

In the other study, McCrae, Yik, Trapbell, Bond, and Paulhus (1998) focused on the sizable differences that have been observed when an extensive personality inventory developed by McCrae and colleagues (NEO-PI-R; Costa & McCrae, 1992) is administered to persons of Chinese and European descent. As compared to European-descent norms, Chinese often appear (among other things) to be more introverted, more vulnerable, less competent, and less likely to engage in cognitive and emotional activities. Overall, this pattern is consistent with the ethnic difference in self-esteem examined by Heine and Lehman (1998), indicating that Asians appear to be lower in self-esteem and the perceived likelihood of engaging in volitional activities. In order to determine the degree to which this ethnic difference could be accounted for by an exposure to different cultural contexts, McCrae et al. (1998) tested three groups of Chinese Canadians (i.e., Canadian-born Chinese Canadians, Chinese Canadians who immigrated before 1986, and those who immigrated after 1986), and compared their personality scores with the North American norms.

As in the Heine and Lehman study, McCrae and colleagues found a remarkable acculturation effect, such that the ethnic differences, which were quite sizable for the recent immigrants became very small (although they were rarely eliminated entirely) for the Canadian-born Chinese Canadians. On the basis of this evidence, the researchers concluded that most of the ethnic differences "seem to be the result of cultural influences, because they are affected by length of residence in Canada" (p. 1052). Thus, personality as conceptualized narrowly as dispositions appears to have an inherent limitation. What appear to be properties of a person may well be a constellation of response tendencies attuned to cultural affordances.

Self-Criticism and Relational Self-Improvement

Self-criticism in Japan often entails desirable consequences, because it is embedded in interpersonal and motivational processes of self-improvement. In the Japanese cultural context, which is organized in terms of the model of the self as interdependent, the primary life task involves fitting in and adjusting to social relationships. In order to achieve the task of fitting in, it may be necessary to identify the ideal image of the self expected by others in a relationship, to find what may be missing or lacking in one's own self in reference to this ideal self, and then to improve on these deficits and problems. This act of (1) reflecting on one's past behavior in reference to socially shared standards of excellence so as to be able (2) to improve and therefore (3) to be part of the relevant social unit is captured by the frequently used and highly elaborated Japanese concept of *hansei*, literally meaning "reflection" (Lewis, 1995). The collectively shared mode of self-making, which is anchored in the practice of hansei, may be called "self-improvement" (Kitayama & Karasawa, 1995; Kitayama, Markus, et al., 1997).

For example, Japanese parents constantly encourage their child to become an *iiko*—a good (*ii*) child (*ko*) (White & LeVine, 1986). *Iiko* is a socially shared ideal image of a child, which consists of a fuzzy set of attributes such as diligence, docility, and spiritfulness. Furthermore, such constant expectations from close others to fit into a socially shared image of the ideal person in a given context will continue throughout the life course, although the nature of the image itself obviously changes as one goes through various familial (good child/father/mother/grandparents), organizational (good student/teacher/manager), and age-graded (good young/old person) social roles and categories.

Because it is practically impossible to achieve the state of perfectly fitting into any relevant expected image of the ideal social role or category, there often results a constant, endless cycle of improving oneself in every domain of life by identifying problems vis-à-vis the pertinent socially shared standards of excellence, and subsequently correcting them. A constant state of struggle, perseverance, or effort toward an image that is closer to the pertinent social ideal is always considered possible; it is both encouraged and highly approved in a variety of daily practices in Japan (Azuma, 1994; DeVos, 1973; Lebra, 1976; Lewis, 1995; Kondo, 1990). For example, as described in detail by Lewis (1995), Japanese school children are required at the end of the day to "reflect on" (*hansei*; see above) where their individual or group performance fell short of class goals. Because self-improvement is anchored in a socially shared standard of excellence, continuously engaging in it is to affirm, both in private and in public, one's commitment to the social unit (e.g., family, classroom, company) from which the standard is derived. Put another way, within the Japanese cultural context, self-improvement is a symbolic act of affirming the value of the relationship of which one is part, thereby fulfilling the sense of the self as a fully interdependent entity. As such, self-improvement can be seen as a collectively held mode of living that simultaneously assures both the cohesion of the community and the identity of the self as interdependent (Kitayama & Karasawa, 1995, 1997; Kitayama, Markus, & Lieberman, 1995).

If self-criticism in Japan is in the service of self-improvement, then it may happen most typically in respect to socially undesirable attributes of the self that call out for effort for improvement. Karasawa (1998) recently investigated this possibility. Japanese college students in a large lecture class were tested in the class setting. First, after being given an assurance of anonymity, the students in the class were asked to list 10 attributes of the self. They were further asked to rate the general social desirability of having each of the attributes on a separate sheet of paper. Next the sets of 10 self-descriptions were collected by the experimenter and then redistributed to the class, so that each student received the set of 10 attributes listed by someone else in the class. Each student then gave the same social desirability ratings to the 10 attributes of the other student (whose identity was kept anonymous) in the same class.

The comparison between the self-ratings and the other-ratings could show that the former were in fact lower than the latter. Such a finding would be consistent with the past studies that have found critical self-judgment effects in Japanese samples. Importantly, however, a self–other discrepancy might also stem from a more generous evaluation of the attributes of someone else in the same class. Karasawa therefore compiled all the attributes generated by the students and showed them to a separate group of students from the same university. The students in this second group were asked to judge the general social desirability of having each of the attributes. They were not given any further information (such as characteristics or even the presence of anyone who supposedly possessed any of the attributes). Subsequently, this consensual rating of social desirability was used to evaluate any judgmental biases that could manifest themselves when one made a judgment of social desirability while acknowledging that a given attribute was either one's own (i.e., self-judgment) or that of someone else in the same class (i.e., other-judgment). Thus, on the one hand, for each attribute the consensual-judgment rating was subtracted from the self-judgment rating to yield an index for a bias in self-evaluation; on the other hand, the consensual-judgment rating was subtracted from the other-judgment rating to yield an index of a bias in other-judgment. In both indices, positive scores indicated a relatively generous, enhancing bias in judgment, whereas negative scores indicated a critical bias. Furthermore, in order to test the hypothesis that self-criticism should be more pronounced for socially undesirable attributes, attributes were divided into two sets—either high or low in social desirability as assessed by the consensual ratings.

The results are summarized in Figure 8.6. In support of the hypothesis that self-criticism should be most pronounced for those attributes that call for efforts at improvement, the self-judgment was biased in the critical direction only for those attributes that were consensually judged to be socially undesirable. Interestingly, for those attributes that were consensually judged to be socially desirable, there was no bias in self-judgment; however, other-judgment manifested a significant bias toward enhancement. It appears, then, that Japanese individuals hold a critical stance in respect to undesirable attributes of themselves, but a more generous, enhancing stance in respect to desirable attributes of *others* in some relationship. This other-enhancement effect for desirable attributes may also be seen as an element in the relational self-improvement process, insofar as other individuals in relationships may well provide a standard toward which individuals work to improve them-

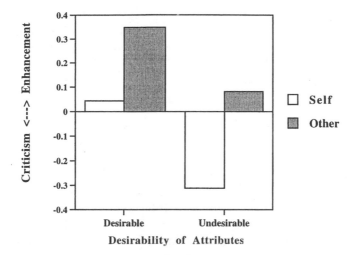

FIGURE 8.6. Self-criticism and other-enhancement in Japanese constructions of the self. The data are from Karasawa (1998).

selves. It is also possible that this effect is a manifestation of sympathetic orientations supposedly held by a majority of Japanese individuals to others in relationships.

Within this experiment, then, we can discern a microcosm of a Japanese cultural system whereby (1) a person focuses on his or her own shortcomings for self-improvement purposes, and, simultaneously, (2) others in the same relationship respond sympathetically to the first person, drawing the person's attention to his or her more desirable aspects, which supposedly not only (3) provide the person with some degree of reassurance about him- or herself, but also (4) serve for these others as an opportunity to recognize what is missing or lacking in themselves, and thus to initiate an effort toward self-improvement. In this analysis, then, self-criticism and other-enhancement may be expected to be closely related and can be seen as two sides of the same coin—or *yin* and *yang* of the social, interpersonal dynamic configured with the model of the self as interdependent.

Finally, self-criticism in Japan is in fact related closely to future achievement. To begin with, if self-criticism is in the service of future improvement of one's own performance in a given domain, it may become stronger when there is a chance of self-improvement in that domain and that domain is important. In support of this analysis, Kitayama (1997) found that critical perceptions of the self became more pronounced when individuals were predicting their own and others' performance in an ability task that was allegedly quite important. In a more recent study, Heine, Kitayama, Lehman, and Takata (1998) used an intrinsic-motivation paradigm and showed that Japanese respondents persisted in a task longer when left alone in a room with an option to work on an ability task if they had failed in a similar task than if they had succeeded—a pattern that was diametrically opposite to the one observed for Canadian respondents.

Implicit Self-Attachment

Given the logic of personal consistency, those who are critical of the self and thus vigilant to their own shortcomings and weaknesses may be expected to dislike the self (Heider, 1958) and to be low in self-esteem (Baumeister, 1993), pessimistic (Seligman, Abramson, Semmel, & Von Baeyer, 1979), and maladjusted (Taylor & Brown, 1988). Even though the criticism may lead to an achievement in the short run, it may well be accompanied by a considerable psychological cost of lowered self-esteem. Nevertheless, despite the fact that the vast majority of the Japanese do show self-criticism, little evidence exists that they are maladjusted. Indeed, recent evidence indicates that along with self-criticism, there is present in Japan a covert, yet quite reliable and strong, sense of attachment to the self.

Kitayama and Karasawa (1997) have obtained evidence for such an implicit sense of self-attachment among the Japanese by assessing it implicitly, without evoking any awareness that the self was being judged. Specifically, these researchers asked Japanese respondents to report how much they liked each of the letters in the Japanese alphabet (Study 1). In order to control for any effects of baseline attractiveness of the letters, for each letter the ratings of those who did not have this letter in their names were averaged to yield a consensual level of attractiveness. Subsequently, for each respondent the pertinent consensual-attractiveness score was subtracted from the score of each of the name letters. Positive difference scores would indicate a greater preference for one's own name letters. As summarized in Figure 8.7, such an effect was very robust. Moreover, this effect was most pronounced for those letters that were seemingly most closely associated with the self—the initials of the first names for female respondents, but those of family names for male respondents. Similar effects have been observed in many cultures both in the West (Johnson, 1986, cited in Greenwald & Banaji, 1995; Nuttin, 1985, 1987) and in the East (i.e., Thailand; Hoorens, Nuttin, Herman, & Pavakanun, 1990).

Kitayama and Karasawa (1997, study 2) also examined likings for numerals and found that they were better liked if they constituted one's birthdate than if they did not. Importantly, Kitayama and Uchida (1998) showed that the name letter effect and the birthdate number effect were significantly correlated with one another for college undergraduates ($r = .35$), suggesting that they are reliable as a measure of implicit self-attachment. Recently, Blass, Schmitt, Jones, and O'Connell (1997) used the Kitayama and Karasawa procedure and examined the birthdate number effect among U.S. undergraduates. Their data suggest that U.S. respondents show a much

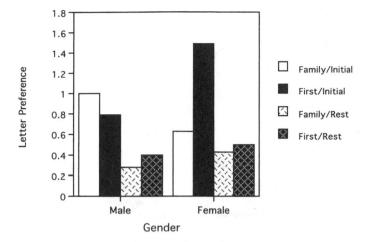

FIGURE 8.7. Implicit self-attachment in Japan: The name letter effect is most pronounced for those letters that were most closely associated with the self. The data are from Kitayama and Karasawa (1997).

stronger tendency to prefer the numerals in their birthdates than do Japanese respondents. It may be the case that the U.S. tendency toward self-enhancement augments the effect.

Implicitly Liking the Self That One Explicitly Criticizes

We are now left with fascinating questions: Where does this implicit self-attachment come from, and how can it fit with the pervasive tendency of the Japanese to be self-critical? In other words, how can we resolve the apparent paradox of implicitly liking the self that one explicitly criticizes? As we have indicated above, Japanese selves are multiperspectival, and two primary perspectives involved in them are associated with the "official" and "personal" frames. Self-criticism geared toward self-improvement is likely to be a psychological tendency in the self in the official frame. In many domains of life, Japanese individuals do operate within the official frame. In these circumstances, representations of the self as defined within the alternative, personal frame do exist. But they are likely to be objectified and thus reflected upon from the perspective of the ongoing, official frame.

This state of the self is schematically illustrated in Figure 8.8. The official frame, which serves as the ongoing system of self-regulation or as a working self-concept (Markus & Wurf, 1987), is highlighted with a thicker circle. The relationship of this official self to other selves, including the ones defined in the personal frame, may take various forms. The personal self may occasion-

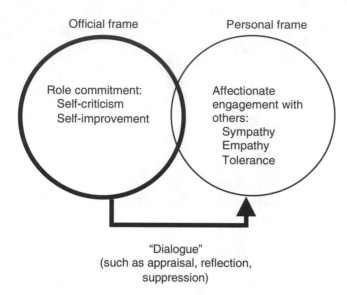

FIGURE 8.8. Japanese constructions of the self within the official frame: Individuals seek to improve themselves via critically appraising themselves. The self defined within the alternative, personal frame may become an object of the critical appraisal. More typically, however, individuals operating within the official frame suppress any thoughts and feelings associated with the personal frame. Hence the self constructed within the personal frame tends to recede temporarily into the background.

ally become the object of critical self-appraisal. Yet, most of the time, the official self may be preoccupied with duties, obligations, interpersonal expectations, and social rules, while suppressing personal affects and feelings. Accordingly, it may be the case that more often than not, the personal self is bound to be suppressed, relegated to the periphery of self-awareness when the official self predominates.

The self defined in terms of the official discourse is only one of its two aspects. Thus the person may switch to the personal frame to configure the self in a very different mode, whereby affectionate, sympathetic engagement with others is highlighted and elaborated. Even when the person is engaging in social activities within the official frame, he or she may occasionally switch to the other frame and take, if only briefly and temporarily, a personal perspective. When this happens, the self is temporarily redefined and reconfigured within the personal frame; as a consequence, the preparedness of the self to engage affectionately with others is brought back to the conscious experience. As shown in Figure 8.9, the official representation of the self recedes into the background, or otherwise is objectified, and appraised from the alternative, personal perspective. The self being constructed in the official

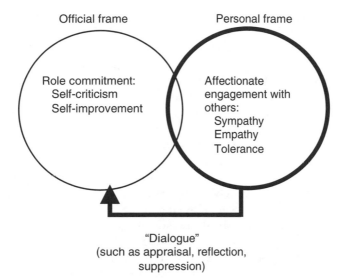

Official frame   Personal frame

Role commitment: Affectionate
Self-criticism   engagement with
Self-improvement   others:
                                          Sympathy
                                          Empathy
                                          Tolerance

"Dialogue"
(such as appraisal, reflection,
suppression)

FIGURE 8.9. Japanese constructions of the self within the personal frame: Individuals are prepared to engage affectionately with others, including their own past, current, and future selves. The frame switch can happen "on-line" so that the ongoing representation of the self constructed within the official frame may be temporarily suppressed, objectified, reflected upon, and appraised from the alternative, personal frame, when the perspective is switched from the former frame to the latter, causing warm feelings of self-attachment to accrue. But once the frame is switched back to the official frame, the feelings may disappear.

frame is seen as someone with whom the personal self has a dialogue, and, furthermore, this dialogue is framed in terms of sympathy, empathy, and tolerance. When this happens, warm feelings of sympathy may accrue, especially if the objectified self—the self being constructed within the official frame—is burdened with difficulties, deficits, and miseries.

This analysis helps explain why Japanese often show a strong self-critical tendency if self-evaluation is assessed explicitly, but show self-attachment if it is assessed implicitly. When individuals evaluate themselves explicitly, knowingly doing so within an experimental setting or on a questionnaire, they are likely to take an official perspective, insofar as the participation in psychological studies is seen as a typical social, public activity, rather than as anything akin to personal, affectionately motivated conduct. The individuals therefore are likely to operate within the official mode, hence taking a strongly critical stance toward themselves.

By contrast, when individuals evaluate themselves implicitly, they are not aware that their responses reveal anything about the self. Instead, they are asked to report their evaluations of stimuli that are seemingly unrelated to the self. Stimuli are chosen so that some of them are in fact associated closely with the self (e.g., name letters) and the rest are not (e.g., non-name letters). We suggest that in this procedure, when self-relevant stimuli (e.g., name letters) are presented, a representation of the self is activated. Although rarely is this activation consciously noted or recognized (Nuttin, 1985), it is nonetheless likely to activate affective responses associated with the representation as well. These implicitly activated affective responses may in turn color the evaluation of the stimuli. And there is reason to believe that these affective responses tend to be relatively positive.

To illustrate, suppose the stimulus "hi" is presented to a Japanese man called Hiroshi. Our analysis begins with the assumption that "hi" is a strong enough cue to activate Hiroshi's representations of himself. With those representations are associated a variety of affective responses. Some of these affective responses may well have been self-generated. That is, they may be residues of the explicit evaluations made by the person himself as he contemplated himself in the past. Some of them may be negative, especially if they were generated when the person evaluated himself within the official frame; yet even in these cases, the negative responses are likely to be counteracted by the sympathetic, warm feelings that are likely to accrue when the act of self-criticism is evaluated from the perspective defined by the alternative, personal frame.

Affective responses associated with the self-representations may also include those generated and communicated to Hiroshi by others around him. They therefore may serve as a "sociometer" (Leary, Tambor, Terdal, & Downs, 1995). These responses are likely to be predominantly positive, if only because individuals make personal connections with those who provide more or less positive, affirming feedback (Baumeister & Leary, 1995). If Hiroshi had accomplished something, then he may have received applause or praise; but even if he had failed, he may have received sympathy. The very fact that self-criticism is encouraged by one of the two dominant cultural frames of Japan (i.e., the official frame) implies that engaging in self-criticism should be associated more with positive responses from others than with negative ones (see Muramoto, 1998, for evidence).

Together, focal stimuli are likely to be colored with a glow of warm feelings, resulting in an implicit self-attachment effect. Furthermore, this effect should increase with the strength of the association between each letter and the self-representations—a prediction consistent with the Kitayama and Karasawa (1997) finding that the effect was strongest for the initials of first names for females, but those of family names for males.

CONCLUSIONS

In this chapter, we have proposed two alternative ways in which personality coherence is culturally constructed; one is grounded in the notion of consistency and is pervasive in the West, the other is based on the idea of balance and is widespread in the East. Although preliminary, our analysis challenges one assumption that has been hegemonic in personality research from its inception, has been shared throughout its history, and is currently upheld regardless of specific theoretical stances, whether dispositional or social-cognitive. This assumption is the idea that personal consistency is a key marker of personhood and therefore is *the* criterion for personality coherence. Furthermore, the discipline of personality psychology has been narrowly focused on personal and interpersonal processes. Of course, there is nothing wrong with psychologists' studying these processes. Yet we believe that studying them necessarily involves articulating in as much detail as possible the social and cultural history of these processes. To understand personality coherence across a wide spectrum of cultures, one must examine the cultural and historical underpinnings of the social and cognitive processes for both consistency and balance.

We have argued that the emphasis on personal consistency in the analysis of personality is grounded in a view of the self as independent, composed of and defined primarily in terms of a set of attributes within it. To the degree that there exists an independent, bounded individual detached from the surrounding, there may arise an urgent need to maintain personal consistency. This possibility has been taken very seriously through the development of Western cultures. But given an alternative, interdependent view of the self, it is the relational context that is bound to define the self. To the degree that there are many relational contexts in one's life space, there arises the need to maintain a balance among them. And it is this possibility that has been elaborated extensively over the course of the historical development of Eastern cultures.

The maintenance of a balance across different domains of the self is made possible through organizing each of the seemingly contradictory aspects of the self (e.g., self-criticism and self-attachment) as being required by and requiring, or as being afforded by and affording, one another. Thus self-criticism is an aspect of the self that invites self-attachment when one's perspective is switched from one frame (the official frame) to the other (the personal frame); conversely, self-attachment may provide a secure base on which to engage in criticizing oneself, thereby improving it.

Although we believe that the dynamics of personality balance sketched here are more common and better appreciated by Asian cultures and people, we also suspect that similar dynamics may exist in other cultural contexts as well, but in forms that by themselves are culture-bound. For example, it has been suggested that self-enhancement is a culturally established means to fend off the existential anxiety of eventual death (Becker, 1973; Solomon, Greenberg, & Pyszczynski, 1991). Similarly, many Freudian notions, such as rationalization, defense, and projection, assume the presence of "dark instincts" or id, which are to be suppressed by "rational" means or ego (Greenwald, 1980). The suggestion is that the balance or equilibrium between

these two forces lends itself to a "normal" and "adaptive" personality functioning. One important feature in these theories should be noted, however. In
these theories, a balance is assumed among different "layers" of personality—say, between the domain of "conscious reason" and the domain of
"unconscious affect." The conscious ego, some important constituents of
which include self-esteem and linear rationality, is considered to regulate and
control the unconscious animal desires or fateful anxieties by exercising a
force that counteracts the effect of the latter, thus creating a balance between
the two opposing entities (Greenberg et al., 1992).

So it might be speculated that any forms of personality require the
invention of a counter force somewhere to maintain the integrity of the personality itself. Thus, in the East Asian, interdependent selves, such a system
of equilibrium or balance may be typically established among different
domains of life and attendant facets of the self. Equilibrium is made possible
through mutual affordances, negotiation, and cooperation among the various
participants in the system. By contrast, in European-American, independent
selves, it may more typically be created between the self and the structure
that exists outside of it and yet that fuels its functionings by virtue of its role:
to instigate, challenge, and even conspire against the self. Equilibrium is
made possible through the creation of tension and antagonism between the
self itself and the structure outside. These two forms of construction, we suggest, are fundamentally cultural and social: they are enabled by practices and
meanings, such as lay theories, conventions, icons, images, and conversa-
tional scripts, that have been historically invented, elaborated, and preserved
in the different cultural contexts. Nevertheless, the two forms of the self are
likely to constitute psychological entities through development, socialization,
and enculturation, and thus they become subjectively real, unavoidable, and
thus seemingly natural. Indeed, the exploration of this cultural construction
of the natural mode of being is the central agenda of the cultural psychology
of personality.

REFERENCES

Aoki, T. (190). [Change in "Japanologies": Cultural identities of post-war Japan]. Tokyo:
    Chuohyoronsya. (In Japanese)
Ajzen, I. (1996). The social psychology of decision making. In E. T. Higgins & A. W.
    Kruglanski (Eds.), Social psychology: Handbook of basic principles (pp. 297–325).
    New York: Guilford Press.
Ames, P. T., Dissanayake, W., & Kasulis, T. P. (Eds.). (1994). Self as person in Asian theory
    and practice. Albany: State University of New York Press.
Asch, S. (1952). Social psychology. Englewood Cliffs, NJ: Prentice-Hall.
Azuma, H. (1994). Discipline and education in Japan. Tokyo: Tokyo University Press.
Bachnik, J. M. (1992a). Kejime: Defining a shifting self in multiple organizational

modes. In N. R. Rosenberger (Ed.), *Japanese sense of self* (pp. 152–172). Cambridge, England: Cambridge University Press.

Bachnik, J. M. (1992b). The two "faces" of self and society in Japan. *Ethos, 20,* 3–32.

Bachnik, J. M. (1994). *Uchi/Soto*: Challenging our conceptualizations of self, social order, and language. In J. M. Bachnik & C. J. Quinn, Jr. (Eds.), *Situated meaning: Inside and outside in Japanese self, society, and language* (pp. 3–37). Princeton, NJ: Princeton University Press.

Bachnik, J. M., & Quinn, C. J., Jr. (Eds.). (1994). *Situated meaning: Inside and outside in Japanese self, society, and language.* Princeton, NJ: Princeton University Press.

Bandura, A. (1982). Self-efficacy: Mechanism in human agency. *American Psychologist, 37,* 122–147.

Barnlund, D. C. (1989). *Communicative styles of Japanese and Americans: Images and realities.* Belmont, CA: Wadsworth.

Bartlett, F. A. (1932). *Remembering: A study in experimental psychology.* Cambridge, England: Cambridge University Press.

Baumeister, R. F. (1987). How the self became a problem: A psychological review of historical research. *Journal of Personality and Social Psychology, 52,* 163–176.

Baumeister, R. F. (1993). Understanding the inner nature of low self-esteem: Uncertain, fragile, protective, and conflicted. In R. F. Baumeister (Ed.), *Self-esteem: The puzzle of low self-regard* (pp. 201–218). New York: Plenum Press.

Baumeister, R. F., & Leary, M. .R. (1995). The need to belong: Desire for interpersonal attachments as a fundamental human motivation. *Psychological Bulletin, 117,* 497–529.

Bateson, G. (1972). *Steps to an ecology of mind.* New York: Ballantine Books.

Becker, E. (1973). *The denial of death.* New York: Free Press.

Befu, H. (1986). The social and cultural background of child development in Japan and the United States. In H. Stevenson, H. Azuma, & K. Hakuta (Eds.), *Child development and education in Japan* (pp. 13–27). New York: Freeman.

Bellah, R. N., Madsen, R., Sullivan, W. M., Swindler, A., & Tipton, S. M. (1985). *Habits of the heart: Individualism and commitment in American life.* Berkeley: University of California Press.

Bem, D. J. (1967). Self-perception: An alternative interpretation of cognitive dissonance. *Psychological Review, 74,* 183–200.

Bem, D. J., & Allen, A. (1974). On predicting some of the people some of the time: The search for cross-situational consistencies in behavior. *Psychological Review, 81,* 506–520.

Benedict, R. (1946). *The chrysanthemum and the sword.* Boston: Houghton Mifflin.

Berger, P., & Luckmann, T. (1967). *The social construction of reality: A treatise on the sociology of knowledge.* Garden City, NY: Doubleday.

Berline, I. (1992). *The crooked timber of humanity: Chapters in the history of ideas.* New York: Random House.

Blass, T., Schmitt, C., Jones, E., & O'Connell, M. (1997). *The own-birthday effect: From Japan to the United States.* Paper presented at the annual meeting of the American Psychological Association, Chicago.

Bourdieu, P. (1976). *Outline of a theory of practice* (R. Nice, Trans.). Cambridge, England: Cambridge University Press.

Brown, D. E. (1991). *Human universals.* New York: McGraw-Hill.

Bruner, J. (1990). *Acts of meaning.* Cambridge, MA: Harvard University Press.

Bruner, J. (1996). *The culture of education.* Cambridge, MA: Harvard University Press.

Buruma, I. (1984). *A Japanese mirror: Heroes and villains of Japanese culture.* Harmondsworth, England: Penguin Books.

Cantor, N. (1994). Life task problem-solving: Situational affordances and personal needs. *Personality and Social Psychology Bulletin, 20,* 235–243.

Cantor, N., & Kihlstrom, J. (1987). *Personality and social intelligence.* Englewood Cliffs, NJ: Prentice-Hall.

Clancy, P. M. (1986). The acquisition of communicative style in Japanese. In B. B. Schieffelin & E. Ochs (Eds.), *Language socialization across cultures* (pp. 213–250). Cambridge, England: Cambridge University Press.

Cole, M. (1996). *Cultural psychology.* Cambridge, MA: Harvard University Press.

Costa, P. T., Jr., & McCrae, R. R. (1992). *The Revised NEO Personality Inventory (NEO-PI-R) and NEO Five-Factor Inventory (NEO-FFI) professional manual.* Odessa, FL: Psychological Assessment Resources.

Cousins, S. D. (1989). Culture and selfhood in Japan and the U.S. *Journal of Personality and Social Psychology, 56,* 124–131.

Crook, J. & Rabgyas, T. (1988) The essential insight: A central theme in the philosophical training of Mahayanist monks. In A. C. Paranjpe, D. Y. Ho, & R. W. Rieber (Eds.), *Asian contributions to psychology* (pp. 149–183). New York: Praeger.

Deaux, K. (1996). Social identification. In E. T. Higgins & A. W. Kruglanski (Eds.), *Social psychology: Handbook of basic principles* (pp. 777–798). New York: Guilford Press.

Deci, E. L., & Ryan, R. M. (1987). The support of autonomy and the control of behavior. *Journal of Personality and Social Psychology, 53,* 1024–1037.

Deci, E. L., & Ryan, R. M. (1995). Human autonomy: The basis for true self-esteem. In M. H. Kernis (Ed.), *Efficacy, agency, and self-esteem* (pp. 31–49). New York: Plenum Press.

Dodge, K. A. (1993). Social-cognitive mechanisms in the development of conduct disorder and depression. *Annual Review of Psychology, 44,* 559–584.

DeVos, G. A. (1973). *Socialization for achievement: Essays on the cultural psychology of the Japanese.* Berkeley: University of California Press.

DeVos, G. A. (1985). Dimensions of the self in Japanese culture. In A. J. Marsella, G. DeVos, & F. L. K. Hsu (Eds.), *Culture and self: Asian and Western perspectives* (pp. 141–182). London: Tavistock.

Doi, T. (1971). *The anatomy of dependence.* Tokyo: Kodansha.

Doi, T. (1986). *The anatomy of self.* Tokyo: Kodansha.

Durham, W. H. (1991). *Coevolution: Genes, cultures, and human diversity.* Stanford, CA: Stanford University Press.

Dweck, C. S. (1993). Implicit theories: Individual differences in the likelihood and meaning of dispositional inference. *Personality and Social Psychology Bulletin, 19,* 644–656.

Dweck, C. S., & Leggett, E. L. (1988). A social-cognitive approach to motivation and personality. *Psychological Review, 95,* 256–273.

Edwards, P. (1996). Honour, shame, humiliation, and modern Japan. In O. Leaman (Ed.), *Friendship East and West: Philosophical perspectives* (pp. 32–55). Surrey, England: Curzon.

Epstein, S. (1979). The stability of behavior: On predicting most of the people much of the time. *Journal of Personality and Social Psychology, 37,* 1097–1126.

Farr, R. M. (1991). Individualism as a collective representation. In A. Aebischer, J. P. Deconchy, & M. Lipiansky (Eds.), *Ideologies et representations sociales* (pp. 129–143). Cousset (Fribourg), Switzerland: Delval.

Fazio, R. H., & Zanna, M. P. (1981). Direct experience and attitude–behavior consistency. In L. Berkowitz (Ed.), *Advances in experimental social psychology* (Vol. 14, pp. 162–203). New York: Academic Press.

Feningstein, A., Scheier, M. F., & Buss, A. (1975). Public and private self-consciousness: Assessment and theory. *Journal of Consulting and Clinical Psychology, 43,* 522–527.

Festinger, L. (1957). *A theory of cognitive dissonance.* Stanford: Stanford University Press.

Fiske, A. P., Kitayama, S., Markus, H. R., & Nisbett, R. E. (1998). The cultural matrix of social psychology. In D. T. Gilbert, S. T. Fiske, & G. Lindzey (Eds.), *Handbook of social psychology* (4th ed., pp. 915–981). New York: McGraw-Hill.

Funder, D C., & Ozer, D. J. (Eds.). (1997). *The pieces of the personality puzzle.* New York: Norton.

Geertz, C. (1973). *The interpretation of culture: Selected essays.* New York: Basic Books.

Gergen, K. J. (1973). Social psychology as history. *Journal of Personality and Social Psychology, 26,* 309–320.

Gibson, J. J. (1966). *The senses considered as perceptual systems.* Boston: Houghton Mifflin.

Giddens, A. (1984). *The constitution of society.* Oxford: Polity Press.

Gilbert, D. T., & Malone, P. S. (1995). The correspondence bias. *Psychological Bulletin, 117,* 21–38.

Giorgi, L., & Marsh, C. (1990). The Protestant work ethic as a cultural phenomenon. *European Journal of Social Psychology, 20,* 499–517.

Goffman, E. (1959). *The presentation of self in everyday life.* Garden City, NY: Doubleday.

Goffman, E. (1967). *Interaction ritual.* Garden City, NY: Doubleday/Anchor.

Goldberg, L. R. (1993). The structure of phenotypic personality traits. *American Psychologist, 48,* 26–34.

Gollwitzer, P. (1993). Goal achievement: The role of intentions. In W. Stroebe & M. Hewstone (Eds.), *European review of social psychology* (Vol. 4, pp. 141–185). Chichester, England: Wiley.

Greenberg, J., Solomon, S., Pyszczynski, T., Rosenblatt, A., Burling, J., Lyon, D., Simon, L., & Pinel, E. (1992). Why do people need self-esteem?: Converging evidence that self-esteem serves an anxiety-buffering function. *Journal of Personality and Social Psychology, 63,* 913–922.

Greenfield, P. M. (1997). Culture as process: Empirical methods for cultural psychology. In J. W. Berry, Y. H. Poortinga, & J. Pandey (Eds.), *Handbook of cross-cultural psychology* (Vol. 1, pp. 301–346). Needham Heights, MA: Allyn & Bacon.

Greenwald, A. G. (1980). The totalitarian ego: Fabrication and revision of personal history. *American Psychologist, 35,* 603–618.

Greenwald, A. G., & Banaji, M. R. (1995). Implicit social cognition: Attitudes, self-esteem, and stereotypes. *Psychological Review, 102,* 4–27.

Greenwald, A. G., & Pratkanis, A. R. (1984). The self. In R. S. Wyer & T. K. Srull (Eds.), *Handbook of social cognition* (Vol. 3, pp. 129–178). Hillsdale, NJ: Erlbaum.

Heckhausen, J., & Schulz, R. (1995). A life-span theory of control. *Psychological Review, 102,* 284–304.

Heider, F. (1958). *The psychology of interpersonal relations.* New York: Wiley.

Heine, S. J., Kitayama, S., Lehman, D. R., & Takata, T. (1998). *Divergent consequences of success and failure in Japan and North America.* Manuscript in preparation, University of Pennsylvania.

Heine, S. J., & Lehman, D. R. (1997). Culture, dissonance, and self-affirmation. *Personality and Social Psychology Bulletin, 23,* 389–400.

Heine, S. J., & Lehman, D. R. (1998). [A meta-analysis of self-esteem studies with Japanese and Canadians]. Unpublished raw data, University of Pennsylvania.

Heine, S. J., Lehman, D. R., Markus, H. R., & Kitayama, S. (1998). *Culture and the need for positive self-regard.* Unpublished manuscript, University of Pennsylvania.

Hendry, J. (1993). *Wrapping culture: Politeness, presentation, and power in Japan and other societies.* Oxford: Clarendon Press.

Hermans, H. J. M. (1996). Voicing the self: From information processing to dialogical interchange. *Psychological Bulletin, 119,* 31–50.

Ho, D. Y. F. (1976). On the concept of face. *American Journal of Sociology, 81,* 867–884.

Hoorens, V., Nuttin, J. M., Herman, I. E., & Pavakanun, U. (1990). Mastery pleasure versus mere ownership: A quasi-experimental cross-cultural and cross-alphabetical test of the name letter effect. *European Journal of Social Psychology, 20,* 181–205.

Jahoda, G. (1986). Nature, culture and social psychology. *European Journal of Social Psychology, 16,* 17–30.

Jahoda, G. (1992). *Cross-road between culture and mind: Continuities and change in theories of human nature.* London: Harvester Wheatsheaf.

Johnson, F. A. (1993). *Dependency and Japanese socialization.* New York: New York University Press.

Jones, E. E. (1979). The rocky road from acts to dispositions. *American Psychologist, 34,* 107–117.

Jones, E. E., & Harris, V. A. (1967). The attribution of attitudes. *Journal of Experimental Social Psychology, 3,* 1–24.

Karasawa, M. (1998). [*The cultural basis of self- and other-perceptions: Self-criticism and other-enhancement in Japan*]. Unpublished doctoral dissertation, Shirayuri College, Tokyo. (In Japanese)

Kashiwagi, K. (1997). [Development of self-regulation of behavior and emotion]. In K. Kashiwagi, S. Kitayama, & H. Azuma (Eds.), [*Cultural psychology: Theory and research*] (pp. 180–197). Tokyo: University of Tokyo Press. (In Japanese)

Kelly, G. A. (1955). *The psychology of personal constructs* (Vols. 1 and 2). New York: Norton.

Kelly, W. (n.d.). *The taut and the empathetic: Antinomies of Japanese personhood.* Unpublished manuscript, Yale University.

Kitayama, S. (1997). *Self-criticism in Japan: Critical self-appraisal or modest self-presentation?* Unpublished manuscript, Kyoto University.

Kitayama, S. (1998). [*The cultural psychology of self and emotion*]. Tokyo: Kyoritsu. (In Japanese)

Kitayama, S., & Ishii, K. (1998). *Word evaluation and vocal emotion in speech processing: Priority of activation in Japan and the United States.* Unpublished manuscript, Kyoto University.

Kitayama, S., & Karasawa, M. (1995). [Self: A cultural-psychological perspective]. [*Japanese Journal of Experimental Social Psychology*], *35*(2), 133–162. (In Japanese)

Kitayama, S., & Karasawa, M. (1997). Implicit self-esteem in Japan: Name letters and birthday numbers. *Personality and Social Psychology Bulletin, 23,* 736–742.

Kitayama, S., & Markus, H. R. (Eds.). (1994). *Emotion and culture: Empirical studies of mutual influences.* Washington, DC: American Psychological Association.

Kitayama, S., Markus, H. R. (in press). The pursuit of happiness and the realization of sympathy: Cultural patterns of self, social relations, and well-being. In E. Diener & E. Suh (Eds.), *Subjective well-being across cultures.* Cambridge, MA: MIT Press.

Kitayama, S., Markus, H. R., & Kurokawa, M. (1998). *Does the nature of good feelings depend on culture? A Japan–United States comparison.* Unpublished manuscript, Kyoto University.

Kitayama, S., Markus, H. R., & Lieberman, C. (1995). The collective construction of self-esteem: Implications for culture, self, and emotion. In J. Russell, J. Wellenkamp, T. Manstead, & J. M. F. Dols (Eds.), *Everyday conceptions of emotions* (pp. 523–550). Dordrecht, The Netherlands: Kluwer Academic.

Kitayama, S., Markus, H. R., Matsumoto, H., & Norasakkunkit, V. (1997). Individual and collective processes of self-esteem management: Self-enhancement in the United States and self-depreciation in Japan. *Journal of Personality and Social Psychology, 72,* 1245–1267.

Kitayama, S., & Masuda, T. (1997). [A cultural-mediation model of social inference: Correspondence bias in Japan]. In K. Kashiwagi, S. Kitayama, & H. Azuma (Eds.), *[Cultural psychology: Theory and research]* (pp. 109–127). Tokyo: University of Tokyo Press. (In Japanese)

Kitayama, S., Matsumoto, H., Takagi, H., & Markus, H. R. (1997). *The collective construction of the self: Perceived agentivity and self-relevant social situations in Japan and the United States.* Unpublished manuscript, Kyoto University.

Kitayama, S., Palm, R. I., Masuda, T., Karasawa, M., & Carroll, J. (1996). *Optimism in the U.S. and pessimism in Japan: Perceptions of earthquake risk.* Unpublished manuscript, Kyoto University.

Kitayama, S., Takagi, H., & Matsumoto, H. (1995). Causal attribution of success and failure: Cultural psychology of Japanese self. *[Japanese Psychological Review],* 38, 247–280. (In Japanese)

Kitayama, S., & Uchida, U. (1998). [Mutual sympathy and implicit self-attachment]. Unpublished raw data, Kyoto University.

Kjuchi, A. (1995). Construction of a scale for independent and interdependent construal of the self and its reliability and validity. *Japanese Journal of Psychology, 66,* 100–106.

Kleinman, A. (1989). *Rethinking psychiatry: From cultural category to personal experience.* New York: Free Press.

Kondo, D. K. (1990). *Crafting selves: Power, gender, and discourses of identity in a Japanese workplace.* Chicago: University of Chicago Press.

Kroeber, A. L. (1917). The superorganic. *American Psychologist, 19,* 163–213.

Kuwayama, T. (1992). The reference other orientation. In N. R. Rosenberger (Ed.), *Japanese sense of self* (pp. 121–151). Cambridge, England: Cambridge University Press.

Kwan, V. S. Y., Bond, M. H., & Singelis, T. M. (1997). Pancultural explanations for life satisfaction: Adding relationship harmony to self-esteem. *Journal of Personality and Social Psychology, 73,* 1038–1051.

Lakoff, G., & Johnson, M. (1980). *Metaphors we live by.* Chicago: University of Chicago Press.

Leary, M. R., Tambor, E. S., Terdal, S. K., & Downs, D. L. (1995). Self-esteem as an interpersonal monitor: The sociometer hypothesis. *Journal of Personality and Social Psychology, 68,* 518–530.

Lebra, T. S. (1976). *Japanese patterns of behavior.* Honolulu: University of Hawaii Press.

Lewin, K. (1935). *A dynamic theory of personality.* New York: McGraw-Hill.

Lewis, C. C. (1995). *Educating hearts and minds.* Cambridge, England: Cambridge University Press.

Lillard, A. (1998). Ethnopsychologies: Cultural variations in theories of mind. *Psychological Bulletin, 112,* 3–32.

Lord, C. G., Ross, L., & Lepper, M. R. (1979). Biased assimilation and attitude polarization: The effects of prior theories on subsequently considered evidence. *Journal of Personality and Social Psychology, 37,* 2098–2109.

Lutz, C. (1988). *Unnatural emotions: Everyday sentiments on a Micronesian atoll and their challenges to Western theory.* Chicago: University of Chicago Press.

Markus, H. R. (1977). Self-schemas and processing information about the self. *Journal of Personality and Social Psychology, 35,* 63–78.

Markus, H. R., & Cross, S. (1990). The interpersonal self. In L. A. Pervin (Ed.), *Handbook of personality: Theory and research* (pp. 576–607). New York: Guilford Press.

Markus, H. R., & Kitayama, S. (1991). Culture and the self: Implications for cognition, emotion, and motivation. *Psychological Review, 98,* 224–253.

Markus, H. R., & Kitayama, S. (1994). A collective fear of the collective: Implications for selves and theories of selves. *Personality and Social Psychology Bulletin, 20,* 568–579.

Markus, H. R., & Kitayama, S. (1998). The cultural psychology of personality. *Journal of Cross-Cultural Psychology, 29,* 32–61.

Markus, H. R., Kitayama, S., & Heiman, R. J. (1996). Culture and basic psychological principles. In E. T. Higgins & A. W. Kruglanski (Eds.), *Social psychology: Handbook of basic principles* (pp. 857–913). New York: Guilford Press.

Markus, H. R., Kitayama, S., Mullally, P., Masuda, T., & Fryberg, S. (1997). *Of selves and selfways: Patterns of individuality and uniformity in identity.* Unpublished manuscript, Stanford University.

Markus, H. R., Mullally, P. R., & Kitayama, S. (1997). Selfways: Diversity in modes of cultural participation. In U. Neisser & D. Jopling (Eds.), *The conceptual self in context* (pp. 13–60). New York: Cambridge University Press.

Markus, H. R., & Wurf, E. (1987). The dynamic self-concept: A social psychological perspective. *Annual Review of Psychology, 38,* 299–237.

McCrae, R. R., & Costa, P. T., Jr. (1997). Personality trait structure as a human universal. *American Psychologist, 52,* 81–90.

McCrae, R. R., Yik, M. S. M., Trapbell, P. D., Bond, M. H., & Paulhus, D. L. (1998). Interpreting personality profiles across cultures: Bilingual, acculturation, and peer rating studies of Chinese undergraduates. *Journal of Personality and Social Psychology, 74,* 1041–1055.

Mead, G. (1934). *Mind, self, and society.* University of Chicago Press.

Miller, J. G. (1984). Culture and the development of everyday social explanation. *Journal of Personality and Social Psychology, 46,* 961–978.

Miller, J. G. (1994). Cultural psychology: Bridging disciplinary boundaries in understanding the cultural grounding of self. In P. K. Bock (Ed.), *Handbook of psychological anthropology* (pp. 139–170). Westport, CT: Greenwood.

Mischel, W. (1973). Toward a cognitive social learning theory of personality. *Psychological Review, 80,* 252–283.

Mischel, W. (1990). Personality dispositions revisited and revised: A view after three decades. In L. A. Pervin (Ed.), *Handbook of personality theory and research* (pp. 111–134). New York: Guilford Press.

Mischel, W., & Shoda, Y. (1995). A cognitive-affective system theory of personality:

Reconceptualizing situation, dispositions, dynamics, and invariance in personality structure. *Psychological Review, 102,* 246–268.

Mischel, W., Shoda, Y., & Rodriguez, M. L. (1989). Delay of gratification in children. *Science, 244,* 933–938.

Misumi, J. (1985). *The behavioral science of leadership: An interdisciplinary approach.* Ann Arbor: University of Michigan Press.

Morris, I. (1975). *The nobility of failure: Tragic heroes in the history of Japan.* New York: Noonday Press.

Morris, M. W., & Peng, K. (1994). Culture and cause: American and Chinese attributions for social and physical events. *Journal of Personality and Social Psychology, 67,* 949–971.

Muramoto, Y. (1998). *Another self-serving bias: The co-presence and meanings of self-effacing and group-serving tendencies in Japanese patterns of attribution.* Unpublished doctoral dissertation, University of Tokyo.

Muramoto, Y., & Yamaguchi, S. (1997). Another type of self-serving bias: Coexistence of self-effacing and group-serving tendencies in attribution in the Japanese culture. *Japanese Journal of Experimental Social Psychology, 37,* 65–75.

Myers, F. R. (1991). *Pintupi country, Pintupi self: Sentiment, place, and politics among Western desert aborigines.* Berkeley: University of California Press.

Nakamura, H. (1989). [*Ways of thinking of Japanese people*]. Tokyo: Shunjyu-sha. (In Japanese)

Nakane, C. (1970). *Japanese society.* Los Angeles: University of California Press.

Newman, L. S., & Uleman, J. S. (1989). Spontaneous trait inference. In J. S. Uleman & J. A. Bargh (Eds.), *Unintended thought* (pp. 155–188). New York: Guilford Press.

Nitobe, I. (1969). *Bushido: The soul of Japan.* Tokyo: Charles E. Tuttle. (Original work published 1905)

Nuttin, J. M., Jr. (1985). Narcissism beyond gestalt and awareness: The name letter effect. *European Journal of Social Psychology, 15,* 353–361.

Nuttin, J. M., Jr. (1987). Affective consequences of mere ownership: The name letter effect in twelve European languages. *European Journal of Social Psychology, 17,* 381–402.

Ochs, E. (1988). *Culture and language development: Language acquisition and language socialization in a Samoan village.* New York: Cambridge University Press.

Ohnuki-Tierney, E. (1984). *Illness and culture in contemporary Japan.* Cambridge, England: Cambridge University Press.

Okazaki, S. (1997). Sources of ethnic differences between Asian American and white American college students on measures of depression and social anxiety. *Journal of Abnormal Psychology, 106,* 52–60.

Paranjpe, A. C. (1988). A personality theory according to Vedanta. In A. C. Paranjpe, D. Y. Ho, & R. W. Rieber (Eds.), *Asian contributions to psychology* (pp. 185–213). New York: Praeger.

Peng, K. (1997). *Beyond the principle of non-contradiction: Naive dialecticism and its effects on reasoning and social judgment.* Unpublished doctoral dissertation, University of Michigan.

Pepitone, A. (1976). Toward a normative and comparative biocultural social psychology. *Journal of Personality and Social Psychology, 34,* 641–653.

Pervin, L. A. (Ed.). (1990). *Handbook of personality: Theory and research.* New York: Guilford Press.

Pervin, L. A. (1994). A critical analysis of current trait theory. *Psychological Inquiry, 5,* 103–113.

Plath, D. W. (1980). *Long engagement: Maturity in modern Japan.* Stanford, CA: Stanford University Press.

Roland, A. (1988). *In search of self in India and Japan.* Princeton, NJ: Princeton University Press.

Rohlen, T. P. (1989). Order in Japanese society: Attachment, authority, and routine. *Journal of Japanese Studies, 15,* 5–40.

Rosenberger, N. R. (Ed.). (1992). *Japanese sense of self.* Cambridge, England: Cambridge University Press.

Ross, L. (1977). The intuitive psychologist and his shortcomings: Distortions in the attribution process. In L. Berkowitz (Ed.), *Advances in experimental social psychology* (Vol. 10, pp. 174–220). New York: Academic Press.

Ross, L., Lepper, M. L., & Hubbard, M. (1975). Perseverance in self-perception and social perception: Biased attribution processes in the debriefing paradigm. *Journal of Personality and Social Psychology, 32,* 880–892.

Ross, L., & Nisbett, R. E. (1991). *The person and the situation: Perspectives of social psychology.* New York: McGraw-Hill.

Saito, A. (1996). Social origins of cognition: Bartlett, evolutionary perspective and embodied mind. *Journal of the Theory of Social Behavior, 26,* 399–421.

Sakita, T. I. (1998). *Reporting discourse in English: Discourse, cognition, and consciousness.* Unpublished doctoral dissertation, Kyoto University.

Sampson, E. E. (1977). Psychology and the American ideal. *Journal of Personality and Social Psychology, 35,* 767–782.

Sampson, E. E. (1988). The debate on individualism: Indigenous psychologies of the individual and their role in personal and societal functioning. *American Psychologist, 43,* 15–22.

Scheier, M. F., & Carver, C. S. (1983). Two sides of the self: One for you and one for me. In J. Suls, & A. G. Greenwald (Eds.), *Psychological perspectives on the self* (Vol. 2, pp. 123–158). Hillsdale, NJ: Erlbaum.

Schutz, A., & Luckmann, T. (1974). *The structure of the life-world* (R. M. Zaner & H. T. Engelhardt, Trans.). London: Heinemann.

Schwartz, B. (1986). *The battle for human nature.* New York: Norton.

Seligman, M. E. P., Abramson, L. Y., Semmel, A., & Von Baeyer, C. (1979). Depressive attributional style. *Journal of Abnormal Psychology, 88,* 242–247.

Sethi, S., & Lepper, M. (1997). *Rethinking the value of choice: A cultural perspective on intrinsic motivation.* Unpublished manuscript, Stanford University.

Shweder, R. A. (1990). Cultural psychology: What is it? In J. W. Stigler, R. A. Shweder, & G. Herdt (Eds.), *Cultural psychology: Essays on comparative human development* (pp. 1–43). Cambridge, England: Cambridge University Press.

Shweder, R. A. (1991). *Cultural psychology: Thinking through cultures.* Cambridge, MA: Harvard University Press.

Shweder, R. A., & Bourne, L. (1984). Does the concept of the person vary cross-culturally? In R. A. Shweder & R. A. LeVine (Eds.), *Culture theory: Essays on mind, self, and emotion* (pp. 158–199). New York:

Shweder, R. A., Goodnow, J., Hatano, G., LeVine, R., Markus, H., & Miller, P. (1998). The cultural psychology of development: One mind, many mentalities. In W.

Damon (Series Ed.) & R. M. Lerner (Vol. Ed.), *Handbook of child psychology: Vol. 1. Theoretical models of human development* (5th ed.). New York: Wiley.

Shweder, R. A., Jensen, L. A., & Goldstein, W. M. (1995). Who sleeps by whom revisited: A method for extracting the moral goods implicit in practice. In J. J. Goodnow, P. J. Miller, & F. Kessel (Eds.), *New directions for child development: No. 67. Cultural practices as contexts for development* (pp. 21–39). San Francisco: Jossey-Bass.

Shweder, R. A., & Sullivan, M. (1993). Cultural psychology: Who needs it? *Annual Review of Psychology, 44,* 497–523.

Singelis, T. M. (1994). The measurement of independent and interdependent self-construals. *Personality and Social Psychology Bulletin, 20,* 580–591.

Smith, R. J. (1983). *Japanese society: Tradition, self, and the social order.* Cambridge, England: Cambridge University Press.

Solomon, S., Greenberg, J., & Pyszczynski, T. (1991). A terror management theory of social behavior: The psychological functions of self-esteem and cultural worldviews. In L. Berkowitz (Ed.), *Advances in experimental social psychology* (Vol. 24, pp. 93–159). San Diego, CA: Academic Press.

Stearns, C. Z., & Stearns, P. N. (1986). *Anger: The struggle for emotional control in America's history.* Chicago: University of Chicago Press.

Stevenson, H. H., & Stigler, J. W. (1992). *The learning gap: Why our schools are failing and what we can learn from Japanese and Chinese education.* New York: Summit Books.

Suh, E., Diener, E., Oishi, S., & Triandis, H. C. (1998). The shifting basis of life satisfaction judgments across cultures: Emotions versus norms. *Journal of Personality and Social Psychology, 74,* 482–493.

Takata, T. (1987). [Self-deprecative tendencies in self-evaluation through social comparison]. *[Japanese Journal of Experimental Social Psychology]*, 27(1), 27–36. (In Japanese)

Takata, T., & Matsumoto, Y. (1995). The structure of self in Japanese culture: Aspects and age differences. *Japanese Journal of Psychology, 66,* 213–218.

Tardif, T. (1996). Nouns are not always learned before verbs: Evidence from Mandarin-speakers' early vocabularies. *Developmental Psychology, 32,* 492–504.

Taylor, C. (1989). *Sources of the self: The making of modern identities.* Cambridge, MA: Harvard University Press.

Taylor, S. E., & Brown, J. D. (1988). Illusion and well-being: A social psychological perspective on mental health. *Psychological Review, 103,* 193–210.

Tobin, J. J., Wu, D. Y. H., & Davidson, D. H. (1989). *Preschools in three cultures: Japan, China, and the United States.* New Haven, CT: Yale University Press.

Trafimow, D., Triandis, H.C., & Goto, S. G. (1991). Some tests of the distinction between private and collective self. *Journal of Personality and Social Psychology, 60,* 649–655.

Triandis, H. C. (1989). The self and social behavior in differing cultural contexts. *Psychological Review, 96,* 506–520.

Triandis, H. C. (1995). *Individualism and collectivism.* Boulder, CO: Westview Press.

Tu, W. (1994). Embodying the universe: A note on Confucian self-realization. In R. T. Ames, W. Dissanayake, & T. P. Kasulis (Eds.), *Self as person in Asian theory and practice* (pp. 177–186). Albany: State University of New York Press.

Turner, J. C., Oakes, P. J., Haslam, S. A., & McGarty, C. (1994). Self and collective: Cognition and social context. *Personality and Social Psychology Bulletin, 20,* 454–463.

Vygotsky, L. (1978). *Mind in society: The development of higher psychological processes* (M. Cole, V. John-Steiner, S. Scribner, & E. Souberman, Eds. & Trans.). Cambridge, MA: Harvard University Press.

Wallach, M. A. & Wallach, L. (1983). *Psychology's sanction for selfishness.* San Francisco: Freeman.

Wang, L. (1998). [Food, medicine and Chinese care: Transmission of folk knowledge among the Fukienese, Philippines]. *Ecosophia, 1,* 88–111. (In Japanese)

Weber, M. (1992). *The Protestant ethic and the spirit of capitalism* (T. Parsons, Trans.). New York: Routledge. (Original work published 1930)

Weisz, J. R., Rothbaum, F. M., & Blackburn, T. C. (1984). Standing out and standing in: The psychology of control in America and Japan. *American Psychologist, 39,* 955–969.

Wertsch, J. V. (1991). *Voices of the mind: A sociocultural approach to mediated action.* London: Harvester Wheatsheaf.

White, G. M. (1994). Emotion and morality. In S. Kitayama & H. R. Markus (Eds.), *Emotion and culture: Empirical investigations of mutual influences.* Washington, DC: American Psychological Association.

White, M. I., & LeVine, R. A. (1986). What is an *Ii ko* (good child)? In H. Stevenson, H. Azuma, & K. Hakuta (Eds.), *Child development and education in Japan* (pp. 55–62). New York: Freeman.

Whiting, J., & Child, I. (1953). *Child training and personality: A cross-cultural study.* New Haven, CT: Yale University Press.

Whiting, R. (1990). *You gotta have wa.* New York: Vintage.

Wierzbicka, A. (1994). Emotion, language, and "cultural scripts." In S. Kitayama & H. R. Markus (Eds.), *Emotion and culture: Empirical studies of mutual influences.* Washington, DC: American Psychological Association.

Winter, L., & Uleman, J. S. (1984). When are social judgments made?: Evidence for the spontaneousness of trait inferences. *Journal of Personality and Social Psychology, 47,* 237–252.

Yamaguchi, S. (1994). Collectivism among the Japanese: A perspective from the self. In U. Kim, H. C. Triandis, C. Kagitcibasi, S.-C. Choi, & G. Yoon (Eds.), *Individualism and collectivism: Theory, method, and applications* (pp. 175–188). London: Sage.

Yeh, C. (1995). *The clinical grounding of self and morality in Japan and the U.S.* Unpublished doctoral dissertation, Stanford University.

Yik, M. S. M., Bond, M. H., & Paulhus, D. L. (1998). Do Chinese self-enhance or self-efface?: It's a matter of domain. *Personality and Social Psychology Bulletin, 24,* 399–406.

Zajonc, R. B. (1960). The process of cognitive tuning in communication. *Journal of Abnormal and Social Psychology, 61,* 159–167.

9

Bottom-Up Explanation in Personality Psychology
The Case of Cross-Situational Coherence

DANIEL CERVONE

Science seeks explanation. The goal of scientific investigation is to explain how phenomena occur (Salmon, 1989). Our phenomenon of interest is personality coherence. This chapter seeks, then, to explain how personality processes function as coherent systems and why people exhibit coherent patterns of experience and action across time and place.

This chapter, and indeed, this volume, focuses more specifically on explanations of personality coherence that derive from social-cognitive theory (Bandura, 1986 and Chapter 7, this volume; Cervone & Williams, 1992; Mischel, 1973; Mischel & Shoda, 1995). Even those who praise its other virtues have faulted social-cognitive theory on this point. Critics see social-cognitive approaches as containing lists of seemingly disconnected personality processes that fail to explain the coherent functioning of the whole person (Carver & Scheier, 1996; Hogan, 1982). Commentators characterize social-cognitive theory as a "situation-based" (Revelle, 1995, p. 317) perspective that overlooks personal factors that contribute to consistent individual differences. Even if one recognizes these critiques as misrepresentations of social-cognitive theory, the onus clearly is on the social-cognitivist to articulate how an analysis of cognitive and affective processes, and their social foundations (Bandura, 1986; Levine, Resnick, & Higgins, 1993), speaks to the coherence of personality functioning.

Given the present state of the discipline, social-cognitive theory cannot be examined in isolation. Trait models predominate in personality psychology. Trait theorists of various stripes claim that trait constructs explain the coherence of personality functioning (Funder, 1991; McCrae & Costa, 1995; Tellegen, 1991). Others, in contrast, contend that trait and dispositional constructs are descriptive labels with no explanatory value (Buss & Craik, 1983; Wright & Mischel, 1987). Commentators writing from a social-cognitive perspective generally conclude that trait approaches fail to incorporate adequate explanatory principles (Mischel, 1993).

I begin, then, with three questions:

1. Can social-cognitive approaches explain the coherence of personality functioning (and, if so, how)?
2. Do trait theories such as the popular five-factor model (Wiggins, 1996) explain personality coherence?
3. Are trait and social-cognitive theories reconcilable?

The third question is important in that some writers see "the integration of these two" perspectives as "one of the major tasks of a new generation of personality theories" (McCrae & Costa, 1996, p. 59; cf. Cervone 1991). In principle, this integration could take various forms. Trait approaches might supply descriptive information for which social-cognitive theories provide an explanation (cf. Buss & Craik, 1983). Trait and social-cognitive approaches might both provide explanations, but at different levels of analysis, with the result that the approaches can be integrated easily (cf. Bolger, 1990; Langston & Sykes, 1997; McCrae & Costa, 1996).

The answers I suggest to these three questions are (1) yes, (2) yes, and (3) no. Social-cognitive theory can explain personality coherence. Trait approaches also provide an explanation of this phenomenon. Yet trait and social-cognitive theories cannot easily be reconciled.

This constellation of answers is unusual. Theorists generally either criticize each other for failing to explain the coherence of personality or work to integrate theoretical perspectives that might jointly explain the phenomenon. I begin by explaining the basis of this position. These answers are reached by considering the following key point, which has received inadequate attention in personality psychology's discussions of scientific explanation. There is more than one way to explain a phenomenon. There exist alternative strategies of scientific explanation (Salmon, 1989; Wylie, 1995).

This chapter, then, reviews alternative strategies of scientific explanation and shows that social-cognitive and nomothetic trait theories exemplify different explanatory forms. It then returns to the three questions. Next, research is reviewed that illustrates how social-cognitive theory can explain a phenomenon that previously has been considered the province of trait theories, namely, cross-situational coherence in psychological response. The chapter concludes by addressing the status of dispositional variables in social-cognitive theory and briefly considering how biologically based temperament factors could fruitfully be integrated into social-cognitive theory to yield a broader framework for understanding personality coherence.

ALTERNATIVE STRATEGIES OF SCIENTIFIC EXPLANATION

In addressing questions of scientific explanation, the personality psychologist need not—and should not—go it alone. Philosophers have devoted considerable attention to questions of scientific explanation (e.g., Kitcher & Salmon, 1989). Investigators in other social sciences have confronted conceptual issues that parallel those of our field (see Wylie, 1995). Since much can be learned from others' experiences (Bandura, 1965), I first review an explanatory controversy in another discipline, namely, archeology. As we shall see, archeological debate features alternative explanatory schemes that bear an uncanny resemblance to those in personality psychology.

Explaining the Spread of Indo-European Languages

Archeological evidence suggests that the family of Indo-European languages spread from areas near the Black Sea to regions as remote as northern Europe during a roughly 1,500-year period (Renfrew, 1989). The fields of archeology and historical linguistics must explain this phenomenon. At least two types of explanation are available. In other words, philosophers of science recognize at least two strategies of archeological explanation (Wylie, 1995).

One strategy is to search for a small set of universal principles that capture overall trends in language spread. The goal here is to provide a simple, parsimonious explanation for what otherwise might be a bewildering diversity of facts about different languages. The distinguished archeologist Colin Renfrew (1989, 1992) has provided such an explanation. The general principle he relies upon involves population growth resulting from the development of farming. When populations adopt agriculture, they grow rapidly. The larger population requires more land to sustain its growth. When a farming population acquires new land, it takes its language with it. It is estimated that agriculture-induced growth forces a population to spread at about 1 km a year (Ammerman & Cavalli-Sforza, 1984). At this rate, it would take about 1,500 years to get from the Black Sea to northern Europe—which corresponds to the historical evidence (Renfrew, 1989).

This is such a tidy explanation that one might wonder why anybody would even seek an alternative. What shortcoming might this explanation have? Although a number of issues have been raised in the archeological literature (see Renfrew, 1988, including commentaries), one in particular concerns us here. The principle of agriculture-induced spread accounts for data in the aggregate. Specifically, it accounts for data that are aggregated in two ways: across languages and across time. The model explains why the Indo-

European languages—in general—spread at a given rate—on average—over 1,500 years. It does not necessarily capture the spread of any individual language during any specific historical period. The model, in other words, can "be held accountable, *not* to individual instances, but to aggregate outcomes characterized in appropriately general terms" (Wylie, 1995, p. 17).

There are two critical points here. The first concerns description. The agriculture-based model may not accurately describe language spread at the level of the individual language. Particular languages at particular times may have spread in a manner that differs widely from agriculture-based expectations. By working at the level of the aggregate, the model presents a descriptive and explanatory idealization that may "not accurately describe all (or any) particular instances" (Wylie, 1995, p. 17). As it turns out, numerous specific instances fail to accord with the model's expectations (Barker, 1988). Sometimes languages have spread very quickly, or very slowly, or in the absence of marked population growth. The second point concerns explanation. If the descriptions fail at the level of the individual case, then the accompanying explanatory principles cannot be applied there. The model thus does not "establish grounds for . . . claims about underlying causal processes" (Wylie, 1995, p. 17).

What is the alternative strategy of explanation? In the alternative, one's initial goal is not to capture overall trends in the historical data through a small number of overarching principles. Instead, one begins by identifying the potential multiplicity of specific causal processes that could contribute to linguistic spread in any particular time and place.[1] One studies "the process and context of the transition to farming" and "[models] the social processes" (Barker, 1988, p. 449) that produce linguistic change. After a firm understanding of these underlying processes is gained, causal models can be developed to account for both overall trends in language spread and idiosyncratic cases in which a language spread in an atypical manner. Such an approach inevitably would not be "as neat and tidy" (Barker, 1988, p. 448) as one that posits a small number of universal principles. But with the loss of simplicity come significant gains. By drawing on an understanding of specific underlying causal mechanisms, investigators can be more confident that they are not trafficking in statistical abstractions that fail to correspond to individual cases, but that, instead, they are working with processes that actually came into play at particular times and places. A further advantage is that individual languages that deviate from the norm are no longer inexplicable statistical anomalies but well-understood products of atypical arrangements of underlying causal mechanisms. Some archeologists argue that the field should put aside attempts to formulate grand, overarching theoretical unifications and instead should focus on the task of identifying specific causal processes that explain why languages spread (Barker, 1988).

The advantages and disadvantages of these alternative explanations of language spread strikingly parallel those of alternative explanations of personality coherence.

Explaining the Cross-Situational Coherence of Personality Functioning

People exhibit similar psychological characteristics across different situations. Thoughts, feelings, and behavioral tendencies are meaningfully interconnected across time and place. The field of personality psychology must explain this cross-situational coherence in psychological experience. As was the case in archeology, at least two strategies of explanation are available.

One strategy is to search for a small set of universal psychological structures that explain consistent individual differences in psychological experience. The goal here is to provide a simple taxonomic scheme that organizes what otherwise might be a bewildering array of individual-difference tendencies. McCrae and Costa (1995, 1996, 1997) provide a particularly prominent scheme of this sort. Personality coherence derives from psychological structures that manifest themselves as dispositional tendencies. Dispositions shape thoughts and feelings and thereby foster coherent patterns of response that are evident across contexts. Investigators identify these dispositions by analyzing large populations of individuals, each of whom has been described in terms of a large number of personality tendencies. One searches for personality tendencies that intercorrelate, or that form factors. Once a factor is reliably identified, its existence is explained in a straightforward manner. The statistical factor is assumed to correspond directly to a psychological structure that is present in each individual. These structures are seen to constitute "the universal raw material of personality" (McCrae & Costa, 1996).

An advantage of this strategy is its simplicity. A set of only five psychological constructs—that is, five basic dispositional tendencies—explains a substantial amount of the variability in personality tendencies in the population. These five tendencies are identifiable across different techniques of personality assessment and in different cultures (McCrae & Costa, 1987, 1997).

This is such a tidy explanatory system that one might wonder why anybody would even seek an alternative. What shortcoming might this explanation have? Although a number of issues have been raised in the literature (Block, 1995; Pervin, 1994, including commentaries), one in particular is of concern here. The five-factor model accounts for personality tendencies in the aggregate. Specifically, it accounts for data that are aggregated in two ways: across people and across contexts. The model explains why consistent variation—in the population—is found in tendencies to perform—on average—behaviors representative of various dispositional categories. Let us consider these two forms of aggregation more carefully. Regarding aggregation across persons, the factors are statistical properties of populations, not individual persons. Of concern here is that there is no guarantee that population-level constructs will apply at the level of the individual. Recent years have seen wider recognition of this critical point (Revelle, 1995). Rorer (1990) notes that to assume that population-level constructs apply at the level of the individual is to commit an error of logic. Nesselroade and Molenaar (in press) explain that the statistical technique of aggregating data "over individuals who [may be] qualitatively different from each other," can "[distort] the aggregate into an entity that has no parallel in the group" (p. 2). Paraphrasing Wylie (1995), then, the five-factor model may not accurately describe all (or any) particular individuals. Regarding aggregation across contexts, the factors correspond to tendencies to perform a particular class of action on average across the various circumstances of one's life. They thus cannot explain systematic situation-to-situation variations in behavioral tendencies that may uniquely characterize the individual (Mischel & Shoda, 1995).[2]

Once again, problems of both description and explanation arise. Descriptively, there is no guarantee that the five-factor model will capture the dispositional tendencies of individual persons. Indeed, a number of recent findings reveal individual-level phenomena that do not accord with population-level factors (see Cervone & Shoda, Chapter 1, this volume; McAdams, 1995, 1996b). Self-knowledge and situational beliefs foster patterns of cross-situational coherence that do not correspond to population-level individual-difference categories (Cervone, 1997). Variability in response with respect to a given dispositional category, an important "signature of personality" (Mischel & Shoda, 1995), cannot be captured by dispositional models, which correspond to mean levels of response. Finally, factor analyses conducted at the level of the individual suggest that the factor structure of individual tendencies may not correspond to the structure found in analyses of the population. As part of their intensive time-series analyses of individual cases, Nesselroade and Molenaar (in press) have developed a technique for formally assessing the appropriateness of pooling data from individuals. A test of the appropriateness of pooling covariance functions computed on each of 31 research participants found that 10 individuals' functions met the criterion for pooling. Ten participants, in other words, were similar enough to be describable by an aggregate population-level statistic. This means, of course, that 21 were not. The large majority of persons could not be fit into any aggregate model. This finding indeed is "troubling to researchers who pool information across multiple subjects with no apparent concern about its appropriateness or no way to muster statistical support for their actions" (Nesselroade & Molenaar, in press, p. 14).

Regarding explanation, if the factors identified in analyses of populations do not accurately capture personality coherence identified in analyses of the individual, then theories of personality that are based on population-level constructs (e.g., McCrae & Costa, 1996) lose explanatory force at the level of the individual case. This is a most significant loss. Personality psychologists may disagree on many points, but they must agree that the explanatory constructs of a personality theory must apply at the level of the individual person. Explaining the actions of the individual by reference to population-level dispositional constructs (McCrae & Costa, 1995) requires that one be able to identify the dispositional constructs reliably when analyzing the individual case. For the five-factor model, such evidence is completely lacking. Contradictory evidence is beginning to emerge (Fleeson, 1998).

What, then, is an alternative strategy for explaining cross-situational coherence in response? One alternative is to begin by inquiring about specific psychological mechanisms that cause responses to cohere across contexts. Rather than searching for a minimal set of descriptive principles or taxonomic categories, one might seek to identify the potential multiplicity of underlying processes that contribute to cross-situational coherence. Once a basic understanding of these processes is gained, one could develop specific causal models to account for both recurring patterns of cross-situational coherence and idiosyncratic instances in which a person's pattern of coherence deviates from statistical norms.

Social-cognitive theory adopts this strategy. Social-cognitive theory is a theory of the psychological processes underlying personality coherence. It is a theory of "personal determinants" (Bandura, 1991, p. 119) of psychosocial functioning. This "reconceptualization of personality" (Mischel, 1973) is a rethinking of the basic units of analysis that are necessary for explaining personality functioning. Rather than building around an abstract set of dispositional tendencies, the social-cognitivist chooses to ground a personality theory in an understanding of dynamic, causal psychological mechanisms.

Specifically, social-cognitive explanations are built upon two key principles (Cervone & Williams, 1992). The first is that psychological functioning is understood by reference to a set of interacting cognitive and affective processes. These include the individual's capacity to store declarative and procedural knowledge, to use this knowledge to assign meaning to events and to anticipate future contingencies, to plan courses of action, to react evaluatively to one's ongoing performance, and to reflect upon oneself and one's relation to the world. These social-cognitive mechanisms give individuals significant capacity to regulate their behavior and emotional life. The theoretical goal is to understand how these psychological mechanisms, in isolation and in concert (e.g., Bandura & Cervone, 1986; Cervone, Jiwani, & Wood, 1991; Scott & Cervone, 1998), give rise to the coherent patterns of action and experience that are the hallmark of personality.

The second principle is that of reciprocal determinism. Personality processes and structures evolve in reciprocal interaction with the social and cultural environment (Bandura, 1978; also see Baltes, Linderberger, & Staudinger, 1998; Kelly, 1968; Kitayama, Markus, Matsumoto, & Norasakkunit, 1997). In social-cognitive theory, environmental factors play two key roles. They shape the development of personality structures, and they activate psychological structures that have been developed (Cervone & Williams, 1992).[3] The environment, however, is not an ultimate causal agent (Skinner, 1971) but a facet of an interacting causal system. People causally contribute to their own experiences and personal development. Agentic properties of the self-system give rise to much of the coherence of personality functioning (Bandura, Chapter 7, this volume). People create coherent, meaningful life experiences by setting personal goals that serve to organize actions across multiple contexts and extended periods of time.

This contextualized analysis of reciprocal relations among social-cognitive structures and processes, the environment, and social behavior admittedly does not yield as simple an explanatory scheme as do contemporary trait theories. But with the loss of simplicity come significant gains. By focusing on well-specified psychological mechanisms, social-cognitivists are able to draw upon both correlational and experimental sources of evidence. Further, they are able to capture psychological tendencies not only in the population at large, but among particular subsets of persons (e.g., Dweck & Leggett, 1988) and particular individuals (e.g., Cervone, 1997). Indeed, individuals who do not fit population-level categories are not treated as inexplicable statistical anomalies. Instead, they are understood within a theoretical system that contains nomothetic processes but that treats psychological content idiographically (Higgins, 1990). Social-cognitivists thus can be confident that they are not trafficking in mere statistical abstractions, but instead that they have identified psychological processes that actually come into play at particular times for particular individuals.

Top-Down and Bottom-Up Explanation

The obvious similarity between theoretical alternatives in archeology and in personality psychology reflects a highly general principle. Theoretical debate in both areas illustrates a basic distinction between alternative strategies of scientific explanation. The contrasting approaches illustrate the distinction between "top-down" and "bottom-up" explanatory strategies (Kitcher, 1985; Salmon, 1989).

Top-Down Explanation

Top-down explanations organize information about the world (Kitcher, 1985). Particular facts are explained by fitting them within a simple, overarching, organizational framework. This framework provides a preexisting system within which new facts can be anticipated and understood. By organizing and anticipating facts, the high-level framework can be seen to have a form of explanatory power (Kitcher, 1985). Using our above examples, the facts that (1) a particular Indo-European language may have spread 300 km in 300 years, (2) that its population of native speakers grew rapidly during this period, and (3) that the speakers were agriculturalists do not have to be construed as isolated bits of information. Instead, they can be organized and explained by reference to the overarching principle of agriculture-induced linguistic spread. In personality psychology, the facts that a particular individual is observed to be (1) highly reliable in some contexts, (2) hardworking in others, and (3) is often self-reliant do not have to be construed as isolated bits of biography. Instead, they can be organized and explained by reference to the high-level personality construct "conscientiousness."

Top-down explanations relieve investigators from grappling with large numbers of explanatory principles and numerous details about individual instances. Individual cases are "fit within" (Salmon, 1989, p. 182) a simple, overarching explanatory system that "[reduces] the number of independent phenomena we have to accept as ultimate or given" (Friedman, 1974, cited in Wylie, 1995, p. 1).

Top-down explanatory systems can be formulated in the absence of knowledge about underlying causal mechanisms (Salmon, 1989). In principle, one could posit laws or taxonomic categories of broad scope without necessarily being able to identify the processes underlying one's basic principles. Even without this knowledge, the top-down scheme can explain events by subsuming them "under some kind of lawful regularity" (Salmon, 1989, p. 128).

In psychology, the five-factor model of personality (McCrae & Costa, 1996) is a prototypical case of top-down explanation. The model organizes the diversity of individual-difference constructs and thereby relieves investigators from grappling with an overwhelming number of potential distinct personality variables. It provides a simple explanation of the individual case by fitting the person into a common system. As is typical of top-down explanation, five-factor theorists formulate explanatory schemes in ignorance of the causal processes underlying the explanatory constructs; decades after its initial formulation, the "structures and processes underlying [the five factors] remain to be explicated" (John, 1990, p. 95).

Bottom-Up Explanation

As explained by Salmon (1989), "bottom-up" explanatory strategies seek to uncover "the underlying mechanisms . . . that produce the phenomena we want to explain" (p. 134). The goal is not to formulate overarching principles that correspond to average or recurring trends in data, but to identify specific underlying mechanisms that actually come into play in particular instances. One seeks to identify "the internal workings . . . the hidden mechanisms" (Salmon, 1989, p. 134) that give rise to observed phenomena. Bottom-up causal analyses are designed to account not only for recurring trends, but for individual instances that may violate statistical norms (Salmon, 1989).

Although simplicity is a valuable aspect of any causal model, simplicity is not the overriding consideration in a bottom-up approach. The fundamental goal is to identify the causal mechanisms that actually are at work in a given domain, or that truly "are operative in our world" (Salmon, 1989, p. 150). A seemingly parsimonious explanatory framework that fails to correspond to facts about underlying causal processes would, of course, be rejected.

Social-cognitive theory is a prototypical case of bottom-up explanation in personality psychology. Social-cognitive theory does not seek to explain personality coherence by fitting individuals into a system of high-level individual-difference categories. Instead, the social-cognitivist seeks to understand the underlying psychological mechanisms that give rise to coherence in psychological experience and action. Social-cognitive theory is a theory of "the internal workings" (Salmon, 1989, p. 134) that produce personality coherence. As is prototypical of bottom-up explanation, social-cognitive theory seeks to explain not just average, aggregated dispositional tendencies, but unique patterns of response exhibited by potentially unique individuals (Cervone, 1997; also see Shadel, Niaura, & Abrams, in press; Shoda, Chapter 6, this volume; Zelli & Dodge, Chapter 7, this volume).

A Caveat

Before proceeding, a potential misreading of the present argument must be addressed. As used throughout this chapter, the terms "top-down" and "bottom-up" refer to strategies of scientific explanation, just as they do in the philosophical literature (Kitcher & Salmon, 1989). The terms, then, are *not* equivalent to the notions of data-driven versus theory-driven information processing, a meaning these terms acquire within information-processing models of thought (e.g., Simon, 1979). Used in this very different way, the terms "bottom-up" and "top-down" do not characterize trait and social-cognitive models whatsoever. Five-factor approaches were formulated through data-driven statistical methods (Goldberg, 1993). Social-cognitive models posit that theory-driven information processing contributes to personality coherence (Cantor & Kihlstrom, 1987). Trait and social-cognitive models are "top down" and "bottom up" only in the sense that the terms are used here. Nomothetic trait approaches are "top-down" in that they explain coherence in an individual's personality functioning by locating the person within a system of high-level constructs that are said to influence lower-level psychological processes and actions. Social-cognitive models are "bottom-up" in that they explain personality coherence by reference to interactions among underlying causal mechanisms that give rise to coherence in experience and action.

The distinction between bottom-up and top-down approaches is related to Lewin's (1931, 1935) distinction between Aristotelian and Galilean explanatory concepts in psychology. An Aristotelian model, as Lewin explained, considers "abstractly defined classes as the essential nature of [an] object and hence as the explanation of its behavior" (Lewin, 1935, p. 15). Contemporary trait approaches such as the five-factor model, then, are prototypically Aristotelian, as McAdams (1996a) has noted. Lewin called for psychologists to adopt Galilean paradigms, in which explanation involves specifying dynamic processes through which phenomena come about. As Lewin noted, the Galilean perspective does not seek abstract essences that are invariant across circumstances (also see Kagan, 1988). Instead, it explains action by reference to both individual characteristics and the environmental context in which action occurs.

Two Additional Principles

Two additional principles further clarify the social-cognitive strategy and distinguish it from trait approaches. The first is a general principle of scientific explanation. The scientific constructs used to explain a given property or attribute should not themselves contain that attribute. "A fundamental explanation of [a] property . . . will not refer to other things with that very same property; the possession and functioning of that property is what is to be explained" (Nozick, 1981, p. 632). "What requires explanation cannot itself figure in the explanation" (Hanson, 1958, p. 120). Hanson (1958) provides an illustration in the physical sciences: "If the colors of objects are to be explained by atoms, then atoms cannot be colored" (p. 121). Nozick (1981) provides an illustration in the behavioral sciences: "If there is to be an explanation of" free choice, creativity, or love, it must be in terms of "components which don't themselves make free choices," "aren't themselves creative," and "aren't themselves 'in love' " (p. 633). Causal mechanisms should lack the feature one is trying to explain.

Social-cognitive theory embraces this explanatory principle. While recognizing that some people are friendly and others are disagreeable, social-cognitive theory does not posit psychological mechanisms that themselves "are friendly" or "are disagreeable." Instead, these properties are explained by reference to interactions among multiple underlying psychological processes, no one of which directly corresponds to the phenomenon to be explained.

Trait approaches violate this explanatory principle. Investigators working within both idiographic and nomothetic trait models commonly posit explanatory constructs that possess the very qualities that are to be explained. In Allportian approaches, trait constructs "refer to two things at the same time: (1) a complex pattern of behavior from which the trait is inferred, and (2) the psychological structures and processes that are the source of the pattern" (Funder, 1991, p. 32). In the five-factor model, traits are "dimensions of individual differences in tendencies to show consistent patterns of thoughts, feelings, and actions . . . [and] also . . . a property of an individual that accounts for his or her placement along this trait dimension" (McCrae & Costa, 1995, p. 235). By positing constructs that simultaneously possess and explain a given property, trait theories violate a basic principle of scientific explanation (cf. Wiggins, 1973/1997).

Secondly, bottom-up explanation in general, and the social-cognitive strategy of explaining personality coherence in particular, have a close affinity to principles of organization in dynamic, nonlinear, complex systems (e.g., Barton, 1994; Bak & Chen, 1991; Fogel, Lyra, & Valsiner, 1997). Dynamic systems that contain large numbers of interacting elements tend to achieve stable patterns of organization. This organization, however, is achieved "without prespecification" (Lewis, 1997, p. 193). In other words, no a priori, fixed structure exerts its influence throughout the course of development. No preexisting structure determines that exact final form of the system. Instead, organization and stability are achieved gradually. The exact final form of the system may not be predictable. A complex systems view of psychological development, for example, sees distinct cognitive and affective processes as reciprocally interacting and gradually becoming linked to one another. "Processes develop over time into more complex and stable organizations" (Caprara, 1997, p. 20). The psychological system thus self-organizes. This self-organization can, for the individual, take on any of a large variety of final forms; "developmental self-organization [tends] to dig its own idiosyncratic trenches" (Lewis, 1997, p. 196).

Disciplines outside of personality psychology provide many examples of psychological phenomena that arise from interactions among a complex system's multiple elements, no one of which directly corresponds to the phenomenon to be explained. The phenomenon, in other words, is an "emergent property" of the system. In connectionist models of cognition (Rumelhart & McClelland, 1986), the phenomenon of word detection is explained through interactions among simple units, no one of which is "a word detector." In the neurosciences, the phenomenon of long-term episodic memory can be understood by reference to interconnected neural systems, no one of which independently stores a complete episodic memory (Schacter, 1996). In the study of group dynamics, the fact that individuals with similar attitudes tend to be "clustered" near one another in social space can be explained by reference to dynamic interactions among individuals, no one of whom has the intention of forming attitudinally consistent spatial clusters (Latané & L'Herrou, 1996). Inside of personality psychology, computer simulations by Shoda and Mischel (1997; Mischel & Shoda, 1995) show how stable mean levels of a dispositional tendency can be explained by a theoretical system in which no individual units correspond to a mean behavioral tendency.

With these two principles and the distinction between top-down and bottom-up strategies of explanation in mind, we return to the three questions with which we began our discussion.

Questions of Explanation and Integration

Can Social-Cognitive Approaches Explain the Coherence of Personality Functioning (and, If So, How)?

In retrospect, this question only arose because, in a superficial analysis, social-cognitive theory appears to be lacking something. It lacks "personality variables" (as this term is commonly used). That is, it does not have any theoretical constructs that directly correspond to broad consistencies in social behavior.

As we have seen, the absence of traditional "personality variables" does not prevent one from explaining coherence in psychological response. Instead, it leads one to a particular type of explanation in which personality coherence is seen as a product of interactions among multiple psychological processes, no one of which is independently responsible for a broad response pattern. So, "yes," in principle, social-cognitive models can explain cross-situational coherence in response. For them to do so, the social-cognitivist must specify mechanisms that cause responses to cohere, assess those mechanisms, and search for resulting patterns of coherence. This is the goal of a research program (Cervone, 1997) described below.

Do Trait Theories Such as the Five-Factor Model Explain Personality Coherence?

Five-factor theorists (McCrae & Costa, 1997) claim that dispositional variables provide an explanation of action: "Suppose Jane declines a social invitation: One might offer as an explanation the fact that Jane is an introvert and the generalization that introverts prefer to avoid parties" (McCrae & Costa, 1995, p. 234). McCrae and Costa (1995) find it "hard to understand why it should be problematic" to conclude that "traits as underlying tendencies cause and thus explain the consistent patterns of thoughts, feelings, and actions one sees" (pp. 236–237).

The distinction between top-down and bottom-up explanation yields a clear answer to our second question. Trait theorists are correct. Dispositional constructs *do* offer an explanation of personality coherence. They offer a top-down explanation (Kitcher, 1985). They explain coherent patterns of action by fitting individuals and their acts into high-level frameworks that organize, anticipate, and, in this sense, "explain" behavior.

The question to ask about dispositional explanations is not "are they explanations" but "are they *good* explanations," that is, do they provide an adequate explanatory foundation for a scientific theory of personality? As we have seen, nomothetic dispositional theories may fail to capture coherence at the level of the individual. They violate a basic principle of scientific explanation by positing constructs that possess the attributes that require explanation. They generally fail to identify causal mechanisms that produce psychological phenomena of interest. These are considerable shortcomings. They raise serious problems for those who seek to base a scientific explanation of individual's experiences and actions on any set of inferred nomothetic dispositional structures.

Are Trait and Social-Cognitive Theories Easily Reconcilable?

Some investigators answer this question in the affirmative. Trait and social-cognitive models are seen to capture different aspects, or levels, of personality. The theories can be integrated by positing that the trait level influences the social-cognitive level, which, in turn, mediates social behavior (McCrae & Costa, 1996).

The problem with this form of integration is revealed by the principles of explanation discussed above. Trait and social-cognitive approaches do not differ simply in that they highlight different aspects of the person. They differ fundamentally, in that they adopt different *strategies* of explanation. In trait theory, dispositional variables have causal status. To the social-cognitivist, dispositional tendencies are not the *causes of* thought or action. Dispositions, construed as the person's characteristic experiential and behavioral tendencies, are the *phenomena* to be explained. The social-cognitivist strives to explain the phenomena by reference to cognitive and affective processes that cause responses to cohere across contexts.

The philosopher Shaffer (1996) has analyzed contemporary developments in personality psychology, including the alternative theoretical paradigms discussed here. Shaffer highlights the implicit goals and assumptions that drive theoretical approaches. She concludes that the goal of factor-analytic trait research (e.g., Goldberg, 1993) "is not to give the causal foundations of observable behavior; it is to find *predictors* of specific behaviors which meet administrative needs in applied settings" (p. S95). Social-cognitive theory, in contrast, assumes that "the goal of . . . research is to give causal models which are empirically adequate to behavior across contexts" (Shaffer, 1996, p. S94). Though differing somewhat from the present analysis, Shaffer's work is similar in that it indicates that the differences between social-cognitive and dispositional approaches are deeper than is generally acknowledged.

The theoretical distinction between top-down and bottom-up explanatory strategies has direct empirical implications. Alternative strategies of explanation suggest alternative strategies of investigation. This relation between theory and research is perhaps most evident in the study of cross-situational coherence, or cross-situational consistency, in psychological response.[4]

TOP-DOWN AND BOTTOM-UP ANALYSES
OF CROSS-SITUATIONAL COHERENCE

One of the most vexing issues in the history of personality psychology is the question of how to identify and explain cross-situational coherence in psychological response. This question endures because the contemporary notion of "personality" (Allport, 1937) rests on the supposition that people tend to exhibit similar styles of thought, feeling, and action across different situations.

The long history of research on this problem has yielded a variety of methodological solutions (reviewed in Kenrick & Funder, 1988; Schmitt & Borkenau, 1992). The seeming diversity of these methods, however, masks the fact that they share a fundamental conceptual similarity. Work on cross-situational coherence has been dominated by a top-down approach to the problem. Investigators have gauged the degree to which populations of individuals behave consistently with respect to high-level trait constructs. The various methodological advances have addressed the questions of what population to study (Bem & Allen, 1974), how to identify valid trait indicators (Jackson & Paunonen, 1985), and how to assess trait indicators reliably (Epstein, 1979). In all cases, however, consistency ultimately has meant consistency with respect to a trait construct that is defined by a fixed set of indicators. Reflecting an implicit top-down conception, investigators gauge the degree to which a group of individuals "fit(s) within" (Salmon, 1989, p. 182) the a priori structure.

These top-down approaches have identified statistically significant levels of response consistency (Kenrick & Funder, 1988). They nonetheless have two significant limitations. They may overlook cross-situational coherence that does not happen to correspond to the investigator's definition of the given trait construct. An individual's responses may cohere across complex, idiosyncratic sets of circumstances. This critical point has been recognized previously (e.g., Allport, 1937; Bem & Allen, 1974; Bowers, 1977; Magnusson & Endler, 1977) but has not been systematically incorporated into research design. Secondly, top-down approaches generally fail to identify the causal mechanisms responsible for any coherence in response that may be observed. It is remarkable that the long history of research and debate in this area has focused almost entirely on methodological solutions while giving scant attention to the question of psychological mechanisms that might cause responses to cohere across contexts.

Social-cognitive theory, and its bottom-up strategy of explanation, suggest an approach to the study of cross-situational consistency that differs fundamentally from a top-down trait strategy. In a social-cognitive approach, one would not begin by selecting a high-level trait construct and identifying a fixed set of trait indicators. Instead, one would start by asking about psychological mechanisms that may cause responses to cohere. A theoretical analysis of underlying causal mechanisms would guide the methodological search for consistency. Cross-situational consistency would be anticipated across those circumstances that activate a common set of underlying social-cognitive mechanisms. Whether these circumstances are shared from one person to another, and whether they correspond to traditional high-level trait categories, would be an empirical question.

More specifically, a social-cognitive analysis of cross-situational coherence might take the following form. First, one would identify a social-cognitive process whose causal impact on social behavior is well established. Next, one would inquire into additional psychological structures and processes that might create cross-situational coherence in the initial social-cognitive variable. The search for coherence, then, would be based on an interacting system of causal mechanisms.

Many different social-cognitive processes may contribute to cross-situational coherence in experience and action. In the following, then, we review what should be understood as one particular instantiation of this bottom-up strategy for analyzing cross-situational coherence in response. We focus on perceived self-efficacy (Bandura, 1977, 1997) and ask whether it qualifies as a social-cognitive process that causally influences behavior. We then look into additional psychological mechanisms that might cause self-efficacy perceptions to generalize cross-situationally.

Perceived Self-Efficacy as a Causal Mechanism

Research on perceived self-efficacy addresses people's appraisals of their capabilities for performance (Bandura, 1997). Self-efficacy perceptions are defined as judgments of one's capability to attain a given type or level of performance in designated settings. Self-efficacy appraisals influence a range of cognitive, affective, and behavioral mechanisms that, in turn, are critical to human adjustment and achievement. People attempt activities for which they judge themselves highly efficacious but avoid valued pursuits they judge they cannot handle (Hackett & Betz, 1995). Once engaged in activities, self-efficacy appraisals influence decisions about how much effort to expend and how long to persevere in the face of setbacks (Bandura & Cervone, 1983, 1986; Cervone & Peake, 1986; Peake & Cervone, 1989; Stock & Cervone, 1990). People who judge themselves efficacious on tasks generally experience less anxiety (Bandura, Cioffi, Taylor, & Brouillard, 1988; Bandura, Reese, & Adams, 1982; Bandura, Taylor, Williams, Mefford, & Barchas, 1985; Williams, 1995). On cognitively complex activities that require detailed strategy formulation (Cervone, 1993; Cervone et al., 1991; Cervone & Wood, 1995), people with a low sense of personal efficacy exhibit impaired cognitive performance. Through these multiple mechanisms, people's appraisals of their efficacy for coping with life events significantly influence physical and mental health. The effect of self-efficacy perceptions on long-term health outcomes such as recovery from physical setbacks (Ewart, 1995), adjustment to stressful life events (Cozzarelli, 1993; Major et al., 1990; Mueller & Major, 1989), coping with pain (O'Leary, 1995), and success in overcoming addictions (Borrelli & Mermelstein, 1994; Marlatt, Baer, & Quigley, 1995) and phobias (e.g., Williams, Kinney, & Falbo, 1989) is well established (reviewed in Bandura, 1997; Cervone & Scott, 1995; Maddux, 1995; Williams & Cervone, 1998).

Since people's perceptions of their coping capabilities may vary considerably across situations and behavioral domains, perceived self-efficacy is defined and assessed contextually. Self-efficacy measures tap people's confidence in their capabilities to perform specified actions in designated settings (Bandura, 1977, 1997; Cervone, 1985). These contextualized assessments often prove to be highly correlated with subsequent performance within the designated contexts.

Much evidence indicates that the relation between self-efficacy and action is not merely correlational, but causal. Two research strategies directly address the causal impact of self-efficacy judgment. One gauges efficacy—action relations while statistically controlling for potential "third variables." One important variable to control for is past performance. By assessing self-efficacy perceptions between trials of a multitrial task, one can assess the impact of self-efficacy perception on future performance while controlling for past accomplishments. On complex decision-making tasks, people with a higher sense of efficacy are better able to develop task strategies and to achieve higher levels of performance, even after controlling for the effects of past performance on that task (Cervone et al., 1991; Cervone & Wood, 1995). On physically effortful tasks, appraisals of self-efficacy influence changes in effort over time (Bandura & Cervone, 1983, 1986). Other factors to control for are alternative cognitive processes that might mediate behavioral change. In studies of phobic behavior, self-efficacy measures predict therapeutic change even after one controls for people's expectations of environmental threat or personal harm (Williams, 1995; Williams & Cervone, 1998). Beliefs in personal efficacy commonly predict behavior more strongly than do expectations of environmental rewards and punishments (Cervone & Scott, 1995).

The second research strategy is to manipulate self-efficacy judgment experimentally. The strongest tests of self-efficacy theory derive from work that manipulates self-efficacy judgment without introducing any factors that might influence people's actual capabilities on a task. Self-efficacy perceptions can be manipulated, for example, through the use of subtle situational cues that bias the processes through which people form judgments of their capabilities. Self-efficacy perceptions are reliably influenced by having people consider apparently random anchor values that represent high or low levels of performance (Cervone & Peake, 1986; Cervone & Palmer, 1990), varying the order in which subjects consider hypothetical levels of future performance (Berry, West, & Dennehey, 1989; Peake & Cervone, 1989), and varying the cognitive availability of personal and situational factors that might help or hinder one's efforts (Cervone, 1989). Variations in self-efficacy stemming from these judgmental biases correspondingly affect subsequent motivation (Cervone, 1989; Cervone & Peake, 1986; Peake & Cervone, 1989). In other words, even when people's high- or low-self-efficacy perceptions stem from trivial factors—such as their having received a high or low anchor value by chance (Cervone & Peake, 1986)—variations in perceived self-efficacy still affect subsequent behavior. This experimental evidence, combined with related experimental work (Holroyd et al., 1984; Litt, 1988) and the correlational strategy outlined above, provides firm evidence that self-efficacy perceptions indeed do causally contribute to behavior.

Cross-Situational Generalization in Perceived Self-Efficacy

Having established the context-specific link between self-efficacy perception and behavior, we now turn to the question of whether self-efficacy beliefs generalize across situations. There are two strategies for investigating this question. These approaches embody the top-down and bottom-up strategies outlined above. In a top-down approach, one begins by positing a high-level dispositional variable, "generalized self-efficacy" (Sherer et al., 1982; Tipton & Worthington, 1984). Individuals are fit within this construct. That is, they are assigned a singular location on the linear dimension of generalized self-efficacy. This can be done by specifying a fixed set of situations and behaviors that assess the trait and then aggregating people's responses across these circumstances to yield an overall self-efficacy score. Despite criticism (Bandura, 1997), this strategy remains popular (e.g., Schwarzer, Bäßler, Kwiatek, & Schröoder, 1997).

Although useful for some purposes (see Weitlauf, Smith, & Cervone, 1998), this strategy has significant shortcomings. By positing a high-level, generalized construct, it begs the critical question of whether there actually is enough consistency in self-efficacy beliefs across contexts that a generalized variable is warranted in the first place. By assigning individuals a single self-efficacy score, it disregards the potentially unique patterns of high- and low-efficacy beliefs that distinctively characterize the individual. By focusing on high-level dispositional variables, it deflects attention from critical questions about the underlying psychological mechanisms that may produce cross-situational generalization in self-efficacy appraisals.

The alternative strategy is to begin by focusing directly on these underlying mechanisms. Why might people's appraisals of their coping capabilities in different situations meaningfully interrelate, or cohere? This question can be addressed by considering the processes through which people appraise their efficacy for performance.

In appraising their efficacy within a domain, people may consider both information about the domain and information about themselves (Cervone, 1989). Both self-knowledge and situational beliefs, in other words, may influence self-efficacy appraisal in any given context. Students judging their capability to earn an A, for example, may dwell upon both course demands and personal attributes such as intelligence or a tendency to get anxious (e.g., during tests). Particularly salient aspects of self-knowledge may come to mind in diverse settings. Knowledge of one's anxious tendencies, for example, may come to mind and lower self-efficacy appraisals in various academic, work, or social activities. These salient aspects of self-knowledge, then, may foster cross-situational coherence in self-efficacy appraisal.

Generalizations in self-efficacy, then, may derive in part from highly salient, elaborated concepts about the self, or "self-schemas" (Markus, 1977). Schematic self-knowledge may come to mind in numerous settings and foster a relatively consistent pattern of self-efficacy appraisal. If someone sees herself as "not being a quitter," for example, this salient belief may boost efficacy perceptions across a range of settings that require perseverance in the face of obstacles.

An additional consideration is the relation between self-knowledge and situational beliefs. Even schematic personality attributes may come to mind and influence self-efficacy appraisal only within situations that are judged to be relevant to the attribute. Self-knowledge may be "applicable" (Higgins, 1996; Higgins, Chapter 3, this volume) to some situations but not others.

Work in social cognition reveals that the content of both self- and situational knowledge may be highly idiosyncratic (Cantor & Kihlstrom, 1987; Higgins, King, & Mavin, 1982). People possess unique schemas and constructs about the self and may possess idiosyncratic beliefs about how these attributes relate to social circumstances.

These considerations suggest that consistently high- and low-self-efficacy perception may be found across sets of functionally interrelated situations and that these circumstances may vary from one individual to the next. Consistency should be found across sets of situations that are related in that they are applicable to the same aspect of self-knowledge. High- (or low-) self-efficacy appraisals should be found across sets of situations that are linked to positive (negative) self-schemas. In the relevant situations, the schematic self-knowledge should come to mind and foster a relatively consistent level of self-efficacy beliefs. The processes of knowledge activation and applicability, then, would explain cross-situational coherence in efficacy beliefs. The fact that both self-knowledge and situational beliefs may be highly idiosyncratic dictates that the search for cross-situational consistency in self-efficacy appraisal must proceed idiographically.

A Social-Cognitive Search for Cross-Situational Consistency

Recent work (Cervone, 1997) has explored cross-situational coherence in self-efficacy appraisal in the manner suggested above. In this research, participants take part in three experimental sessions scheduled over approximately a 1-month period. The first two sessions are designed to assess schematic personal attributes and people's beliefs about the contexts in which these attributes are relevant. Perceived self-efficacy for handling a wide range of circumstances is assessed in session 3. Information from sessions 1 and 2 is used to identify clusters of situations across which people are predicted to have relatively high versus low perceptions of self-efficacy.

This work does not attempt to fit individuals into an a priori template of personality attributes or to identify a fixed set of trait indicators for any given attribute. Instead, personal attributes and situational beliefs are assessed idiographically. Schematic attributes are identified using two techniques. In a free-response method, subjects write brief narratives describing their "personal strengths" and "personal weaknesses" and then identify one attribute from each narrative that is most self-descriptive. In a more structured method, participants assess themselves on a series of bipolar trait dimensions and then rate the personal importance of each attribute (cf. Markus, 1977); the singular attribute categorized as "most important" is selected as a third schematic characteristic (Cervone, 1997).

To assess situational beliefs, participants categorize the relevance of 81 social situations to each of a series of personality attributes. This task, then, identifies the potentially idiosyncratic sets of situations in which people believe a given personality attribute might be manifested. Verb phrases describe a general type of situation and a potentially challenging behavior (e.g., "Actively participate in class discussion sections," "Avoid saying anything critical about a boyfriend's driving if he makes some mistakes," "Turn off the TV and stick to studying for an exam, even if a favorite show is on"). Participants judge the relevance of these circumstances to each of their three schematic attributes from session 1 and also to two common personality characteristics (e.g., helpful, creative, lazy, irritable), one positive and one negative. These latter characteristics, referred to as the "experimenter-provided traits," are chosen to be unrelated to the three schematic traits. They provide an internal control that enables us to test the prediction that cross-situational coherence will only be found with respect to personality attributes that are cognitively salient to the individual.

In the last session, participants complete a multidomain self-efficacy questionnaire. Items assess their confidence in performing specific behaviors in specific contexts. Each question presents a concrete situation and asks people to indicate their confidence in being able to perform a designated act. The concrete situational descriptions are systematically linked to the somewhat more general content of the session 2 items. For example, in session 2, participants judge the applicability of personality attributes to the situation "Actively participate in class discussion sections." In session 3, they complete the self-efficacy item "If you're in a class that has weekly discussion sections, how confident are you that you can actively participate in the discussion by making at least three or four comments in class every week?" The 81 self-efficacy items are designed to range across diverse personality dispositions and social contexts. Most of the items were based upon Botwin and Buss's (1989) analysis of 11 act categories associated with the five-factor model (McCrae & Costa, 1987) of personality dispositions. We constructed items representing each of five interpersonal settings—same-sex friend, opposite-sex friend, authority figure, group of peers, or stranger—for each category (e.g., "If a guy you have just met is interested in the arts, impress him by talking about contemporary art or classical music" is a cultured/opposite sex item and "If you're driving and someone cuts you off in traffic, avoid getting angry or yelling at them; instead, just concentrate fully on your driving" is an emotional stability/stranger item). Remaining items represented academic, athletic, and interpersonal activities of relevance to college student populations (Fisher-Beckfield & McFall, 1982).

A primary question is whether perceived self-efficacy was consistently high and low in situations judged as particularly relevant to the schematic attributes. The data in Figure 9.1 speak to this issue. For the schematic personality characteristics, self-efficacy appraisals varied significantly as a function of situational relevance. Participants had consistently higher and lower beliefs in their efficacy for performance across groups of situations that they linked to positive and negative schematic attributes. We were able to identify these situations by considering subjects' unique construals of their personal characteristics and the circumstances that draw upon them.

Perceived self-efficacy did not vary as a function of situational relevance when we examined the experimenter-provided personality characteristics (see Figure 9.1). Unlike the schematic attributes, self-efficacy levels did not differ in situations judged most relevant to positive versus negative generic traits. Thus, for these common personality traits, we could not predict consistent patterns in self-efficacy appraisal even when we identified the specific situations that individuals judged most relevant to the attributes.

These findings illustrate the shortcoming inherent in characterizing people as "high" or "low" on a trait of generalized self-efficacy. In this work, we identify *for each person* separate clusters of situations in which we predict high- versus low-self-efficacy perceptions. The success of these predictions reveals that much information about the person would be lost by collapsing diverse high- and low-self-efficacy beliefs into a single score. The aggregate score would be a statistical abstraction that does not correspond to any meaningful attribute of the individual.

Although a trait of generalized self-efficacy cannot account for these results, it is possible that some other nomothetic scheme would be useful. In principle, once one knows the person's schematic attributes, one might be able to predict consistencies in self-efficacy appraisal across situations that are identified nomothetically, rather than idiographically. This possibility was tested by examining perceived self-efficacy in the 10 situations that were nomothetically relevant to the individual's self-schematic strength and weakness. To do this, each schematic attribute was mapped onto a dimension of

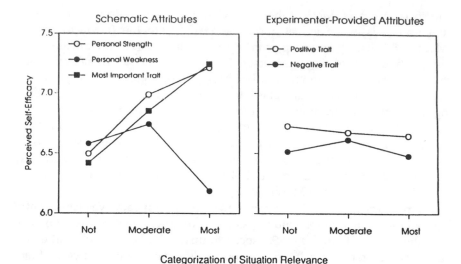

FIGURE 9.1. Mean strength of perceived self-efficacy as a function of situation categorizations for schematic and experimenter-provided personality attributes. From Cervone (1997). Copyright 1997 by Blackwell Publishers. Reprinted by permission of Cambridge University Press.

the five-factor model, and the 10 situations that nomothetically tapped that dimension were examined. To illustrate, suppose a self-described strength is "hard working." "Hard working" is a component of conscientiousness (McCrae & Costa, 1987). The particularly "hard working" individual thus may be seen as relatively conscientious and may be expected to be relatively efficacious across behaviors and situations that tap into conscientiousness. For such an individual, then, the 10 nomothetic situations would be the 10 questionnaire items related to conscientiousness.

Results reveal that the idiographic identification of situations is critical to our findings (Figure 9.2). When situations were identified idiographically, levels of self-efficacy differed significantly in situations related to the positive and negative attributes. When a nomothetic, top-down classification was used, they did not.

Why was it so important to assess self-knowledge and situational beliefs idiographically? Analyses of individual cases answer this question. Consider subject 10 (Figure 9.3), who saw herself as "determined" (her personal strength), having a "bad temper" (personal weakness), and being "warm" (most important trait). Focusing on her personal strength, she judged as relevant to "determined" a diverse collection of circumstances that do not fit into any standard nomothetic framework. These included personal achievements that might be captured in a nomothetic analysis of "determined" (e.g., losing

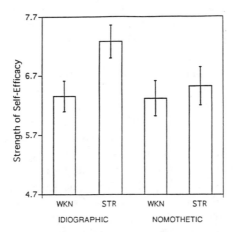

FIGURE 9.2. Mean strength of perceived self-efficacy for circumstances relevant to schematic personal strengths ("STR") and weaknesses ("WKN"), with situational relevance defined either idiographically or nomothetically. From Cervone (1997). Copyright 1997 by Blackwell Publishers. Reprinted by permission of Cambridge University Press.

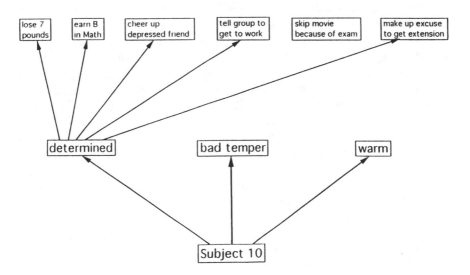

FIGURE 9.3. One research participant's schematic personal attributes and the circumstances the individual linked to her personal strength, "determined." See text for details. From Cervone (1997). Copyright 1997 by Blackwell Publishers. Reprinted by permission of Cambridge University Press.

weight, earning a good grade in a difficult class), circumstances that would seem peripheral to the nomothetic act category "determined" (e.g., cheering up a depressed friend), and yet other circumstances that would be judged as irrelevant to "determined" but highly relevant to some other personality attribute in a nomothetic approach. For example, convincing a professor "to grant an extension on a paper by making up some 'good excuse' for why a little extra time is needed" might be seen, in general, as a "calculating" act (cf. Botwin & Buss, 1989). Subject 10, however, saw it as a reflecting "determination." Finally, a traditional hallmark of determination among college students—"Tell friends who are going to a movie that you won't be able to go out with them because of an important exam coming up in a couple of days"—was seen as irrelevant to this attribute by this individual.

Our bottom-up search for personality coherence often directly violated the structure of top-down trait categories. Consider the following two circumstances: "On a job interview, tell a lively story to the interviewer" and "On a long trip, keep a lively conversation going with a quiet male friend." Generally, these circumstances might be grouped together as exemplars of the high-level trait of "extraversion." Idiographically, however, such circumstances may get pulled apart. Consider subject 7 (Figure 9.4). For this individual, the seemingly similar "extraversion" indicators were part of different, opposing categories. He judged the telling of a lively story to an interviewer as relevant to his personal strength, "skilled at public relations," but irrelevant to his personal weakness, shyness. Maintaining a lively conversation with a friend was judged relevant to shyness but not public relations skills.[5]

The idiosyncratic nature of these situational construals explains why, in the earlier group-level analyses, cross-situational coherence was found only when the situations were defined idiographically. Individuals' subjective categorizations of social circumstances commonly violated the structure of nomothetic act categories. As a result, even if we had known the particular attributes that were most relevant to the individual, we would have failed to identify cross-situational coherence in response if we had forced the individual into a common template of trait indicators. We succeeded in identifying consistent response tendencies by disregarding high-level nomothetic constructs. We sometimes predicted to circumstances that seemed unrelated to a given personal attribute, ignored circumstances that seemed prototypical of an attribute, and clustered together and split apart circumstances in a manner that violated the dictates of any traditional high-level scheme. This bottom-up approach revealed cross-situational coherence that a top-down analysis would have missed (Cervone, 1997).

Recent data, involving a larger population of participants, has replicated these basic findings. This larger sample also has enabled us to address some new issues, two of which are briefly reviewed here.

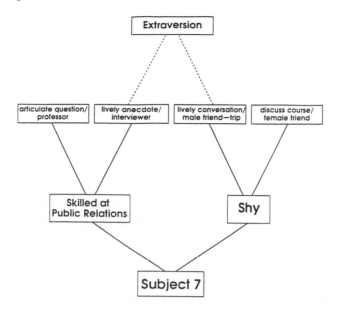

FIGURE 9.4. One research participant's schematic personal strength and personal weakness, and an illustration of how circumstances that typically are grouped together in nomothetic analyses of a high-level personality trait (extraversion) became split apart in analyses with this individual.

Schema Level and Importance

Assessments of schematic personality attributes often suffer from a methodological limitation (Burke, Kraut, & Dworkin, 1984; Nystedt, Smari, & Boman, 1991). When a combination of self-rated trait level and trait importance are used to identify schematic attributes, level and importance are generally confounded. More extreme self-ratings are found on more important attributes.

In our data set, level, and importance can be unconfounded. We identify a subset of participants who (1) rate themselves as having a very high level on one of the experimenter-provided traits, but (2) judge that trait to be unimportant to their self-concept. We then compare this high-level, unimportant trait to the participants' high-level, highly important schematic attribute. This analysis reveals that ratings of trait importance are an important component of self-schema assessments. For the schematic attributes, levels of perceived self-efficacy differed significantly in situations judged most relevant versus not relevant to the attribute. For the high-level, aschematic attributes, no such differences were found (Cervone, 1998).

Cognitive Complexity and Variability in Self-Efficacy Appraisal across Contexts

The results reviewed above examined schematic attributes in isolation. Another approach is to examine how interrelations among multiple attributes give rise to cross-situational coherence. One approach to this problem focuses on cognitive complexity in self-schemas and associated situational construals.

Work by Linville (1985, 1987) reveals that cognitive complexity buffers individuals against extreme reactions to stress. People high in cognitive complexity vary less in their emotional reactions from one circumstance to the next. A complex cognitive framework enables people to see things from many different perspectives (Kelly, 1955), which reduces the extremity of emotional response.

Cognitive complexity might relate to perceived self-efficacy in a similar manner. People with a complex system of situational and self-knowledge may be more capable of seeing both the possibilities and the challenges inherent in any given situation. They therefore may be less prone to either extreme overconfidence or a complete lack of confidence when facing a particular challenge. In contrast, a less complex knowledge system may predispose people to judge situations in a more black-and-white manner. Low cognitive complexity, then, should predict greater extremes, that is, greater variability, in self-efficacy appraisal across situations.

Cognitive complexity can be indexed in our paradigm by evaluating the multiple situational categorizations made in the second experimental session. People who provide relatively unique situational categorizations for each schematic attribute, that is, people whose situational profiles are relatively uncorrelated from one attribute to the next, can be seen to be employing a more complex knowledge system. People who repeatedly sort situations in the same manner with respect to purportedly different attributes can be seen to be employing a less complex system. Analyses reveal that this index of complexity predicts overall situation-to-situation variability on the self-efficacy questionnaire (Cervone, 1998). People with greater cognitive complexity are less prone to extreme situation-to-situation swings in efficacy appraisal.

I conclude the review of this research program by highlighting two points. First, our findings violate a common stereotype of social-cognitive research on personality. Traditionally, social-cognitivists have highlighted situational specificity in response (Mischel, 1968). They have done so, in part, to demonstrate that dispositional variables are not an adequate foundation for a personality theory. However, social-cognitive mechanisms do not only produce situational specificity. Knowledge and appraisal processes may give rise to significant cross-situational consistency in response. Social-cognitive theory, then, does not argue against cross-situational coherence. It merely suggests that this phenomenon cannot be adequately identified or explained from a top-down trait perspective. Our bottom-up social-cognitive analysis identified meaningful coherence in response that a top-down approach would have missed.

The point of this research program is not that cross-situational consistency in response is the singularly definitive yardstick for gauging personality characteristics. Response consistency is only one expression of coherence in personality functioning. Changes in response across time and contexts also can reveal coherence in underlying personality systems, as other chapters in this volume illustrate. My points are that social-cognitive theory is capable of explaining not only variability but also consistency in response and that social-cognitive theory's bottom-up explanation is simultaneously truer to the individual and more acceptable on grounds of explanatory adequacy than accounts provided by nomothetic trait theory. The ability of social-cognitive theory to capture cross-situational consistency in response is particularly interesting, of course, because such consistencies are what led previous investigators to infer trait variables in the first place (Allport, 1937).

Second, cross-situational coherence did not derive from any singular psychological mechanism. People did not display generalized high- or low-self-efficacy perceptions. Both high and low self-appraisals were identified for each person. Coherence was not predictable from assessments of self-schemas alone. We needed also to consider participants' situational beliefs. Situational construals did not uniformly predict self-efficacy appraisals. They did so only for schematic attributes. No singular psychological mechanism functioned in the manner of a trait variable. No social-cognitive processes independently produced or corresponded to coherence in response. Instead, cross-situational coherence was understood by reference to interactions among multiple causal mechanisms, no one of which directly corresponded to the phenomenon to be explained (cf. Hanson, 1958; Nozick, 1981).

TWO CONCLUDING ISSUES

Throughout, I have cautioned against a simple integration of social-cognitive and trait theories, that is, an integration in which individual-difference factors are conceived as universal psychology structures that causally influence social-cognitive processes. This integration was shown to be conceptually problematic and empirically unnecessary. It overlooks the fact that social-cognitive and trait approaches differ fundamentally in that they embrace different strategies of scientific explanation. Empirically, social-cognitive analyses were shown to be capable of identifying cross-situational coherence in response (Cervone, 1997), the very phenomenon that initially motivated psychologists to infer traits as causal agents (Allport, 1937).

The arguments advanced here inherently raise two questions that must be addressed in closing. These concern the conceptual status of dispositional variables (from a social-cognitive perspective) and the potential for expanding social-cognitive analyses to consider more explicitly determinants of personality coherence that thus far have received little attention in this approach.

Dispositional Constructs: A Social-Cognitive Perspective

Our first question can be phrased bluntly. How can the social-cognitivist ignore the many advances in trait research? Don't these empirical advances force everyone to conclude that individual-difference factors constitute the core structure of personality? Don't they force theorists in other conceptual camps to integrate their approaches with the doctrine of traits? Stated more formally: What, in social-cognitive theory, is the conceptual status of dispositional constructs?

The empirical evidence cited by trait-based investigators is substantial. It includes (1) the reliable identification of trait variables in factor analyses of self- and peer-reports, (2) the stability of trait scores over substantial periods of time, (3) the convergence of self-ratings and peer ratings on personality traits, (4) the ability of trait assessments to predict (albeit modestly) (Pervin, 1994) significant life outcomes, (5) the relatively greater correspondence in trait scores among monozygotic (MZ) versus dizygotic (DZ) twins, suggesting a genetic basis to personality traits, and (6) the existence of "biological markers" of traits; that is, people who score high versus low on some trait dimensions are found to differ physiologically or anatomically. Shouldn't this evidence lead everyone to accept personality traits as high-level, universal psychic structures that causally influence lower-level psychological mechanisms and behavior?

The problem with drawing this conclusion about the psyche is made evident by an analogy to the soma. Suppose one were to survey individual differences in physical attributes. In addition to questions about qualities such as size or appearance ("Is your hair darker than most people's?"; "Are most of your acquaintances shorter than you?"; "Do friends consider you handsome?"), one might include questions tapping physical fitness ("Are you generally in good health?"; "Do you consider yourself to be a sickly individual?"; "Do you feel 'run down' much of the time?"). In principle, these latter items might intercorrelate so highly that (1) they are reliably identified as a unique statistical factor—one that might be labeled "healthiness." Further, (2) healthiness scores may be stable over substantial periods of time (if only due to a small number of individuals with a chronic disease); (3) self-ratings and peer ratings of healthiness may converge; (4) healthiness scores might predict important life outcomes (health care costs, longevity); (5) MZ twin scores might correlate more highly than DZ scores (due to inherited diseases); and (6) people with low healthiness scores might differ from those who are high in healthiness on one or more biological markers (oxygen-carrying capacity of the cardiovascular system, immune system functioning, percentage of body fat, genetic abnormalities, presence of gastrointestinal viruses, etc.).

No matter how strong this evidence, biologists are unlikely to conclude that "healthiness" is a unitary structure or system that is universally present in everyone's body and that causally influences other "lower-level" biological mechanisms. The notions that "Healthiness causes abnormal cell growth which makes one predisposed to cancer" or that "Possessing low amounts of healthiness causes inadequate development of the lungs which, in turn, makes one susceptible to cardiovascular disease" would be misguided. Indeed, the conclusion that "healthiness" is a unitary, universal biological structure would itself be misguided. No matter what the evidence on the six points above, we reject the conclusion that healthiness corresponds to a unitary biological structure or system because we know that high versus low scores on this descriptive dimension may reflect many *different* underlying systems—that is, systems that are truly distinct, both structurally and functionally. People who obtain the same healthiness score may differ biologically in any of an enormous variety of ways.

The construct "healthiness" might have applied value. It might "meet administrative needs in applied settings" (Shaffer, 1996, p. S95). "Healthiness," for example, might be a useful screening tool. Insurers might reject policy applicants who score in the unhealthy range. Organizers of groups who must forego access to health care services for extended periods (e.g., a wilderness trek) might screen out unhealthy scorers. Change scores also might be of interest. Public health interventions could be assessed by examining change in a population's healthiness self-reports. Despite this practical utility, an inferred biological structure of "healthiness" could not serve as a foundation for a science of human biology or medicine.

Personality dispositional constructs similarly have much utility. We might screen out PhD applicants who score in the extremely low range of "openness to experience." We might not hire employees who score two standard deviations below the mean on conscientiousness. Much might be learned by analyzing changes in a dispositional construct as a function of social experiences (see Roberts, 1994). This practical utility, however, does not imply that dispositional constructs can be granted causal status or that they can provide an adequate foundation for a scientific theory of personality.

Temperament and Social-Cognitive Theory

An analysis of social-cognitive processes is necessary to understanding the coherence of personality across circumstances and across time (Huesmann & Guerra, 1997). However, it may not be sufficient. Inherited temperamental factors also contribute to personality coherence (Halverson, Kohnstamm, & Martin, 1994). Individuals differentially inherit physiological mechanisms whose psychological ramifications are evident early in life and across the life course (Caspi, 1998). Our final question, then, is whether social-cognitive theory can incorporate this important source of personality coherence.

The issue here is not whether temperamental factors are important, but how to conceptualize their nature and role in personality functioning. Many investigators suggest that temperament can be described according to a small number of broad individual-difference dimensions. These dimensions include factors such as attentional self-regulation (Ahadi & Rothbart, 1994), activity level, and reactivity to stimuli (Strelau & Plomin, 1992), and tendencies toward approach, withdrawal, and inhibition (Gray, 1991).

Kagan (1994) reviews each of these approaches and draws a conclusion that is congruent with the arguments presented here. "One problem with all of these approaches is that they are top-down. Their creators begin with a theoretical ambition to keep the number of constructs at a minimum, without a persuasive rationale for that choice" (p. 48). Although a simple system of high-level temperamental dimensions may have certain conceptual advantages, it also may have a serious drawback. "Children with similar surface profiles can belong to different groups"; they may have "different histories and [be] in possession of different physiologies" (Kagan, 1994, p. 122). Top-down categories, in other words, may not map onto underlying causal mechanisms. Different underlying mechanisms give rise to similar phenotypic profiles.

Temperament can be studied, instead, from the bottom up. In Kagan's analysis, temperament constructs refer to well-specified physiological systems. These systems give rise to distinct affective profiles when activated by particular environmental contexts. In this approach, then, temperament mechanisms are not construed as traits in the traditional sense of the word. They are not equated with a broad range of phenotypic tendencies. They cannot be assessed by an interchangeable mix of self-report and peer-report methods (Kagan, 1994). They are not high-level causes of lower-level cognitions and actions. Instead, temperament mechanisms are contextually activated physiological systems that give rise to specific affective reactions.

This bottom-up analysis of temperament and affect indeed could be integrated with social-cognitive theory's bottom-up analysis of cognitive mechanisms in personality functioning. Temperament factors may be one of a number of variables that contribute to the formation of social-cognitive structures (cf. Contrada, Leventhal, & O'Leary, 1990; Mischel & Shoda, 1995). The temperamentally inhibited child (Kagan & Snidman 1991), for example, may develop fewer skills for coping with novel social circumstances and lower self-efficacy beliefs for activities involving strangers. An interesting possibility is that, in the adult, such social-cognitive variables might be causally responsible for emotional or behavioral tendencies whose parallel, in the child, is a direct product of inherited physiological systems. People commonly avoid threatening circumstances in the absence of physiological arousal (Bandura, 1977). Social-cognitive mechanisms, then, would become functionally autonomous (cf. Allport, 1937) from the temperament systems that partly contributed to their development.

An enhanced understanding of interactions among biological temperament, cognitive processes, and the social environment may prove an important step toward the comprehensive model of the person that all personality psychologists seek.

ACKNOWLEDGMENT

I thank my colleagues Gian Vittorio Caprara, Jim Kelly, Bill Shadel, and Arnaldo Zelli for their helpful comments on an earlier draft of this chapter.

NOTES

1. In addition to the gradual spread of a population resulting from agriculture, other causal factors might involve sudden shifts of an entire population or invasions of a population by an outside group (Coleman, 1988).
2. Recent findings by Caprara, Barbaranelli, and Zimbardo (1997) suggest that a third type of aggregation is important to the five-factor model: aggregation across targets. A large sample of raters, using a pool of trait adjectives, assessed the personalities of a small number of targets, namely, well-known politicians. Rather than a five-factor model, only two to three factors were required to describe politicians' personalities. This result raises the general point that the five-factor model could be obtained when analyzing observer-ratings of a population of targets even if the ratings of individual targets do not correspond to the model.
3. The study of reciprocal causal influences distinguishes social-cognitive theory from the five-factor model of personality, which posits that personality variables are inherited structures that are in no way influenced by social experience; in the five-factor approach, causal influences "lead out from personality traits, but not in" (McCrae & Costa, 1996, p. 72). This rejection of reciprocal influences is puzzling in light of the compelling evidence of reciprocal processes in personality development (Baltes et al., 1998; Caprara & Cervone, in press; Lerner, 1998), including evidence that social experience shapes brain mechanisms (Edelman, 1992; Sapolsky, 1996).
4. For purposes of linguistic convenience, the terms "cross-situational coherence" and "cross-situational consistency" are used somewhat interchangeable in this chapter. However, in more precise definitions, "cross-situational coherence" would refer to an interconnection among responses exhibited in different settings. "Cross-situational consistency" refers to a tendency to exhibit a similar type of response in different contexts. Consistency, then, is one manifestation of coherence. Coherence in response might also be manifested by systematic patterns of high- versus low-response tendencies in different settings (Mischel & Shoda, 1995).
5. Note that this person's spontaneous self-descriptions include attributes that might be judged semantically inconsistent (cf. Hampson, 1997; Hampson, John, &

Goldberg, 1986). A recent study reveals that, even in spontaneous self-descriptions, semantic and evaluative inconsistencies are surprisingly common (White & Cervone, 1998).

REFERENCES

Ahadi, S. A., & Rothbart, M. K. (1994). Temperament, development, and the big five. In C. F. Halverson, Jr., G. A. Kohnstamm, & R. P. Martin (Eds.), *The developing structure of temperament and personality from infancy to adulthood* (pp. 189–207). Hillsdale, NJ: Erlbaum.

Allport, G. (1937). *Personality: A psychological interpretation.* New York: Holt, Rinehart, & Winston.

Ammerman, A. J., & Cavalli-Sforza, L. L. (1984). *The neolithic transition and the genetics of populations in Europe.* Princeton, NJ: Princeton University Press.

Bak, P., & Chen, K. (1991). Self-organized criticality. *Scientific American, 262,* 92–99.

Baltes, P. B., Linderberger, U., & Staudinger, U. M. (1998). Life-span theory in developmental psychology. In W. Damon (Series Ed.) & R. M. Lerner (Vol. Ed.), *Handbook of child psychology: Vol. 1. Theoretical models of human development* (5th ed., pp. 1029–1144). New York: Wiley.

Bandura, A. (1965). Vicarious processes: A case of no-trial learning. In L. Berkowitz (Ed.), *Advances in experimental social psychology* (Vol. 2, pp. 1–55). New York: Academic Press.

Bandura, A. (1977). Self-efficacy: Toward a unifying theory of behavioral change. *Psychological Review, 84,* 191–215.

Bandura, A. (1978). The self-system in reciprocal determinism. *American Psychologist, 33,* 344–358.

Bandura, A. (1986). *Social foundations of thought and action: A social cognitive theory.* Englewood Cliffs, NJ: Prentice-Hall.

Bandura, A. (1991). The changing icons in personality psychology. In J. H. Cantor (Ed.), *Psychology at Iowa: Centennial essays* (pp. 117–139). Hillsdale, NJ: Erlbaum.

Bandura, A. (1997). *Self-efficacy: The exercise of control.* New York: Freeman.

Bandura, A., & Cervone, D. (1983). Self-evaluative and self-efficacy mechanisms governing. *Journal of Personality and Social Psychology, 45,* 1017–1028.

Bandura, A., & Cervone, D. (1986). Differential engagement of self-reactive influences in cognitive motivation. *Organizational Behavior and Human Decision Processes, 38,* 92–113.

Bandura, A., Cioffi, D., Taylor, C. B., & Brouillard, M. E. (1988). Perceived self-efficacy in coping with cognitive stressors and opioid activation. *Journal of Personality and Social Psychology, 55,* 479–488.

Bandura, A., Reese, L., & Adams, N. E. (1982). Microanalysis of action and fear arousal as a function of differential levels of perceived self-efficacy. *Journal of Personality and Social Psychology, 43,* 5–21.

Bandura, A., Taylor, C. B., Williams, S. L., Mefford, I. N., & Barchas, J. D. (1985). Catecholamine secretion as a function of perceived coping self-efficacy. *Journal of Consulting and Clinical Psychology, 53,* 406–414.

Barker, G. (1988). Review of C. Renfrew, *Archaeology and language: The puzzle of Indo-European origins. Current Anthropology, 29,* 448–449.

Barton, S. (1994). Chaos, self-organization, and psychology. *American Psychologist, 49,* 5–14.

Bem, D. J., & Allen, A. (1974). On predicting some of the people some of the time: The search for cross-situational consistencies in behavior. *Psychological Review, 81,* 506–520.

Berry, J. M., West, R. L., & Dennehey, D. M. (1989). Reliability and validity of the memory self-efficacy questionnaire. *Developmental Psychology, 25,* 701–713.

Block, J. (1995). A contrarian view of the five-factor approach to personality description. *Psychological Bulletin, 117,* 187–215.

Bolger, N. (1990). Coping as a personality process: A prospective study. *Journal of Personality and Social Psychology, 59,* 525–537.

Borrelli, B., & Mermelstein, R. (1994). Goal setting and behavior change in a smoking cessation program. *Cognitive Therapy and Research, 18,* 69–83.

Botwin, M. D., & Buss, D. M. (1989). Structure of act-report data: Is the five-factor model of personality recaptured. *Journal of Personality and Social Psychology, 56,* 988–1001.

Bowers, K. S. (1977). There's more to Iago than meets the eye: A clinical account of personal consistency. In D. Magnusson & N. S. Endler (Eds.), *Personality at the crossroads* (pp. 65–82). Hillsdale, NJ: Erlbaum.

Burke, P. A., Kraut, R. E., & Dworkin, R. H. (1984). Traits, consistency, and self-schemata: What do our measures measure? *Journal of Personality and Social Psychology, 47,* 568–579.

Buss, D. M., & Craik, K. H. (1983). The act frequency approach to personality. *Psychological Review, 90,* 105–126.

Cantor, N., & Kihlstrom, J. F. (1987). *Personality and social intelligence.* Englewood Cliffs, NJ: Prentice-Hall.

Caprara, G. V. (1997). Structures and processes in personality psychology. *European Psychologist, 1,* 14–26.

Caprara, G. V., Barbaranelli, C., & Zimbardo, P. G. (1997). Politician's uniquely simple personalities. *Nature, 385,* 493.

Caprara, G. V., & Cervone, D. (in press). *Personality: Determinants, mechanisms, and potentialities.* New York: Cambridge University Press.

Carver, C. S., & Sheier, M. F. (1996). *Perspectives on personality* (3rd ed.). Boston: Allyn & Bacon.

Caspi, A. (1998). Personality development across the life course. In W. Damon (Series Ed.) & N. Eisenberg (Vol. Ed.), *Handbook of child psychology: Vol. 3. Social, emotional, and personality development* (5th ed., pp. 311–388). New York: Wiley.

Cervone, D. (1985). Randomization tests to determine significance levels for microanalytic congruences between self-efficacy and behavior. *Cognitive Therapy and Research, 9,* 357–365.

Cervone, D. (1989). Effects of envisioning future activities on self-efficacy judgments and motivation: An availability heuristic interpretation. *Cognitive Therapy and Research, 13,* 247–261.

Cervone, D. (1991). The two disciplines of personality psychology. *Psychological Science, 2,* 371–377.

Cervone, D. (1993). The role of self-referent cognitions in goal setting, motivation, and performance. In M. Rabinowitz (Ed.), *Cognitive science foundations of instruction* (pp. 57–96). Hillsdale, NJ: Erlbaum.

Cervone, D. (1997). Social-cognitive mechanisms and personality coherence. *Psychological Science, 8,* 43–50.

Cervone, D. (1998, July). Explaining the coherence of personality: A social-cognitive perspective. In G. V. Caprara & D. Cervone (Chairs), *Personality and social cognition.* Symposium conducted at the 9th European Conference on Personality, Surrey, UK.

Cervone, D., Jiwani, N., & Wood, R. (1991). Goal-setting and the differential influence of self-regulatory processes on complex decision-making performance. *Journal of Personality and Social Psychology, 61,* 257–266.

Cervone, D., & Palmer, B. W. (1990). Anchoring biases and the perseverance of self-efficacy beliefs. *Cognitive Therapy and Research, 14,* 401–416.

Cervone, D., & Peake, P. K. (1986). Anchoring, efficacy, and action: The influence of judgmental heuristics on self-efficacy judgments and behavior. *Journal of Personality and Social Psychology, 50,* 492–501.

Cervone, D., & Scott, W. D. (1995). Self-efficacy theory of behavioral change. In W. O'Donohue & L. Krasner (Eds.), *Theories of behavior therapy* (pp. 349–383). Washington, DC: American Psychological Association.

Cervone, D., & Williams, S. L. (1992). Social cognitive theory and personality. In G. V. Caprara & G. L. Van Heck (Eds.), *Modern personality psychology: Critical reviews and new directions* (pp. 200–252). New York: Harvester Wheatsheaf.

Cervone, D., & Wood, R. (1995). Goals, feedback, and the differential influence of self-regulatory processes on cognitively complex performance. *Cognitive Therapy and Research, 19,* 521–547.

Coleman, R. (1988). Review of C. Renfrew, *Archaeology and language: The puzzle of Indo-European origins. Current Anthropology, 29,* 449–453.

Contrada, R. J., Leventhal, H., & O'Leary, A. (1990). Personality and health. In L. A. Pervin (Ed.), *Handbook of personality: Theory and research* (pp. 638–669). New York: Guilford Press.

Cozzarelli, C. (1993). Personality and self-efficacy as predictors of coping with abortion. *Journal of Personality and Social Psychology, 65,* 1224–1236.

Dweck, C. S., & Leggett, E. L. (1988). A social-cognitive approach to motivation and personality. *Psychological Review, 95,* 256-273.

Edelman, G. M. (1992). *Bright air, brilliant fire: On the matter of the mind.* New York: Basic Books.

Epstein, S. (1979). The stability of behavior: I. On predicting most of the people much of the time. *Journal of Personality and Social Psychology, 37,* 1092–1126.

Ewart, C. K. (1995). Self-efficacy and recovery from heart attack: Implications for a social-cognitive analysis of exercise and emotion. In J. E. Maddux (Ed.), *Self-efficacy, adaptation, and adjustment: Theory, research, and application* (pp. 203–226). New York: Plenum Press.

Fischer-Beckfield, D. F., & McFall, R. M. (1982). Development of a competence inventory for college men and evaluation of relationships. *Journal of Consulting and Clinical Psychology, 50,* 697–705.

Fleeson, W. (1998). Across-time within-person structures of personality: Common and individual traits. In G. V. Caprara & D. Cervone (Chairs), *Personality and social cognition.* Symposium conducted at the 9th European Conference on Personality, Guildford, UK.

Fogel, A., Lyra, M. C. D. P., & Valsiner, J. (Eds.). (1997). *Dynamics and indeterminism in developmental and social processes.* Mahwah, NJ: Erlbaum.

Funder, D. C. (1991). Global traits: A neo-Allportian approach to personality. *Psychological Science, 2,* 31–39.

Goldberg, L. R. (1993). The structure of phenotypic personality traits. *American Psychologist, 48,* 26–34.

Gray, J. A. (1991). Neural systems, emotion and personality. In J. Madden IV (Ed.), *Neurobiology of learning, emotion and affect.* New York: Raven Press.

Hackett, G., & Betz, N. (1995). Self-efficacy and career choice and development. In J. E. Maddux (Ed.), *Self-efficacy, adaptation, and adjustment: Theory, research, and application* (pp. 249-280). New York: Plenum Press.

Halverson, C. F., Jr., Kohnstamm, G. A., & Martin, R. P. (1994). *The developing structure of temperament and personality from infancy to adulthood.* Hillsdale, NJ: Erlbaum.

Hampson, S. (1997). Determinants of inconsistent personality descriptions: Trait and target effects. *Journal of Personality, 65,* 249–290.

Hampson, S., John, O. P., & Goldberg, L. R. (1986). Category breadth and hierarchical structure in personality: Studies of asymmetries in judgments of trait implications. *Journal of Personality and Social Psychology, 51,* 37–54.

Hanson, N. R. (1958). *Patterns of discovery: An inquiry into the conceptual foundations of science.* Cambridge, UK: Cambridge University Press.

Higgins, E. T. (1990). Personality, social psychology, and person–situation relations: Standards and knowledge activation as a common language. In L. A. Pervin (Ed.), *Handbook of personality: Theory and research* (pp. 301–338). New York: Guilford Press.

Higgins, E. T. (1996). Knowledge activation: Accessibility, applicability, and salience. In E. T. Higgins & A. E. Kruglanski (Eds.), *Social psychology: Handbook of basic principles* (pp. 133–168). New York: Guilford Press.

Higgins, E. T., King, G. A., & Mavin, G. H. (1982). Individual construct accessibility and subjective impressions and recall. *Journal of Personality and Social Psychology, 43,* 35–47.

Hogan, R. (1982). On adding apples and oranges in personality psychology. *Contemporary Psychology, 27,* 851–852.

Holroyd, K. A., Penzien, D. B., Hursey, D. B., Tobin, D. L., Rogers, L., Holm, J. E., Marcille, P. J., Hall, J. R., & Chila, A. G. (1984). Change mechanisms in EMG biofeedback training: Cognitive changes underlying improvements in tension headache. *Journal of Consulting and Clinical Psychology, 52,* 1039–1053.

Huesmann, L. R., & Guerra, N. G. (1997). Children's normative beliefs about aggression and aggressive behavior. *Journal of Personality and Social Psychology, 72,* 408–419.

Jackson, D. N., & Paunonen, S. V. (1985). Construct validity and the predictability of behavior. *Journal of Personality and Social Psychology, 49,* 554–570.

John, O. P. (1990). The "Big Five" factor taxonomy: Dimensions of personality in the natural language and in questionnaires. In L. A. Pervin (Ed.), *Handbook of personality: Theory and research* (pp. 66–100). New York: Guilford Press.

Kagan, J. (1988). The meaning of personality predicates. *American Psychologist, 43,* 614–620.

Kagan, J. (1994). *Galen's prophecy.* New York: Basic Books.

Kagan, J., & Snidman, N. (1991). Infant predictors of inhibited and uninhibited profiles. *Psychological Science, 2*, 40–44.

Kelly, G. (1955). *The psychology of personal constructs.* New York: Norton.

Kelly, J. G. (1968). Towards an ecological conception of preventive interventions. In J. W. Carter, Jr. (Ed.), *Research contributions from psychology to community mental health* (pp. 75–99). New York: Behavioral Publications.

Kenrick, D. T., & Funder, D. C. (1988). Profiting from controversy: Lessons from the person–situation debate. *American Psychologist, 43*, 23–34.

Kitayama, S., Markus, H. R., Matsumoto, H., & Norasakkunit, V. (1997). Individual and collective processes in the construction of the self: Self-enhancement in the United States and self-criticism in Japan. *Journal of Personality and Social Psychology, 72*, 1245–1267.

Kitcher, P. (1985). Two approaches to explanation. *Journal of Philosophy, 82*, 632–639.

Kitcher, P. & Salmon, W. C. (Eds.). (1989). *Minnesota studies in the philosophy of science: Vol. XIII. Scientific explanation.* Minneapolis: University of Minnesota Press.

Langston, C. A., & Sykes, W. E. (1997). Beliefs and the Big Five: Cognitive bases of broad individual differences in personality. *Journal of Research in Personality, 31*, 141–165.

Latané, B., & L'Herrou, T. (1996). Spatial clustering in the conformity game: Dynamic social impact in electronic groups. *Journal of Personality and Social Psychology, 70*, 1218–1230.

Lerner, R. M. (1998). Theories of human development: Contemporary perspectives. In W. Damon (Series Ed.) & R. M. Lerner (Vol. Ed.), *Handbook of child psychology: Vol. 1. Theoretical models of human development* (5th ed., pp. 1–24). New York: Wiley.

Levine, J. M., Resnick, L. B., & Higgins, E. T. (1993). Social foundations of cognition. *Annual Review of Psychology, 44*, 585–612.

Lewin, K. (1931). The conflict between Aristotelian and Galileian modes of thought in contemporary psychology. *Journal of General Psychology, 5*, 141–177. Reprinted in K. Lewin (1935), *A dynamic theory of personality: Selected papers.* New York: McGraw-Hill.

Lewis, M. D. (1997). Personality self-organization: Cascading constraints on cognition–emotion interactions. In A. Fogel, M. C. D. P. Lyra, & J. Valsiner (Eds.), *Dynamics and indeterminism in developmental and social processes* (pp. 193–216). Mahwah, NJ: Erlbaum.

Linville, P. W. (1985). Self-complexity and affective extremity: Don't put all of your cognitive eggs in one basket. *Social Cognition, 3*, 94–120.

Linville, P. W. (1987). Self-complexity as a cognitive buffer against stress-related illness and depression. *Journal of Personality and Social Psychology, 52*, 663–676.

Litt, M. D. (1988). Self-efficacy and perceived control: Cognitive mediators of pain tolerance. *Journal of Personality and Social Psychology, 54*, 149–160.

Maddux, J. E. (Ed.). (1995). *Self-efficacy, adaptation, and adjustment: Theory, research, and application.* New York: Plenum Press.

Magnusson, D., & Endler, N. S. (1977). Interactional psychology: Present status and future prospects. In D. Magnusson & N. S. Endler (Ed.), *Personality at the crossroads* (pp. 3–31). Hillsdale, NJ: Erlbaum.

Major, B., Cozzarelli, C., Schiacchitano, A. M., Cooper, M. L., Testa, M., & Mueller, P. M. (1990). Perceived social support, self-efficacy, and adjustment to abortion. *Journal of Personality and Social Psychology, 59*, 452–463.

Markus, H. (1977). Self-schemata and processing information about the self. *Journal of Personality and Social Psychology, 35,* 63–78.

Marlatt, G. A., Baer, J. S., & Quigley, L. A. (1995). Self-efficacy and addictive behavior. In A. Bandura (Ed.), *Self-efficacy in changing societies.* New York: Cambridge University Press.

McAdams, D. P. (1995). What do we know when we know a person? *Journal of Personality, 63,* 365–396.

McAdams, D. P. (1996a). *The person as a differentiated region of the life space.* Paper presented at the Society for Personality and Social Psychology Preconference to the annual meeting of the American Psychological Association, San Francisco, CA.

McAdams, D. P. (1996b). Personality, modernity, and the storied self: A contemporary framework for studying personality. *Psychological Inquiry, 7,* 295–321.

McCrae, R. R., & Costa, P. T., Jr. (1987). Validation of the five-factor model of personality across instruments and observers. *Journal of Personality and Social Psychology, 52,* 81–90.

McCrae, R. R., & Costa, P. T., Jr. (1995). Trait explanations in personality psychology. *European Journal of Personality, 9,* 231–252.

McCrae, R. R., & Costa, P. T., Jr. (1996). Toward a new generation of personality theories: Theoretical contexts for the five-factor model. In J. S. Wiggins (Ed.), *The five-factor model of personality: Theoretical perspectives* (pp. 51–87). New York: Guilford Press.

McCrae, R. R., & Costa, P. T., Jr. (1997). Personality trait structure as a human universal. *American Psychologist, 52,* 509–516.

Mischel, W. (1968). *Personality and assessment.* New York: Wiley.

Mischel, W. (1973). Toward a cognitive social learning reconceptualization of personality. *Psychological Review, 80,* 252–283.

Mischel, W. (1993). *Introduction to personality* (5th ed.). Fort Worth, TX: Harcourt, Brace, Jovanovich.

Mischel, W., & Shoda, Y. (1995). A cognitive-affective system theory of personality: Reconceptualizing situations, dispositions, dynamics, and invariance in personality structure. *Psychological Review, 102,* 246–286.

Mueller, P., & Major, B. (1989). Self-blame, self-efficacy, and adjustment to abortion. *Journal of Personality and Social Psychology, 57,* 1059–1068.

Nesselroade, J. R., & Molenaar, P. C. M. (in press). Pooling lagged covariance structures based on short, multivariate time-series for dynamic factor analysis. In R. Hoyle (Ed.), *Research strategies for small samples.*

Nozick, R. (1981). *Philosophical explanations.* Cambridge, MA: Belknap Press of Harvard University Press.

Nystedt, A., Smari, J., & Boman, M. (1991). Self-schemata: Ambiguous operationalizations of an important concept. *European Journal of Personality, 5,* 1–14.

O'Leary, A., & Brown, S. (1995). Self-efficacy and the physiological stress response. In J. E. Maddux (Ed.), *Self-efficacy, adaptation, and adjustment: Theory, research, and application* (pp. 227–246). New York: Plenum Press.

Peake, P. K., & Cervone, D. (1989). Sequence anchoring and self-efficacy: Primacy effects in the consideration of possibilities. *Social Cognition, 7,* 31–50.

Pervin, L. A. (1994). A critical analysis of current trait theory. *Psychological Inquiry, 5,* 103–113.

Renfrew, C. (1988). Précis to *Archaeology and language: The puzzle of Indo-European Origins. Current Anthropology, 29,* 437–441.

Renfrew, C. (1989). The origins of Indo-European languages. *Scientific American, 261,* 106–114.

Renfrew, C. (1992). Archaeology, genetics, and linguistic diversity. *Man, 27,* 445–478.

Revelle, W. (1995). Personality processes. *Annual Review of Psychology, 46,* 295–328.

Roberts, B. W. (1994). *A longitudinal study of the reciprocal relation between women's personality and occupational experience.* Unpublished doctoral dissertation, University of California, Berkeley.

Rorer, L. G. (1990). Personality assessment: A conceptual survey. In L. A. Pervin (Ed.), *Handbook of personality: Theory and research* (pp. 693–720). New York: Guilford Press.

Rumelhart, D. E., & McClelland, J. L. (1986). *Parallel distributed processing: Explorations in the microstructure of cognition: Vol. 1. Foundations.* Cambridge, MA: MIT Press/ Bradford Books.

Salmon, W. C. (1989). Four decades of scientific explanation. In P. Kitcher & W. C. Salmon (Eds.), *Minnesota studies in the philosophy of science: Vol. XIII. Scientific explanation.* Minneapolis: University of Minnesota Press.

Sapolsky, R. M. (1996). Why stress is bad for your brain. *Science, 273,* 749–750.

Schacter, D. L. (1996). *Searching for memory: The brain, the mind, and the past.* New York: Basic Books.

Schmitt, M., & Borkenau, P. (1992). The consistency of personality. In G. V. Caprara & G. L. Van Heck (Ed.), *Modern personality psychology: Critical reviews and new directions* (pp. 29–55). New York: Harvester Wheatsheaf.

Schwarzer, R., Bäßler, J., Kwiatek, P., & Schröoder, K. (1997). The assessment of optimistic self-beliefs: Comparisons of the German, Spanish, and Chinese versions of the general self-efficacy scale. *Applied Psychology: An International Review, 46*(1), 69–88.

Scott, W. D., & Cervone, D. (1998). *The influence of negative affect on self-regulatory cognition.* Unpublished manuscript, University of Miami.

Shadel, W. G., Niaura, R., & Abrams, D. B. (in press). An idiographic approach to understanding personality structure and individual differences among smokers. *Cognitive Therapy and Research.*

Shaffer, D. (1996). Understanding bias in scientific practice. *Philosophy of Science, 63*(Suppl.), 89–97.

Sherer, M., Maddux, J. E., Mercandante, B., Prentice-Dunn, S., Jacobs, B., & Rogers, R. W. (1982). The self-efficacy scale: Construction and validation. *Psychological Reports, 51,* 663–671.

Shoda, Y., & Mischel, W. (1997). Personality as a stable cognitive-affective activation network: Characteristics patterns of behavior variation emerge from a stable personality structure. In S. Read & L. Miller (Eds.), *Connectionist models of social reasoning* (pp. 175–208). Mahwah, NJ: Erlbaum

Simon, H. (1979). Information processing models of cognition. *Annual Review of Psychology, 30,* 363–396.

Skinner, B. F. (1971). *Beyond freedom and dignity.* New York: Knopf.

Stock, J., & Cervone, D. (1990). Proximal goal-setting and self-regulatory processes. *Cognitive Therapy and Research, 14,* 483-498.

Strelau, J., & Plomin, R. (1992). A tale of two theories of temperament. In G. V. Caprara & G. L. Van Heck (Ed.), *Modern personality psychology: Critical reviews and new directions* (pp. 327–351). New York: Harvester Wheatsheaf.

Tellegen, A. (1991). Personality traits: Issues of definition, evidence, and assessment. In W. M. Grove & D. Cicchetti (Eds.), *Thinking clearly about psychology: Vol. 2. Personality and psychopathology* (pp. 1–35). Minneapolis: University of Minnesota Press.

Tipton, R. M., & Worthington, E. L. (1984). The measurement of generalized self-efficacy: A study of construct validity. *Journal of Personality Assessment, 48,* 545–548.

Weitlauf, J. C., Smith, R. E., & Cervone, D. (1998). *Effects of coping skills acquisition on task-specific self-efficacy, generalized self-efficacy, and global personality variables: A study of self-defense training for women.* Unpublished manuscript, University of Washington, Seattle.

White, T. R., & Cervone, D. (1998). *Identifying personality trait inconsistencies in open-ended self-descriptions.* Paper presented at the annual convention of the Midwestern Psychological Association, Chicago, IL.

Wiggins, J. S. (Ed.). (1996). *The five-factor model of personality: Theoretical perspectives.* New York: Guilford Press.

Wiggins, J. S. (1997). In defense of traits. In R. Hogan, J. Johnson, & S. Briggs (Eds.), *Handbook of personality psychology* (pp. 95–115). San Diego, CA: Academic Press. (Original work published 1973)

Williams, S. L. (1995). Self-efficacy, anxiety, and phobic disorders. In J. Maddux (Ed.), *Self-efficacy, adaptation, and adjustment: Theory, research, and application* (pp. 69–107). New York: Plenum Press.

Williams, S. L., & Cervone, D. (1998). Social cognitive theory. In D. Barone, M. Hersen, & V. B. Van Hasselt (Eds.), *Advanced personality* (pp. 173–207). New York: Plenum Press.

Williams, S. L., Kinney, P. J., & Falbo, J. (1989). Generalization of therapeutic changes in agoraphobia: The role of perceived self-efficacy. *Journal of Consulting and Clinical Psychology, 57,* 436–442.

Wright, J. C., & Mischel, W. (1987). A conditional approach to dispositional constructs: The local predictability of social behavior. *Journal of Personality and Social Psychology, 53,* 1159–1177.

Wylie, A. (1995). Unification and convergence in archaeological explanation: the agricultural "wave of advance" and the origins of Indo-European languages. *Southern Journal of Philosophy* (Suppl.: *Explanation in the Human Sciences*), 34, 1–30.

IV

Goals and Life Tasks
as a Source
of Personality Coherence

10

A Goal Analysis of Personality and Personality Coherence

HEIDI GRANT

CAROL S. DWECK

Let me observe that if I know the goal of a person I know in a general way what will happen. . . . We must remember that the person under observation would not know what to do with himself were he not oriented toward some goal.

—ADLER (1927/1964)

Personality theorists have time and again faced the "personality paradox" (Mischel & Shoda, 1995), or the inability to reconcile the stable, coherent nature of personality with the variation in an individual's behavior across situations. Trait theories have predominantly addressed the more static, invariant elements of personality through the assessment of individual differences in average levels of behavior (e.g., *agreeableness*). In contrast to the primarily descriptive nature of trait theory, and its inability to account for within-individual variability, social-cognitive theories have taken a more process-oriented approach. This approach is aimed at revealing the underlying *mechanisms* of personality and accounting for variability in human behavior.

In exploring and documenting the richness and complexity of personality, however, social-cognitive theorists have often sacrificed the parsimony characteristic of the more static approaches. Thus the challenges ahead for social-cognitive theorists of personality are to delineate in a concise manner the basic elements of personality and to specify how they generate (1) coherence within individuals, (2) variation in an individual across situations, and (3) differences among individuals.

We believe that the answer to this challenge lies in according *motivation* a central role in process-oriented theories of personality. Motivation is missing or underemphasized in many current accounts of personality and personality coherence, despite the rich history of motivational concepts in the field. We contend in this chapter that motivational principles are fundamental to understanding personality—that we cannot begin to comprehend how a system functions without taking into account the individual's *goals*.

We begin by briefly reviewing the history of motivation in personality psychology. Next, we discuss evidence for the utility of a central motivational construct—*goals*—in personality and social psychology and suggest that goals can be used to predict and explain personality coherence, individual differences, and within-individual variation in a wide variety of domains. For example, we show how chronic goal selection provides a powerful source of cross-situational personality coherence and at the same time creates systematic individual differences. We go on to propose that goals can best bring order and parsimony to the field if we identify *basic classes* of goals that are few in number but that capture the diversity of human striving. Finally, we argue that goals can provide a common language for personality psychologists and a common ground between personality and other areas of psychology.

A BRIEF HISTORY OF MOTIVATION IN PERSONALITY

Motivational principles were at the very heart of many of the earliest theories of personality. Freud (1933/1964) believed that personality was shaped by the ability or the failure to attain two basic needs or goals in childhood, namely the hedonic goals of attaining pleasure and avoiding pain. Freud's theory of personality had both dynamic and static elements, in that it was composed largely of needs and drives (which are dynamic forces), with an emphasis on typologies and dispositions (which are relatively static). Later theorists in the psychodynamic tradition maintained an emphasis on motivation but shifted dramatically from a focus on hedonic goals, to more abstract, higher-order goals, often involving the self and relationships (e.g., *superiority, identity, self-realization*) (Adler, 1927; Erikson, 1959; Horney, 1945).

These neo-Freudians, as well as the humanist personality theorists (Maslow, 1954/1970; Rogers, 1961), all took as fundamental to personality the question of what individuals are striving for, or what end their behavior is directed toward. Their answers naturally varied a great deal, from the need for *self-actualization* (Horney, 1945; Maslow, 1954/1970; Rogers, 1961) to the need for *autonomy* and *intimacy* (Erikson, 1959). Nonetheless, these theories, like Freud's, grew up around the idea that satisfying or failing to satisfy a need has far-reaching implications for subsequent personality and behavior. Personality was thus characterized by the type of goal and level of goal one typically sought and the success that one had encountered in meeting it.

The problem with these theories, however, lies in the difficulty one encounters when trying to operationalize constructs such as "self-actualization" and to observe their workings in a rigorous fashion. In addition, with their reliance upon typology to capture individual differences, classic theories of personality were not able to identify precisely those mechanisms underlying current behavior and as a result were also unable to predict and explain variability in behavior across situations.

Taking a different tack, behaviorism maintained that "personality," or individual differences, is the result of different histories of reinforcement. Interestingly, even this, perhaps the most conceptually sterile approach to personality, had motivation at its core. Ironically, cognitive theorists, in their attempts to redress the blackbox sterility of behaviorism, began by largely ignoring motivational principles in favor of social-cognitive constructs such as expectancies, encodings, and schemas.

While the field of personality has certainly been enriched by the social-cognitive approach, what has often been lacking is the more classic emphasis on motivation. Understanding the important cognitive elements that direct behavior is of course critical, but *how* do these elements affect behavior? How is behavior driven? How is it selected? How are affect, cognition, and behavior organized? The challenge is thus to understand the how and why of an individual's behavior—how cognition, affect, and behavior work in concert to accomplish something. Otherwise, as Pervin (1989) noted, "[It is] as if people only collect maps but never go on trips."

AN EXAMPLE FROM THE SOCIAL-COGNITIVE APPROACH TO PERSONALITY: MISCHEL AND SHODA'S CAPS MODEL

To illustrate the ways in which social-cognitive models of personality can benefit from a renewed emphasis on motivation, let's look at an example that contains, but is not organized around, motivational elements.

Mischel and Shoda's (1995) ground-breaking cognitive-affective personality system (CAPS) identifies *goals/subjective values* as one of five types of relatively stable person variables (along with encodings, expectancies, self-regulatory strategies, and competencies). According to this theory, individuals differ in how they encode features of situations and how these encodings interact with other person variables. The organization of person variables within the individual (their strength and connections to one another) provides cross-situational stability, while allowing for variation in behavior elicited by features of different situations.

Mischel and Shoda (1995) have provided compelling evidence for their theoretical approach, identifying striking "situation–behavior profile patterns" that characterize both the stability and variability of an individual's behavior over time. These profiles take the form of *if...then...* statements (i.e.,

"If Johnny is taunted by peers, then he will be aggressive"), illustrating the contingent nature of behavior upon situation, while allowing for the particular content of the *if...then...* to be stable and tailored to fit the individual. We believe that such an approach has done a great deal to solve the riddle of the "personality paradox" and has given personality theorists a valuable tool for understanding and predicting human behavior that is grounded in sound cognitive principles of knowledge activation and use (see Higgins, 1996).

However, how can we best characterize the *organization* among elements in the CAPS model? Are there systematic ways in which cognitive-affective units tend to be regularly linked and activated? Is it possible to identify commonly shared pathways or groupings of units on the basis of sound psychological principles of functioning? We believe that motivation (in particular, a goal analysis) can bring such organization to the cognitive-affective system approach, by identifying distinct groupings of cognitive-affective elements organized around particular classes of goals. In other words, in our view, goals are not simply one of many person variables interacting with one another. The aim of this chapter is to show instead that goals drive, select, energize, and direct the activation and use of *all* of the person variables that, working in concert, produce specific behaviors.

CURRENT GOAL THEORIES OF PERSONALITY

Let's now turn to social-cognitive models of personality that *are* organized around goal constructs and to the ways in which these models do and do not address our criticisms of nonmotivational approaches. We examine the kinds of goals these models invoke and the cognitive, affective, or behavioral patterns predicted by each model. We also suggest that while these models document nicely the utility of the goal construct in understanding personality, none have fully realized the potential of the goal approach.

In recent years, a motivational analysis of personality had reemerged and enjoyed a new popularity, relying heavily on goal-related constructs (Cantor & Kihlstrom, 1989; Carver & Scheier, 1982; Dweck & Leggett, 1988; Emmons, 1986; Ford, 1992; Klinger, 1977; Little, 1989; Pervin, 1983; Read & Miller, 1989). Several prominent theories of personality, including Cantor and Kihlstrom's *social intelligence* approach and Emmons's *personal strivings* approach, are explicitly goal-based, positing that our most meaningful and significant thoughts, feelings, and behaviors occur in relation to the things we value and strive for and that much of our action is in the service of the attainment of valued goals.

Cantor and her colleagues (Cantor & Kihlstrom, 1989; Cantor, Norem, Niedenthal, Langston, & Brower, 1987) have used the term *life task* to describe the important goals that people pursue in daily life, often specific to a particular stage or time and context in the life span. In addition to examining differences in life task content among individuals, Cantor and colleagues have looked at *how* people pursue life tasks, and interesting patterns of goal striving have emerged. They have found that people formulate particular strategies for goal attainment and that these strategies are used discriminatively within life task contexts. For example, some students, "defensive pessimists," use a strategy of anticipating negative outcomes from academic tasks and ruminating in detail about how to cope with the task itself. Interestingly, this strategy generally results in better performance (but higher levels of test anxiety) than more "optimistic" strategies, even when past performance is held constant. Students who are defensive pessimists with respect to academic life tasks, however, do not necessarily utilize the same strategy with respect to social life tasks (Cantor et al., 1987). This particular finding illustrates well how motivational constructs, like goals and strategies of goal pursuit, can give us insight into both the stability and variability in behavior over time and across situations.

Emmons's (1989) emphasis, not unlike Cantor and Kihlstrom's (1989), is on *personal strivings*, or the typical kinds of goals a person is likely to have in different situations. Personal strivings are coherent patterns of goal pursuit, which are grouped by their content into thematically relevant categories. Examples of personal strivings include: "Get to know new people," "Make a good impression," and "Avoid arguments when possible." Strivings can also be characterized along several more structural dimensions, including value, commitment, and expectancy for success.

Emmons has found that the experience of positive affect over time is predicted by the value, importance, and past fulfillment of personal strivings. Moreover, conflict between strivings or ambivalence predicts negative affect and low life satisfaction, as well as neuroticism and depression. These findings illustrate the ways in which the setting of and striving for goals can influence our experience of affect and overall well-being.

Cantor and Kihlstrom's (1989) and Emmons's (1989) goal approaches, along with those of Klinger (*current concerns*; 1977) and Little (*personal projects*; 1989), are examples of the way in which theorists can utilize the goal concept to capture the nature of personality. However, the facts that each focuses on people's self-articulated, content-laden goals, and that these goals vary across different levels of abstraction, raise problems. Indeed, in the field as a whole, there is clearly a need for principled distinctions among types of goals beyond their content, as well as for principled distinctions with respect to the appropriateness of using one level of goal abstraction over another. Thus these approaches, although they have dramatically demonstrated the utility of the goal construct for understanding the dynamics of personality, have not offered needed parsimony to the field. Knowing a person's goal tells us little about that individual's patterns of striving. Are there ways of identifying goals where knowing the goal can tell us much about the cognitions, affects, and behaviors that will characterize goal pursuit? Is there a way to classify goals into meaningful categories that cut across content areas? Can these categories of goals help us make clear, precise predictions about how people will think, feel, and act?

Before we attempt to answer these questions, we provide further evidence (much from our own research) to support our claim that goals are powerful organizers and predictors of behavior. This evidence also begins to suggest a different way of classifying goals.

GOALS PREDICT COHERENT PATTERNS ACROSS DOMAINS

To illustrate the utility of the goal construct for understanding personality processes, we briefly examine some of the uses of goals in understanding social phenomena, such as withdrawal, aggression, and intimate relationships, beginning with our own use of the goal approach in the study of achievement motivation. Further, we will suggest how the same kinds of goals can be used to predict patterns of behavior across these different domains, specifically, by means of two types or classes of goals: *judgment* goals and *development* goals.

"Judgment" refers to the goal of seeking to judge or validate an attribute. The attribute can be an attribute of oneself (e.g., one's intelligence, personality, moral character, physical attractiveness), or it can be an attribute of other people or groups of people. When the attribute that is being judged is one's own, this goal will often take the form of seeking positive judgment and seeking to avoid negative judgment (these "performance goals" are a subset of judgment goals).

"Development" refers to the goal of seeking to develop an attribute. When the attribute that is being developed is one's own, this goal will often take the form of seeking to acquire new skills or knowledge (these "learning goals" are a subset of development goals).

Everyone pursues both classes of goals—both are natural and important in our everyday lives. But which goal one pursues in a given situation or which goal one tends to pursue in a given domain will give the goal striving a unique, predictable, and coherent character. As we show, these two types of goals are each linked to meaningful patterns of behavior that are similar or analogous across domains.

Achievement

Dweck and colleagues have amassed considerable evidence to suggest that achievement motivation, and particularly patterns of responding to failure, can be understood in terms of the different goals individuals bring to the achievement context (Elliott & Dweck, 1988; see also Heyman & Dweck, 1992, for a review).

In a series of studies with late grade-school-age children conducted by Diener and Dweck (1978, 1980), two different cognitive, affective, and behavioral patterns of responding to failure were documented. The first pattern was marked by an increase in strategy generation and use, a highly positive prognosis for future performance, spontaneous expressions of constructive cognitions, and positive affect. The second pattern, in stark contrast, was marked by students' spontaneous assertions of low ability, a negative prognosis for future performance, significant negative affect, and deterioration of problem-solving strategies. Diener and Dweck referred to these distinct, coherent patterns of responding as mastery-oriented and helpless patterns, respectively. These particular patterns have been described by other researchers as well (Ames & Archer, 1988; Boggiano et al., 1992; Elliot & Church, 1997; Nichols, 1984; Weiner, 1985).

In an attempt to understand why helpless children react to failure in an achievement situation as if it is diagnostic of ability or intelligence, while mastery-oriented children react as if it is an opportunity for learning and challenge, Elliott and Dweck (1988; Dweck & Elliot, 1983) hypothesized that the patterns were being generated by the different kinds of goals that the children were bringing to the same situation. These particular kinds of goals affected the *meaning* of the situation, thereby leading to highly discrepant ways of responding to it.

Specifically, Elliott and Dweck (1988; Dweck & Elliot, 1983) proposed two kinds of goals in the achievement domain—*performance goals*, where the purpose is to attain favorable judgments of one's competence (i.e., to display and validate one's competence; a judgment goal), and *learning goals*, where the aim is to acquire new knowledge or skills (i.e., to increase one's competence; a development goal). They reasoned that approaching a situation with the goal of documenting your ability would lead you to use your performance as a measure of the level of your ability. Thus a failure could readily be interpreted as meaning that you have low ability, and a helpless reaction could result. In contrast, if you approach a situation with the goal of learning or of developing a skill, a failure is more likely to be seen as information about your learning strategy and an opportunity for improvement in the future.

The hypothesis that approaching a situation with a performance goal leads to a vulnerability to helpless responses to failure while approaching a situation with a learning goal leads to mastery-oriented responses to failure, has been tested and supported in several studies (see Dweck & Elliott, 1983; Elliott & Dweck, 1988; Dweck & Leggett, 1988). In Elliott and Dweck (1988), goals were experimentally induced in order to substantiate the posited *causal* relationship between goals and responses. In Dweck and Leggett (1988), naturally existing differences in goal selection provided further evidence in support of the hypothesis that particular kinds of goals produce meaningful patterns of behavior.

Judgment and development goals not only predict different and unique patterns of coping with failure but also different patterns of task selection and goal striving before feedback. For example, children with judgment goals will knowingly sacrifice an opportunity to learn if offered an alternative task on which they are likely to perform better (Elliott & Dweck, 1988).

Nichols (1984) has made a distinction similar to our own, between *ego-involved* and *task-involved* goals, and Ames and Archer (1988) distinguish between *ability-evaluative* goals and *task-mastery* goals. Taken together, a considerable body of evidence exists to suggest that what an individual will do in an achievement situation depends a great deal on what he or she is trying to accomplish—more specifically, whether he or she is seeking favorable judgment or skill development.

Social Withdrawal

What, if any, role do goals play in people's responses to social failure? Several researchers have looked at children's social goals and their reactions to social setbacks (e.g., rejection) (Erdley, Cain, Loomis, Dumas-Hines, & Dweck, 1997; cf. Goetz & Dweck, 1980).

Goetz and Dweck (1980) documented two patterns of responding to such social failures, directly analogous to the helpless and mastery-oriented patterns in the achievement domain. The first pattern was characterized by decreased effort, withdrawing from the social encounter, and blaming of the self for lack of social ability. The second pattern, in sharp contrast, was marked by increased social efforts, persistence (e.g., continued attempts to overcome rejection), and a lack of self-blame for the failure. (Social failure was often attributed to unstable sources, such as another person's bad mood or a misunderstanding.)

These patterns of responding to social setbacks are strikingly similar to the helpless and mastery-oriented patterns documented by Dweck and colleagues (Diener & Dweck, 1978, 1980; Elliott & Dweck, 1988; Dweck & Elliott, 1983) in the achievement domain. Do different types of goals predict these patterns? Furthermore, do the *same* types of goals predict helplessness and mastery-oriented behavior in the domains of social interaction and achievement?

A study by Erdley et al. (1997), using the paradigm developed by Goetz and Dweck (1980), addressed these questions by manipulating children's social goals and observing their responses to a social setback. Erdley and colleagues informed a group of fourth- and fifth-grade children that they would be participating in a "pen-pal tryout." The children were asked to write a letter to a potential pen-pal and believed that this letter was transmitted to a peer rater, who would decide if the child could join the pen-pal club. After transmitting the letter, each child was told that the rater was "not sure whether to have you in the club" and would like the child to write another letter. After the second letter, all children were told that they had been accepted.

Before writing the first letter, however, each child was told either that "We'd like to see how good you are at making friends," setting up a judgment goal, or that "This is a chance to practice and improve how you make friends," establishing a development goal. The postrejection second letter was coded by independent raters, who found that letters written by children with judgment goals, when compared to those written by children with development goals, showed decreased effort and withdrawal from the task. This was evidenced among children with judgment goals by a decrease in the number of strategies used by the writer, a decrease in over-all message length, and a decrease in the amount of information about the writer contained in the letter. The judgment group was also more likely than the development group to attribute the initial social setback to uncontrollable factors.

These results illustrate how goals can influence the way in which a social setback is interpreted by an individual and how goals are linked to coherent, meaningful patterns of responding in a social interaction. They also support the claim that there are types or classes of goals that cut across domains and predict analogous patterns of behavior.

Aggression

Can this goal analysis be used to illuminate the causes of aggressive behavior? Much of the research on adolescent aggression has focused on the kinds of thoughts and expectations that aggressive individuals may have, rather than what aggressive individuals are trying to *do*. For example, Dodge's (1993) social information-processing approach to understanding aggression and conduct disorder has emphasized how one's expectancies about being the target of aggressive or antisocial behavior shape one's own behavior toward others. In other words, aggressive youths are aggressive because they expect to be rejected or treated with hostility, and they react to even ambiguous events as hostile provocations.

From our point of view, the chronic selection of inappropriate goals, as well as inappropriate goal strategies, could result in an "aggressive personality," perhaps moderating the effects of having a particular expectancy. For example, expecting that peers will be hostile and aggressive toward you might have a different impact on an adolescent with the primary interpersonal goal of being validated or judged positively by others (or of not being rejected or undermined by others), than it would on one whose primary interpersonal goal is to understand and develop relationships with others over time. One can easily see how the former goal type might lead to defensiveness and hostility in the service of "saving face" or protecting one's self from rejection and negative evaluation.

Do the interpersonal goals of aggressive children in fact differ in some systematic way from those of nonaggressive children? Evidence exists to suggest that they do. La Greca, Dandes, Wick, Shaw, and Stone (1988) found that rejected-aggressive children fear and wish to avoid the negative evaluation of others, and Taylor and Asher (1989) found that rejected-aggressive children worry significantly more about avoiding future negative outcomes. Also consistent with this hypothesis, Taylor and Asher (1989) found that the more these adolescents endorsed judgment goals, the more aggressively they behaved.

Why might some children with judgment social goals respond to a social failure with aggression, whereas others respond by withdrawing from the interaction, as in the Erdley et al. (1997) study? While there are many possible explanations, we suggest that the difference may lie in the selection of different strategies for coping with social conflict and failure. For example, aggressive behavior may be the result of the presence of retaliation strategies (i.e., "getting back" at the perceived aggressor or rejecter) (Dodge, 1980; Dodge & Frame, 1982; Erdley & Asher, 1996). Aggressive children have been shown to believe in the effectiveness of aggressive solutions and to believe in their own ability to carry them out (Erdley & Asher, 1996). In contrast, helpless/withdrawn children have been shown to lack belief in their own ability to find direct solutions and carry them out (Diener & Dweck, 1978, 1980; Erdley et al., 1997). Thus, children with judgment goals in social interactions who meet with a perceived rejection will use strategies that they believe are appropriate, effective, and can be successfully carried out by them.

The classic experiments by Dodge and Frame (1982) can be construed in this goal framework. In these studies, aggressive and nonaggressive boys heard a series of stories about an interaction between two children. For half of the stories, the target of a potentially aggressive behavior was the boy himself, while for the other half of the stories the interaction was between two other peers. It was demonstrated that aggressive boys overattributed hostile intentions to peers when the target was the self but *not* when the behavior was directed toward a second peer rather than the self. In other words, aggressive boys do not overperceive hostile aggression *everywhere*, but rather only when they themselves are involved.

Dodge and Frame suggest that aggressive boys have a greater expectancy of being the target of hostility than other boys and that this leads to subsequent overattribution of hostility. We might suggest that another reason aggressive boys do not overattribute hostile intent when observing the peer–peer exchanges is that their own interpersonal goal system is not engaged. When their goal system *is* engaged, the tendency to perceive hostile acts is heightened by a highly accessible defensive judgment goal, as opposed to a development goal that might lead to more effective problem solving. That is, the expectancy of hostility from others, coupled with the chronically accessible goal of avoiding the negative judgment of others (e.g., being undermined, slighted, treated disrespectfully, etc.), could result in a hypervigilance with respect to hostile acts as well as in the overperception of hostile acts (see Downey & Feldman, 1996).

Intimate Relationships

Can a goal analysis be used to understand the ways in which people interact in intimate relationships? According to Reis and Patrick (1996), the process of intimate interaction begins with the individual's "motives, needs, and goals." But what are the different *kinds* of goals that individuals bring to intimate relationships, and how do they affect behavior?

Some recent work in our lab has attempted to extend the judgment/development distinction that had proved useful in understanding achievement motivation, aggression, and withdrawal into the realm of intimate relationships (Kamins, Morris, & Dweck, 1997). Specifically, Kamins, Morris, and Dweck (1997) looked at the kinds of self-goals that college students have in relationships, and they found that some people tend to seek partners who will make them look good to others and validate their worth, whereas others are more likely to look for partners who help them learn about themselves and challenge them to grow. Interestingly, it was also found that individuals who see their own personality as relatively fixed tend to have more self-validation goals in intimate relationships—that is, they want a partner who will validate their attributes. In contrast, those who see their own personality as something that can develop tend to have more self-development goals in intimate relationships. Thus the judgment versus development distinction may capture an important existing distinction in the domain of intimate relationships as well as achievement striving.

We might expect that the seeking of validation or favorable judgment in the domain of intimacy would lead to behaviors analogous to those reported in the achievement domain (e.g., nonconstructive strategies in the face of conflict or difficulty). Some evidence exists to suggest that this is in fact the case. McAdams (1989), drawing on Murray and McClelland's conceptualizations of the need for affiliation, distinguished between *n*-affiliation and *n*-intimacy. The *intimacy motive* is a desire for positive, growth-promoting relationships. The *affiliation motive* is a more defensive desire for acceptance, security, and social power. Studies suggest that *n*-intimacy predicts increased self-disclosure, greater social support, more positive affect, and less negative affect in ongoing personal relationships, whereas *n*-affiliation has been shown to potentially *undermine* intimacy (Koestner, 1989; Brundage, Derlega, & Cash, 1977). McAdams's *n*-intimacy versus *n*-affiliation distinction seems parallel to our own judgment versus development goals, as does his finding that *n*-affiliation (most analogous to judgment goals) can undermine intimacy, just as judgment goals have been found to undermine the surmounting of social obstacles.

These examples illustrate the utility of using a person's goals to predict and explain the dynamics of intimate interaction. We are also currently exploring the nature of one's goals *toward others,* rather than for the self, in domains such as social judgment and stereotyping. Here we have found evidence suggesting that the judgment class of basic goals may be relevant to stereotyping behavior. For example, Levy, Stroessner, and Dweck (1998) have suggested that persons with the goal of judging, labeling, and categorizing others (a judgment goal toward others) may be prone to endorsing existing stereotypes and forming new ones to a greater extent than those subjects whose primary goal is to understand the dynamics of others' personalities.

Judgment goals may play a part not only in the perception of other persons or social groups, but also in one's behavior toward these persons or groups. For example, Sorich and Dweck (1997) have found evidence suggesting that persons with the goal of judging, labeling, and categorizing others are more likely to endorse the punishment of wrong-doers and less likely to advocate education and rehabilitation for criminals (see also Chiu, Dweck, Tong, & Fu, 1997). Thus basic classes of goals appear to predict meaningful patterns of cognition, affect, and behavior not only with respect to goals for the self but also when another person or group is the target.

In this section we have shown that the kinds of goals that individuals bring to a variety of situations predict the choices they will make and the way in which they will respond. But *how* do goals create behavior? Why does having a certain goal make you more likely to be aggressive, helpless, or withdrawn? In the following sections, we discuss *how* goals can produce coherent patterns of behavior.

HOW DO GOALS DRIVE, SELECT, AND ORGANIZE BEHAVIOR?

Several points should be made with respect to our use of the term "goal" before we proceed. By goal, we mean what an individual is striving to accomplish at a given time in a particular situation—in other words, the individual's *purpose.* Goals in this sense need not be conscious or explicit, though they, no doubt, often are. Goals are fluid and dynamic—they can be activated or inhibited momentarily and replaced or overshadowed by other goals as the situation demands. Everyone has a variety of goals in his or her repertoire, though differences can exist among individuals as to which goals are used and valued more or less than others.

As we discuss in greater detail below, goals often exist in hierarchies, such that one goal acts in the service of other (often more abstract) goals. For example, a person may have the goal of developing his or her knowledge of music and the arts in order to impress a potential romantic partner. Here, the goal of developing knowledge is in the service of another, more ultimate purpose—the judgment goal of being positively evaluated by an admired other. We would therefore not refer to the person's goal in this situation as a development goal, because the development of knowledge is not the primary purpose, but rather a means to an end. Predictions about an individual's behavior are best made in reference to what the individual is ultimately trying to accomplish.

How do goals drive, select, and organize behavior? Dweck and her colleagues have suggested that goals influence the aspects of a situation that are attended to and encoded, as well as the interpretation of elements in the situation, exerting a large influence over the psychological meaning of the situation for the individual (Dweck, 1997; see also Cantor et al., 1991). A similar position has been taken by Dodge (1993), who noted, "The meaning applied to an encoded stimulus array relates the stimulus to an individual's needs and goals." In other words, elements in a situation are encoded and understood with respect to current predominant goals.

For example, it has been shown that a person entering an achievement situation with a judgment goal is likely to pay particular attention to aspects of the situation (e.g., teacher feedback, performance of peers) that will enable that person to gauge or evaluate his or her ability (Mueller & Dweck, 1998). For example, in a study conducted by Mueller and Dweck (1998), students who had either a judgment or development orientation were given an opportunity to look at one of two folders. One folder contained information about the performance of other students on the impending task, while the other contained information about strategies for performing better on the task. Students with a judgment goal were more likely to select the folder containing information about peer performance, so that they might gauge their own ability, than students with a development goal, even when it deprived them of information that might be important for performance.

After failure, students with a judgment orientation are also more likely to interpret certain elements in the situation (e.g., a teacher saying "You didn't do very well") as relevant to and informative about their own underlying ability. Thus the psychological meaning of the situation and outcome (in this case an academic failure or setback), is the conclusion that one has low ability or is not "smart." This pattern of attention and encoding, interpretation, and inference is uniquely predicted by the presence of a judgment goal, as opposed to a development goal, in an achievement situation (see Heyman & Dweck, 1992).

In contrast, students entering an achievement situation with a development goal are likely to pay attention to aspects of the situation that will allow them to improve their skills (e.g., instructions and hints). For example, in the Mueller and Dweck study (1998), students with a development goal were more likely to select the folder containing information about strategy improvement than students with a judgment goal. After failure, they were also more likely to interpret certain elements in the situation (e.g., a teacher saying "You didn't do very well") as a challenge to do better and a signal to reevaluate their strategies. Thus the psychological meaning of the academic failure or setback is that they must alter their behavior to improve and develop their ability. The identical situation and feedback will vary dramatically in its meaning as a function of one's goal.

It is also important to note that goals, as knowledge structures (Kruglanski, 1996), can be activated by salient situational features as well as through chronically high accessibility. This aspect of goal activation enables us to explain how an individual can exhibit relatively stable patterns of behavior over time (chronically accessible goals) as well as variation across situations (situationally activated goals), which we discuss in more detail below.

Specifically, we are suggesting that when a goal is activated, either as the result of situational features or chronically high accessibility, the cognitive, affective, and behavioral units that are strongly linked to the activated goal become highly accessible. For example, as we have seen, judgment goals lead to a pattern of attention and cue selection that can result in negative affect, negative self-evaluation, and helplessness after failure, whereas, development goals lead to a pattern of attention and cue selection that can result in maintained or positive affect, positive self-evaluation, and persistence after failure. Figure 10.1 illustrates how different classes of goals can generate different pathways of cognition, affect, and behavior, providing parsimony in the cognitive-affective approach to personality without sacrificing its richness or complexity.

CHRONIC GOAL ACTIVATION AND PERSONALITY COHERENCE

So far we have suggested that understanding a person's goals is a critical element in understanding his or her personality and that the production of behavior is driven by and organized around an individual's *purpose*. We have shown that possessing a particular goal predicts entire patterns of thought, feeling, and behavior in response to a given situation. We have argued that these patterns are generated by the activation of cognitive, affective, and behavioral constructs that are strongly linked to goals. But what of personality coherence? Why is behavior stable across situations? We suggest that personality coherence is derived from the chronic application of particular kinds of goals and the resulting activation of corresponding cognitive-affective-behavioral elements (as shown in Figure 10.1). Chronic use of a particular kind or class of goals might be the result of a number of influences. Although clearly there are many possible sources of the increased accessibility of a particular goal, Dweck and her colleagues have been most active in studying the ways in which "implicit theories" about the self (see Dweck, 1996) affect chronic goal activation. They have found that people who believe that their personality is trait-like and fixed tend to be more interested in evaluating and validating themselves, whereas people who believe that their personality is

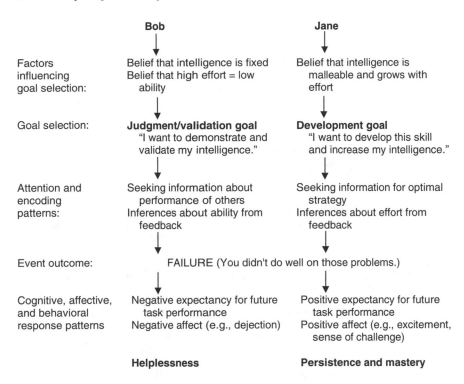

FIGURE 10.1. Different chronic goal dispositions in the achievement domain.

malleable and can be changed over time tend to be more interested in understanding and developing themselves.

To illustrate how chronically activated goals bring about personality coherence, let us take as an example a person for whom judgment goals are chronically accessible in achievement situations (see Figure 10.1, Bob). Bob believes that people have a fixed amount of intelligence and thinks of achievement situations as opportunities to demonstrate or validate his intelligence. We would expect Bob to be more likely to choose tasks that show off his abilities rather than tasks that offer opportunities to learn, and we would also expect Bob to respond to failure across achievement contexts by demonstrating vulnerability to negative affect and self-evaluation, lowered confidence, and poorer future performance. In other words, we would expect to see coherence or stability in Bob's behavior across achievement situations due to the presence of a chronically accessible judgment goal, which organizes and drives a specific pattern of cognitions, affects, and behaviors.

We might, however, see variability in Bob's behavior across situations. For example, as shown in Figure 10.2, Bob believes that personality is

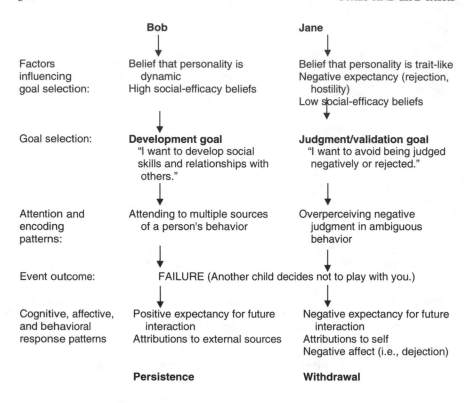

FIGURE 10.2. Different chronic goal dispositions in the social domain.

dynamic and that people can develop their attributes and skills, so he does not focus so much on judgment and validation in social situations and cares more about continuing to develop his social skills and good relationships. Thus we would not expect Bob to exhibit the helpless pattern in response to failure in intimate relationships or social interactions. In other words, a person may chronically approach achievement situations with a judgment goal orientation, while approaching social and intimacy-related situations with a development goal orientation. This domain specificity, in the case of Bob, results in two distinct patterns of coping after failure—negative affect, low self-efficacy, and helplessness in achievement situations, and more positive affect, confidence, and mastery in social interactions.

Jane, on the other hand (see Figures 10.1 and 10.2, Jane), is someone who is very learning-oriented in achievement situations but who worries about being negatively judged in social situations. We would therefore expect to see a different pattern of responding to failure from Jane than we had predicted for Bob. Specifically, we would expect Jane to be more likely to display helplessness in response to setbacks in social interaction, and a more mastery-oriented response to setbacks in achievement situations. Thus goals cannot only help us to capture variation in behavior *within* an individual but also *across* individuals.

But we know that people don't always behave the same way even within a domain. This is in large part, as we noted earlier, because goals can be situationally activated. Thus, although Bob may have chronically accessible judgment goals, a particular achievement setting can promote a development goal (see Figure 10.3, Bob). This could be brought about by feedback ("If you tried harder, you could learn to do this"), or an instruction set ("Don't worry about your performance on this task—it is meant to be a learning experience"). If Bob's primary goal in the situation is a development goal, we would not expect to see helplessness after failure, regardless of the fact that Bob might ordinarily pursue judgment goals in that particular context. In this case, Bob and Jane (see Figure 10.3), although they differ in their chronically accessible goals, will adopt the same goal and exhibit the same cognitive-affective-behavioral pattern.

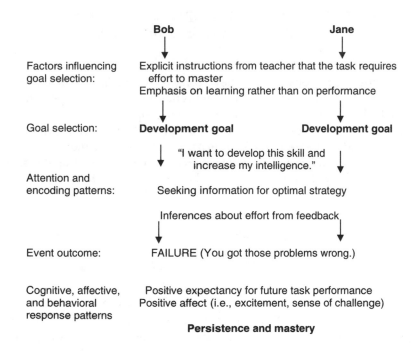

FIGURE 10.3. Situational factors in the achievement domain.

Returning to our earlier challenge to social-cognitive theorists of personality, we have shown how goals can account for the following:

1. Coherence within individuals through the activation of chronically accessible goals and their unique cognitive-affective-behavioral patterns (see Figure 10.1).
2. Variation in an individual across situations through situationally activated goals and through domain specificity of chronic goals (see Figures 10.2 and 10.3).
3. Differences among individuals through variation in the nature and importance of goals and strategies of goal pursuit from individual to individual (see Figures 10.1–10.4).

Why, then, isn't the adoption of a goal analysis even more widespread? We suggested earlier in this chapter that current goal theories of personality often suffer from a lack of parsimony (too many types of goals that are too domain specific) and a lack of agreement on the appropriate level of goal abstraction. We can now attempt to address these issues.

MAXIMIZING THE UTILITY OF A GOAL ANALYSIS THROUGH BASIC CLASSES OF GOALS

At what level of abstraction will goals provide us with insight into and prediction of specific responses? We believe consensus on this issue will further the utility of the goal approach and its acceptance in the field of personality as a whole. It is in this spirit that we make our proposal.

Returning to the work of Diener and Dweck (1978), which documented the helpless and mastery-oriented patterns, we can examine the goals of the students in the experimental situation at three salient levels of analysis. At the highest level of abstraction, there is the need or value to be fulfilled or

	Domain	Goal source	Bob	Jane
(Figure 10.1)	Achievement	Chronic accessibility (individual differences)	Judgment/ validation	Development
(Figure 10.2)	Social interaction	Chronic accessibility	Development	Judgment/ validation
(Figure 10.3)	Achievement	Situational features	Development	Development

FIGURE 10.4. Summary table of goal domains, goal sources, and goal selection.

attained (see Gollwitzer & Moskowitz, 1996; Carver & Scheier, 1982). In this example, both groups of students could be described as striving toward the same value—*competence* ("I want to possess competence"). This is a goal at a level of abstraction such as the goals *self-esteem, relatedness,* or *security.* Clearly, in this case, this level is too abstract to predict specific behaviors, since it does not differentiate between the two groups, and one could easily imagine any number of behaviors arising from a desire to possess *competence* or *self-esteem.*

At the lowest level of abstraction, both groups want to solve the problems given to them by the experimenter. Again, this level of abstraction will not provide us with predictions about specific patterns of responding, but because it is too concrete rather than too abstract.

Between these two levels lies the level of goal abstraction at which the superordinate goal takes a more specific form, and the two groups can be seen to diverge. At this level, the superordinate goal of possessing *competence* takes on a particular nature and determines the particular way in which the individual will self-regulate to achieve the competence goal. In the Elliott and Dweck achievement study (1988), one group's goal was to *demonstrate* competence (judgment goal), while the other's was to *gain* competence (development goal). Once the method of fulfilling the superordinate need is delineated, corresponding behavioral responses to failure can be expected. For example, as noted, at this level, Elliott and Dweck (1988) found that seeking to demonstrate competence can result in a tendency to display helplessness in the face of failure, whereas seeking to gain competence results in a tendency to display a mastery orientation. We propose that this is the level of goal abstraction that is conceptually the most useful in predicting specific behaviors. It is the goal that is both the purpose of the lowest, "nominal" level goal (solving the problems correctly) and the means through which the higher level goal (competence, self-esteem) is achieved.

Our analysis of levels of goal abstraction is analogous to Powers's (1973) model of the hierarchical organization of control systems (see also Carver & Scheier's [1982] description and elaboration of Powers's model). Most germane to our ideas are the highest levels of the nine-level hierarchy. The "system concept" level is the highest level of abstraction, corresponding to goals like self-esteem, relatedness, and identity. The directly subordinate level is the "principle control" level, which specifies the way in which the system concept goal or need can be satisfied. In the case of the system concept "self-esteem," for example, the principle control level goal could be "look good in front of my friends," or "develop a new skill."

In other words, the principle level specifies how people self-regulate with respect to the system level. We suggest that goals at the principle level of abstraction are generally the most useful in predicting an individual's behavior in a particular situation.[1]

By identifying the appropriate level of abstraction for goal analysis, that is, basic classes, goals can provide a greater degree of parsimony in the study of personality. We define "basic classes" as goals grouped together according to a system of classification that *explicitly* cuts across domains.

Often goals have been grouped together according to the need they satisfy (e.g., intimacy goals, achievement goals, power goals). However, we are suggesting that basic classes of goals should instead be based in the *ways* in which these higher-order needs are satisfied, since here we find unique, meaningful patterns of behavior that are similar or analogous across domains.

Our selection of the term "basic classes" was largely influenced by Eleanor Rosch's use of the word "basic" in her description of levels of categorization (Rosch & Mervis, 1975). Rosch described a "basic level category" (e.g., "car") as one whose level of abstraction minimizes within-category differences (e.g., cars, in many respects, are essentially similar to one another) and maximizes between-category differences (e.g., "cars" are very different from "boats").

Similarly, basic classes of *goals* minimize within-goal-type differences, in that a particular class of goal is expected to produce similar or analogous patterns of behavior across situations and domains. Basic classes of goals also maximize between-goal-type differences, in that each basic class of goal predicts *unique* patterns of cognition, affect, and behavior.

Goal typologies based on domain-specific categories (e.g., intimacy goals, achievement goals, social goals, etc.) cannot be said to exist at the *basic level* of analysis. For example, a group of persons can have a wide variety of goals in social situations, including *being popular, making new relationships, understanding others, having fun, being admired,* and *avoiding rejection.* Each of these goals might result in different behaviors in a particular social setting, but each could be described as a "social goal." Therefore, domain-specific goal categories do not minimize within-category differences in behavior.

Similarly, a person may have the goals of looking smart and being praised in school and looking "cool" and being admired among friends. Although the former goal might be considered an "achievement" goal, and the latter a "social" goal, one might expect a rejection or failure in either domain to produce a similar pattern of behavior (e.g., negative affect, lowered confidence, helplessness, and withdrawal). Therefore, domain-specific goal categories do not maximize between-category differences in behavior.

The judgment versus development goal distinction seems to satisfy the requirements of basic classes, and with such a class of basic goals, we can refer to seeking to judge versus to develop in any domain (vis-à-vis the self or others), and we can examine the similarities in behavior patterns across domains.

But are there goals to which basic classes do not apply? The basic classes of goals, as we have described them, do not appear to apply to simple, hedonic goals of approaching pleasure and avoiding pain. For example, one does not generally eat an ice cream cone in order to develop or validate an attribute in the service of some higher-order goal, such as self-esteem or security. One eats an ice cream cone because it tastes good—and wanting to eat an ice cream cone is a simple hedonic goal of attaining pleasure. Hedonic goals, particularly when taken to extremes, can also produce interesting and unique patterns of behavior. Therefore, a fully developed model of goal analysis must distinguish not only among basic classes of goals but also between hedonic goals and goals that serve a more abstract, higher-order psychological purpose, such as self-esteem.

We are currently working on a more thoroughly elaborated, inclusive, and integrative model of goal structure and function in personality. We believe that a principled and parsimonious model based on a goal analysis might help produce greater use of the goal construct among theorists of personality. It may also help to present a more compelling argument for the inclusion of and emphasis on motivation in current nonmotivational accounts of personality.

GOALS AS A COMMON LANGUAGE

In closing, we would like to argue that goals can provide a common language for psychologists working in various subdisciplines. Motivation is an important factor in many areas of psychology, and the use of goal constructs is a way in which findings can be linked from psychobiology to cognition to personality psychology.

As discussed by Dweck (1997), the most obvious connection is between personality and social psychology. Personality psychologists examine individual differences in goals and goal striving, whereas social psychologists concern themselves with situations in which different goals may become salient and goal striving may be facilitated or hindered. Goals, as knowledge constructs, can be chronically or situationally activated, and as such, they are both personality and social psychology variables, respectively.

For example, goals can be used to understand how social information processing is guided by what we want to achieve in social situations, how social information-processing styles can differ among individuals and across situations (Wyer & Srull, 1986; Chaiken, Giner-Sorolla, & Chen, 1996; Dodge 1986; see Gollwitzer & Moskowitz, 1996, for a review). Goals are powerful predictors of our emotional experience (Stein & Levine, 1990; Higgins, 1996; Higgins, Grant, & Shah, in press) and can be used to understand chronic emotional vulnerabilities as well as situationally induced emotional reactions.

The goal analysis is also a useful connection between the already allied areas of personality and abnormal psychology/psychopathology. We suggest that breakdowns in functioning can be the result of inappropriate goals, ineffective goal striving, conflicts among goals, and premature abandonment of goals in the face of difficulty (Dweck, 1997; Emmons, 1989; Pervin, 1983). Because goal selection is also intimately related with a person's beliefs, goal analysis is also compatible with more cognitive, belief-centered systems of understanding impaired psychological functioning (e.g., Beck, 1976).

Classic theorists of personality development (e.g., Erikson, 1959) saw the individual as confronting a series of different tasks throughout the life span, each involving a different kind of goal and different competencies for goal attainment. Recently, some developmental psychologists have turned again to a goal approach, conceptualizing development as a succession of different goals or goal structures. According to these theorists, growth involves the appropriate deemphasis or abandonment of old goals and strategies in exchange for new ones (Baltes & Staudinger, 1996; Damon, 1996; cf. Siegler, 1989). A goal approach to understanding development allows us a more precise, sophisticated conceptualization of adaptive functioning and the factors that influence functioning. For example, we can ask not only what kind of goals and goal strategies are adaptive at particular points in the life span, but also what kinds of socialization lead to the adoption of such goals and strategies. Another significant advantage to the goal approach in developmental psychology is that researchers studying adult personality and those studying personality development would be operating in the same framework and could more easily inform one another's research.

Cross-cultural psychologists refer to the systems of meaning that are created by cultures (Markus & Kitayama, 1991; Morris & Peng, 1994; Shweder, 1991). In other words, they examine the beliefs and values shared by the individuals within a culture, comparing and contrasting them with the beliefs and values of other cultures. This view is highly compatible with a goal analysis for a number of reasons. One could ask how the beliefs and values of a particular culture affect the goals that are selected and the strategic means of goal attainment used by members of the culture. For example, we would expect that some cultures might value a particular kind of goal more than others. Markus and Kitayama (1991) have suggested that the Japanese culture values interdependence and community more than American culture, which values independence and individuality. They also contend that Japanese individuals are more likely to use the strategy of self-criticism than Americans, who tend to favor self-enhancement. Self-criticism can be seen as a strategy that benefits the collective by encouraging development and improvement, whereas self-enhancement can be viewed as a strategy that bolsters or validates the individual, suggesting that these cultures may differ in the particular goals used in particular situations. If, as we have argued, the meaning of a situation is determined by the predominant goals with which one enters it, we should expect a goal analysis to be quite a revealing window into cross-cultural differences.

Finally, goals provide a link from personality to biological psychology.

Motivational processes have long been of interest to psychobiologists and neuroscientists. In a recent book, the neurologist Antonio Damasio (1994) argued for the role of motivational and emotional processes in our ability to make rational decisions, using evidence from neurological case studies and laboratory research. His work has shown that reasoning and rational decision making are intimately dependent upon our ability to set and implement goals; he has done so by demonstrating the deleterious effects of motivational systems gone awry (as, for example, when the wrong goals are given priority or when individuals are unable to unable to select appropriate strategies).

As a field that has long sought to communicate across areas of research, we can truly benefit from the use of a construct that cuts across these research areas.

In this chapter, we have argued that the study of personality and personality coherence can achieve clarity and parsimony through a return to motivation, and specifically, to a focus on purpose. This will be all the more true if goal theorists of personality can agree on the appropriate level of goal abstraction to be used in predicting behavior and on the basic classes of goals that can produce meaningful distinctions among behaviors.

Alfred Adler (1927/1964) once noted, "We cannot think, feel, will, or act without the perception of some goal. . . . All activity would persist in the stage of uncontrolled gropings; the economy visible in our psychic life unattained." We believe that a goal analysis will bring just such "economy" to the study of personality. The goal approach allows us to predict patterns of cognition, affect, and behavior and at the same time to account for coherence of personality within an individual, variation in an individual over time and across situations, and differences among individuals.

NOTE

1. Emmons (1989) has paid careful attention to issues of goal abstraction and has also pointed out that his *personal strivings* could be considered goals at the principle control level of analysis.

REFERENCES

Adler, A. (1927). *The practice and theory of individual psychology.* New York: Harcourt, Brace, & World.

Adler, A. (1964). Individual psychology, its assumptions and its results. In H. M. Ruitenbeek (Ed.), *Varieties of personality theory.* New York: Dutton. (Original work published 1927)

Ames, C., & Archer, J. (1988). Achievement goals in the classroom: Students' learning strategies and motivation processes. *Journal of Educational Psychology, 80,* 260–267.

Baltes, P. B., & Staudinger, U. M. (1996). Interactive minds in a life-span perspective: Prologue. In P. B. Baltes & U. M. Staudinger (Eds.), *Interactive minds: Life-span perspectives on the social foundation of cognition.* New York: Cambridge University Press.

Beck, A. (1976). *Cognitive therapy and the emotional disorders.* New York: International Universities Press.

Boggiano, A. K., Shields, A., Barrett, M., Kellam, T., Thompson, E., Simons, J., & Katz, P. (1992). Helplessness deficits in students: The role of motivation orientation. *Motivation and Emotion, 16*(3), 271–296.

Brundage, L. G., Derlega, V. J., & Cash, T. F. (1977). The effects of physical attractiveness and need for approval on self-disclosure. *Personality and Social Psychology Bulletin, 3,* 63–66.

Cantor, N., & Kihlstrom, J. F. (1989). Social Intelligence and cognitive assessments of personality. In R. S. Wyer & T. K. Srull (Eds.), *Advances in social cognition* (Vol. 2). Hillsdale, NJ: Erlbaum.

Cantor, N., Norem, J. K., Langston, C. A., Zirkel, S., Fleeson, W., & Cook-Flanagan, C. (1991). Life tasks and daily life experience. *Journal of Personality, 59,* 425–451.

Cantor, N., Norem, J. K., Niedenthal, P. M., Langston, C. A., & Brower, A. M. (1987). Life tasks, self-concept ideals, and cognitive strategies in a life transition. *Journal of Personality and Social Psychology, 53,* 1178–1191.

Carver, C. S., & Scheier, M. F. (1982). Control theory: A useful conceptual framework in personality-social, clinical, and health psychology. *Psychological Bulletin, 92,* 111–135.

Chaiken, S., Giner-Sorolla, R., & Chen, S. (1996). Beyond accuracy: Defense and impression motives in heuristic and systematic information processing. In P. M. Gollwitzer & J. A. Bargh (Eds.), *The psychology of action: Linking cognition and motivation to behavior.* New York: Guilford Press.

Chiu, C. Y., Dweck, C. S., Tong, J. Y., & Fu, J. H. (1997). Implicit theories and conceptions of morality. *Journal of Personality and Social Psychology, 73*(5), 923–940.

Damasio, A. R. (1994). *Descartes' error: Emotion, reason, and the human brain.* New York: Putnam.

Damon, W. (1996). The lifelong transformation of moral goals through social influence. In P. B. Baltes & U. M. Staudinger (Eds.), *Interactive minds: Life-span perspectives on the social foundation of cognition.* New York: Cambridge University Press.

Diener, C. I., & Dweck, C. S. (1978). An analysis of learned helplessness: Continuous change in performance and strategy and achievement cognitions following failure. *Journal of Personality and Social Psychology, 36,* 451–462.

Diener, C. I., & Dweck, C. S. (1980). An analysis of learned helplessness II: The processing of success. *Journal of Personality and Social Psychology, 39,* 940–952.

Dodge, K. A. (1980). Social cognition and children's aggressive behavior. *Child Development, 51,* 162–170.

Dodge, K. A. (1986). A social information processing model of social cognition in children. In M. Perlmutter (Ed.), *Minnesota Symposia on Child Psychology: Vol. 18. Cognitive perspectives on children's social and behavioral development.* Hillsdale, NJ: Erlbaum.

Dodge, K. A. (1993). Social-cognitive mechanisms in the development of conduct disorder and depression. *Annual Review of Psychology, 44,* 559–584.

Dodge, K. A., & Frame, C. L. (1982). Social cognitive biases and deficits in aggressive boys. *Child Development, 53,* 620–635.

Downey, G., & Feldman, S. I. (1996). Implications of rejection sensitivity for intimate relationships. *Journal of Personality and Social Psychology, 70,* 1327–1343.

Dweck, C. S. (1996). Implicit theories as organizers of goals and behavior. In P. M. Gollwitzer & J. A. Bargh (Eds.), *The psychology of action: Linking cognition and motivation to behavior.* New York: Guilford Press.

Dweck, C. S. (1997). Capturing the dynamic nature of personality. *Journal of Research in Personality, 30,* 348–362.

Dweck, C. S., & Elliott, E. S. (1983). Achievement motivation. In P. Mussen & E. M. Hetherington (Eds.), *Handbook of child psychology.* New York: Wiley.

Dweck, C. S., & Leggett, E. L. (1988). A social-cognitive approach to motivation and personality. *Psychological Review, 95,* 256–273.

Elliot, A. J., & Church, M. A. (1997). A hierarchical model of approach and avoidance achievement motivation. *Journal of Personality and Social Psychology, 72,* 218–232.

Elliott, E. S., & Dweck, C. S. (1988). Goals: An approach to motivation and achievement. *Journal of Personality and Social Psychology, 54,* 5–12.

Emmons, R. A. (1986). Personal strivings: An approach to personality and subjective well-being. *Journal of Personality and Social Psychology, 51,* 1058–1068.

Emmons, R. A. (1989). The personal striving approach to personality. In L. A. Pervin (Ed.), *Goal concepts in personality and social psychology.* Hillsdale, NJ: Erlbaum.

Erdley, C. A., & Asher, S. R. (1996). Children's social goals and self-efficacy perceptions as predictors of their responses to ambiguous provocation. *Child Development, 67,* 1329–1344.

Erdley, C. A., Cain, K. M., Loomis, C. C., Dumas-Hines, F., & Dweck, C. S. (1997). The relations among children's social goals, implicit personality theories, and responses to social failure. *Developmental Psychology, 33,* 263–272.

Erikson, E. H. (1959). *Identity and the life cycle.* New York: International Universities Press.

Ford, M. E. (1992). *Motivating humans: Goals, emotions, and personal agency beliefs.* Newbury Park, CA: Sage.

Freud, S. (1964). *New introductory lectures on psychoanalysis* (J. Strachey, Trans.). New York: Norton. (Original work published 1933)

Goetz, T. S., & Dweck, C. S. (1980). Learned helplessness in social situations. *Journal of Personality and Social Psychology, 39,* 246–255.

Gollwitzer, P. M., & Moskowitz, G. B. (1996). Goal effects on action and cognition. In E. T. Higgins & A. W. Kruglanski (Eds.), *Social psychology: Handbook of basic principles.* New York: Guilford Press.

Heyman, G. D., & Dweck, C. S. (1992). Achievement goals and intrinsic motivation: Their relation and their role in adaptive motivation. *Motivation and Emotion, 16*(3), 231–247.

Higgins, E. T. (1996). Knowledge activation: Accessibility, applicability, and salience. In E. T. Higgins & A. W. Kruglanski (Eds.), *Social psychology: Handbook of basic principles.* New York: Guilford Press.

Higgins, E. T., Grant, H., & Shah, J. (in press). Self-regulation and subjective well-being: Emotional and non-emotional life experiences. In D. Kahneman, E. Diener, & N. Schwartz (Eds.), *New perspectives on subjective well-being.*

Horney, K. (1945). *Our inner conflicts*. New York: Norton.

Kamins, M. L., Morris, S. M., & Dweck, C. S. (1997). *Implicit theories as predictors of goals in dating relationships*. Poster presented at the Annual Meeting of the Eastern Psychological Association, Washington, DC.

Klinger, E. (1977). *Meaning and void: Inner experience and the incentives in people's lives*. Minneapolis: University of Minnesota Press.

Koestner, R. (1989). *Intimacy, motivation, social support, and subjective well-being*. Unpublished manuscript, McGill University, Montreal, Quebec.

Kruglanski, A. (1996). Goals as knowledge structures. In P. M. Gollwitzer & J. A. Bargh (Eds.), *The psychology of action*. New York: Guilford Press.

La Greca, A. M., Dandes, S. K., Wick, P., Shaw, K., & Stone, W. (1988). Development of social anxiety scale for children: Reliability and concurrent validity. *Journal of Consulting Clinical Psychology, 17*, 84–91.

Levy, S. R., Stroessner, S. J., & Dweck, C. S. (1998). Stereotype formation and endorsement: The role of implicit theories. *Journal of Personality and Social Psychology, 74*(6), 1421–1436.

Little, B. R. (1989). Personal projects analysis: Trivial pursuits, magnificent obsessions, and the search for coherence. In D. M. Buss & N. Cantor (Eds.), *Personality psychology: Recent trends and emerging directions*. New York: Springer-Verlag.

Markus, H., & Kitayama, S. (1991). Culture and the self: Implications for cognition, emotion, and motivation. *Psychological Review, 98*, 224–253.

Maslow, A. H. (1970). *Motivation and personality*. New York: Harper. (Original work published 1954)

McAdams, D. P. (1989). *Intimacy: The need to be close*. New York: Doubleday.

Mischel, W., & Shoda, Y. (1995) A cognitive-affective system theory of personality: reconceptualizing situation, dispositions, dynamics, and invariance in personality structure. *Psychological Review, 102*(2), 246–268.

Morris, M. W., & Peng, K. (1994). Culture and cause: American and Chinese attributions for social and physical events. *Journal of Personality and Social Psychology, 67*, 949–971.

Mueller, C. M., & Dweck, C. S. (1998). Praise for intelligence can undermine children's motivation and performance. *Journal of Personality and Social Psychology, 75*(1), 33–52.

Nichols, J. G. (1984). Achievement motivation: Conceptions of ability, subjective experience, task choice, and performance. *Psychological Review, 91*, 328–346.

Pervin, L. A. (1983). The stasis and flow of behavior: Toward a theory of goals. In M. M. Page (Ed.), *Nebraska Symposium on Motivation*. Lincoln: University of Nebraska Press.

Pervin, L. A. (1989). *Goal concepts in personality and social psychology*. Hillsdale, NJ: Erlbaum.

Powers, W. T. (1973). *Behavior: The control of perception*. Chicago: Aldine.

Read, S. J., & Miller, L. C. (1989) The importance of goals in personality: Towards a coherent model of persons. In R. S. Wyer, Jr. & T. K. Srull (Eds.), *Advances in social cognition: Vol. 2. Social intelligence and cognitive assessments of personality*. Hillsdale, NJ: Erlbaum.

Reis, H. T., & Patrick, B. C. (1996). Attachment and intimacy: component processes. In E. T. Higgins & A. W. Kruglanski (Eds.), *Social psychology: Handbook of basic principles*. New York: Guilford Press.

Rogers, C. R. (1961). *On becoming a person.* Boston: Houghton Mifflin.

Rosch, E., & Mervis, C. B. (1975). Family resemblances: Studies in the internal structure of categories. *Cognitive Psychology, 7,* 573–605.

Shweder, R. (1991). *Thinking through cultures.* Cambridge, MA: Harvard University Press.

Siegler, R. (1989). Mechanisms of cognitive development. *Annual Review of Psychology, 40,* 353–379.

Sorich, L., & Dweck, C. S. (1997). *Implicit theories and endorsement of punishment and reha-bilitation.* Unpublished manuscript, Columbia University, New York.

Stein, N. L., & Levine, L. J. (1990). Making sense out of emotion: The representation and use of goal-structured knowledge. In N. L. Stein, B. Leventhal, & T. Trabasso (Eds.), *Psychological and biological approaches to emotion.* Hillsdale, NJ: Erlbaum.

Taylor, A. R., & Asher, S. R. (1989). *Children's goals in game playing situations.* Paper presented at the Annual Meeting of the American Psychological Association, New York.

Weiner, B. (1985). An attributional theory of achievement motivation and emotion. *Psychological Review, 92,* 548–573.

Wyer, R. S., & Srull, T. K. (1986). Human cognition in its social context. *Psychological Review, 93,* 322–359.

11

A Life Task Perspective on Personality Coherence
Stability versus Change in Tasks, Goals, Strategies, and Outcomes

CATHERINE A. SANDERSON
NANCY CANTOR

Considerable research in personality has been based in the trait model, which focuses on individual-difference dimensions and posits that individuals' distinct traits largely determine their behavior, across both different situations and across time (Caspi, Bem, & Elder, 1989; Costa & McCrae, 1980). For example, individuals who are high on the "agreeableness" dimension of the five-factor model of personality are thought to be more trusting and cooperative in their interpersonal relationships, whereas those who are high on the "openness to experience" dimension are thought to daydream and question authority (McCrae & John, 1992; Watson & Clark, 1992). Although these perspectives provide insight into aspects of the person's needs and motivations, they often pay less attention to the specific social and cultural contexts in which individuals' goals are formed and their behavior is carried out. Such situational factors, however, are likely to influence behavior in a variety of ways, including what broad tasks the person works on and the goals and strategies he or she uses in this pursuit (Erikson, 1950; Havighurst, 1953; Veroff, 1983). Therefore, in considering how personality coheres across the life span, we believe one must take into account not only what individuals themselves are trying to do (e.g., their goals and strategies of task pursuit) but also how their social context influences what they are able to do (e.g., by providing opportunities for the pursuit of tasks with particular valued goals; by discouraging the pursuit of nonnormative tasks).

In this chapter, we present our life task model of personality, which emphasizes the role of cultural, social, and personal factors in influencing task pursuit. First, we examine how individuals' task pursuit is contextualized in several ways, including by their particular age-graded life stage (e.g., the broad tasks they should be working on), their own personal goals (e.g., the particular meanings they bring to these tasks), their own strategies (e.g., how they are working on these goals), and the outcomes of this pursuit (e.g., how the use of particular goals and strategies may be associated with different outcomes during different life periods). We then examine how these various components of personality differ in the extent to which they are associated with personality change versus stability. Specifically, we examine how the taking on of new tasks, with new strategies and potentially new outcomes, across the life span generally acts as a *push* toward personality change, whereas individuals' distinct personal goals generally act as a *pull* towards personality stability. In this way, our approach suggests that personality both changes and coheres across the life course: As people transition from one life period to the next, their tasks and strategies are likely to change, while their underlying goals are likely to remain stable (i.e., a functional continuity). Finally, we propose a number of still unanswered questions about how goal and task pursuit may lead to personality coherence and change in distinct ways for different subcultures, in different daily life situations, and for different people.

A LIFE TASK MODEL OF PERSONALITY

The life task perspective in personality psychology posits that to understand the meaning of individuals' behavior in daily life, one needs to understand both the broader culturally mandated problems or tasks that they are working on and the specific meaning they bring to these tasks (Cantor, 1990; Cantor & Kihlstrom, 1987). As described in Erikson's (1950) psychosocial model of development, sociocultural contexts prescribe particular tasks for individuals to work on in their daily lives during a given life period (Carstensen, 1993; Havighurst, 1953, 1972; Helson & Moane, 1987; Higgins & Eccles-Parsons, 1983; Veroff, 1983). These life tasks are influenced both by their broader macro-level culture as well as by the micro-level situations in their daily lives, and hence represent mid-level units of analysis (Cantor, 1994). For example, making friends, being on your own, and academic achievement are all normative age-graded tasks for adolescents, at least in our Western culture, whereas career advancement and raising a family are normative tasks for midadulthood. These tasks, namely the problems that individuals are attempting to solve in daily life, are widely articulated by families, schools, and the media, and hence they are powerful influences on behavior (Elder, 1975; Havighurst, 1953).

Although sociocultural contexts prescribe the pursuit of certain tasks, individuals are remarkably flexible in how they approach these tasks in line with their own distinct needs and goals (Cantor & Fleeson, 1994; Emmons, 1989; Little, 1989; Veroff, 1983). In other words, individuals can take on the broad valued tasks of their culture with particular personally valued goals. For example, Snyder's work on volunteerism has shown that some individuals take on this task with predominant other-focused goals in mind (e.g., helping those who are less fortunate, making a difference in the world), whereas others pursue this task with a focus on more self-oriented goals (e.g., feeling good about one's self; establishing friendship networks; Omoto & Snyder, 1990; Snyder, 1993). Therefore, although most individuals in a given age-graded subculture take on the socially mandated tasks at periods of life transition, they bring their own personal meaning to these tasks.

Moreover, the particular goals that individuals bring to their life tasks are associated with particular patterns of and strategies for goal pursuit, such as the selection of particular goal-relevant situations in which to spend time and the shaping of interactions in goal-fulfilling ways (e.g., Buss, 1987; Cantor et al., 1991; Emmons, Diener, & Larsen, 1986; Gollwitzer, 1993; Mischel, Cantor, & Feldman, 1996; Snyder, 1981). These strategies are the distinct methods by which individuals are attempting to fulfill their personally valued goals within a culturally valued task. Individuals who pursue the task of volunteering with other-focused motivations, for example, are likely to use particular goal-relevant strategies for working on this goal (e.g., serving as a buddy to an HIV-positive person as opposed to stuffing envelopes for fundraising efforts) (Omoto & Snyder, 1990; Snyder, 1993). Moreover, even when individuals cannot be in a goal-affording situation, they may still be able to flexibly pursue their goals and even compensate for the absence of on-line situations that concretely facilitate goal pursuit (Buss, 1987). For example, those with strong compassion goals in volunteering may work to elicit subjective feedback (e.g., the person claims to feel better even if there are no objective indicators of progress) or erroneously interpret feedback in line with their goals. The distinct personal goals that individuals bring to their tasks are therefore associated in particular ways with their strategies of pursuit.

Finally, adopting a particular goal with particular strategies will have different consequences during different life periods because cultures value the pursuit of normative goals and strategies (Helson, Mitchell, & Moane, 1984). In turn, cultures both provide various affordances for the pursuit of culturally valued tasks and goals and discourage the pursuit of nonnormative ones. For example, the typical portrayal of adolescence is as a time of self-exploration and identity formation (Erikson, 1950), and correspondingly, teenagers are encouraged to approach the normative task of social dating with both a focus on self-reliance and the use of specific strategies of goal pursuit (e.g., dating a series of casual partners, attending large, group social events, etc.). On the other hand, the pursuit of romantic relationships with such self-focused goals during adulthood is likely to be seen more negatively (e.g., as a "midlife crisis") and hence be associated with negative outcomes (e.g., social isolation). Thus, the timing and method of goal pursuit influences its outcome.

IMPLICATIONS OF THIS MODEL FOR PERSONALITY COHERENCE

Our life task model of personality posits that individuals can and do show both change and stability in personality across time, as individuals take on different tasks across the life course. For example, individuals may take on the new tasks of a particular life period with different goals, or alternatively, may maintain the same goal focus across life tasks, but may use different strategies in this pursuit. Moreover, individuals who experience negative outcomes from the pursuit of a particular goal or the use of particular strategies are likely to be motivated to change their methods of goal pursuit in order to experience well-being. Thus, each of these components of personality can be associated with both change and stability, albeit in different ways.

In turn, this raises the tricky issue of what is personality coherence. For example, a trait perspective would posit that if an individual's goals remain consistent over time, personality is stable. However, because our approach is so grounded in the situational factors that influence behavior (e.g., subculture, daily life, outcomes), we believe that goals have different meanings when they have different implications for people's lives (i.e., personal well-being, adaptive outcomes). Although we believe that personal goals can provide a source of personality coherence, we do not want to ignore the real differences in personality that occur over time (i.e., in tasks, strategies, outcomes). Our life task perspective therefore posits that, in some ways, personality shows remarkable coherence over time (in large part due to individuals' predominant goals), whereas in other ways, considerable personality change occurs over time (in large part due to life transitions). Each of these units of personality allows for both change and stability, but they differ in the extent to which they generally facilitate personality change versus encourage personality stability (see Figure 11.1). Thus, this model views the issue of personality coherence versus change as largely gray, or perhaps as a black and white checkerboard, as opposed to all black or all white.

The Role of Life Tasks in Driving Change in Goals

Because cultures emphasize the pursuit of different tasks in different life periods, there are opportunities to change goals as one takes on new challenges

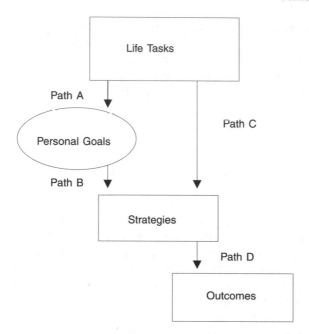

FIGURE 11.1. A life task model of personality change and coherence.

across the life course, as illustrated in Path A of Figure 11.1 (e.g., Helson et al. [1984] "social clock"; see also Erikson, 1950; Havighurst, 1972). In an analysis of data from the longitudinal Terman study of gifted children, Harlow and Cantor (1996) found that individuals who approached one life period with particular goals may take on new life tasks with different goals. For example, a person who has approached career advancement with a focus on self-reliant and instrumental needs has the opportunity to approach productivity during retirement with more interpersonal and expressive goals. Life transitions, such as the transition to college, to parenting, or to retirement, involve substantial changes in the structuring of individuals' daily lives, are salient and important to the individual, and invoke demands on the individual for new behavior and self-conceptions (Stewart, 1982). Times of life transition thereby facilitate changes in goals in several ways.

First, life transitions provide opportunities for self-reflection because individuals' goals are typically most easily articulated during periods of life transition when people face new surroundings and new role demands (Higgins & Eccles-Parsons, 1983). For example, as a student makes the transition to college, he or she may reflect on the goals he or she has pursued during high school and decide to pursue new and different goals (Langston & Cantor, 1989). In fact, a study with college students at three different types of institutions (an Ivy League university, a state teacher's college, and a 2-year community college) revealed that at all three schools students at different years in school were focusing on different types of goals (Stewart, 1982). Specifically, freshmen, who had newly made the transition from high school, scored higher on measures of receptivity (e.g., taking in of new information), whereas seniors scored higher on assertion (e.g., reaching out, expanding) and integration (e.g., relating, committing, connecting). These findings indicate that during times of transition, individuals may be receptive to exploring new goals.

Life transitions can also facilitate the acquisition of new goals by providing a release from previously established routines and habits (Stewart, 1982). Specifically, individuals may be reluctant to change their goal focus and thereby disrupt the structuring of their daily life but should find it considerably easier to implement such changes during natural periods of change. For example, a high school student who typically withdraws from social interactions may have difficulty in changing how he or she approaches the task of building friendships while he or she is still in the high school environment, but may be able to take on this task with more extraverted goals during college. Higgins and Eccles-Parsons (1983) describe how children enter distinct life phases over time, with corresponding changes in the socialization agents (e.g., peers, teachers, youth leaders, etc.), activities and tasks (e.g., intellectual tasks, recreational tasks, socialization tasks, etc.), and social motives and concerns (e.g., appearing competent, making friends, etc.). In turn, these changes in children's social lives may lead to changes in social cognition as well as goals. For example, younger children typically focus on goals related to being liked by teachers and other adults, whereas adolescents are primarily concerned with getting along with peers. During times of transition, individuals experience a loosening of the constraints on a particular type of focus, and hence are more easily able to make change in their overarching goal pursuit.

Periods of transition include not only normative age-graded changes (e.g., going to college, retirement) but also significant life events that lead to opportunities for change (e.g., a divorce, a disabling injury) (Langston & Cantor, 1989; Levinson, 1978; Stewart, 1989). Experiencing a major life event also provides opportunities for self-reflection as well as a freeing of the daily habits and routines, and hence can lead to greater openness to taking on new goals. For example, an individual may pursue intimacy goals in a marital relationship, but following a divorce or death of a spouse, he or she may alternatively focus on more identity goals related to self-exploration and self-reliance. The role of such negative experience with mutuality in a serious relationship in shifting one's goals toward independence and self-reliance is illustrated by this quote from a woman in the Mills College longitudinal study: "I have followed a totally different path than I could have had I stayed married. I'm sure I would not have developed my career or sense of an independent self" (p. 1087, Helson et al., 1984). Similarly, Taylor's research on adaptation to breast cancer demonstrates that many people see the opportunity to reevaluate their priorities and change their goals as one of the positive experiences resulting from a traumatic life event (Taylor, 1983; Taylor & Brown, 1988). As one woman with cancer described, "You take a long look at your life and realize that many things that you thought were important before are totally insignificant. That's probably been the major change in my life," (Taylor, 1983, p. 1163). Thus, research suggests that changes in life circumstances can also prompt individuals to take on new goals.

Moreover, cultures even actively assist people in taking on new tasks with normative and valued goals by providing particular normative prescriptions of "how to act" in these unfamiliar settings as well as providing distinct affordances for goal pursuit (Cantor, Zirkel, & Norem, 1993). For example, couples who are anticipating parenthood often actively seek out information (e.g., from books, doctors, family members) and certainly receive considerable (even unwanted) advice from others on how to prepare for this significant life event (Deutsch, Ruble, Fleming, Brooks-Gunn, & Stangor, 1988). Relatedly, in a longitudinal study of women who had attended a private women's college in the northeastern United States, Stewart (1989) found that those who focused on independence during their 20s as they were building a career were likely to focus on interpersonal relationships during their 30s, perhaps in at attempt to achieve an overall life balance. In turn, it is likely that during this latter time period women find considerable sociocultural support for the pursuit of interpersonal goals. The normative prescriptions of getting married and raising a family are very strong, particularly for women, and those who have not yet focused on this goal may experience normative pressure (e.g., reminders of one's biological clock) to do so. During age-graded life transitions, such as attending college, becoming a parent, and retiring, cultures often provide substantial information about and assistance in taking on these new tasks in "the right way," namely with culturally valued goals.

Cultures also directly assist people in taking on new tasks with normative goals by providing distinct affordances for goal pursuit (Cantor et al., 1993). For example, late adolescence is seen as a time for focusing on independence and identity (Erikson, 1950), and in turn, the college setting provides many daily life situations that afford personal growth (e.g., selecting classes, choosing a major, participating in various political and religious organizations). Moreover, specific subcultures provide distinct opportunities for the pursuit of normative tasks, and thereby individuals in different subcultures may bring a different meaning to such pursuit. For example, Zirkel (1992) examined the pursuit of independence in two groups of college students, namely those who lived in an academic "honors" college and those who lived in a sorority. Although both groups contained students who found the task of developing independence particularly anxiety-provoking, the distinct meaning brought to this task differed as a function of subculture: Those in the honors college brought this anxiety to bear on their academic performance, whereas for those in the sorority sample, this anxiety impacted primarily on social relationships. In this way, the particular affordances of individuals' daily lives influenced their distinct methods of goal pursuit.

The Role of Personal Goals in Driving Personality Stability

Although life transitions provide opportunities for individuals to change their predominant goal focus by setting forth broad tasks for individuals to pursue, there is probably considerable stability in the particular goals that people bring to their valued age-graded tasks. For example, a longitudinal study examined how boys who had been shy in childhood adjusted to major life events across their lives, such as marriage, parenting, and career establishment (Caspi, Elder, & Bem, 1988). These findings indicated that those who had been shy as children entered these new life periods in adulthood approximately 3 to 4 years later than those who had been more outgoing during childhood suggesting that those who are hesitant about entering new social situations early in life maintain their reluctance to take on new social roles as adults. Similarly, studying individuals' adaptation to transition at one life period seems to be a reliable way of predicting their adjustment at other life periods, providing evidence for personality coherence over time: Personality assessments from children ages 11 to 13—namely, during the transition to junior high school—are more predictive of functioning in adulthood than similar measures assessed earlier or later (Livson & Peskin, 1967). Thus, people may feel external pressure to take on new life tasks with particular socially valued goals, but their distinct dispositions, needs, and experiences are likely to lead them to pursue the same goals across time and across tasks.

Considerable research provides evidence that individuals may approach different tasks during the same life period with the same predominant goals in mind. The literature in attachment styles, for example, has shown that individuals with secure working models of attachment approach a variety of interpersonal situations with openness and comfort, which in turn is associated with having more satisfying romantic relationships, friendships, and even work experiences (Hazan & Shaver, 1987; Shaver & Hazan, 1993). For example, in a longitudinal study of adaptation to college, Hazan asked 80 incoming freshmen to complete attachment style questionnaires before arriving on campus and then assessed their adjustment once they arrived at college (Shaver & Hazan, 1993). Not surprisingly, insecurely attached students reported greater loneliness during the summer than securely attached students. Moreover, while both secure and insecure students were somewhat lonely during the initial semester of college, by the end of the first year, secure students had successfully found friends and adjusted to college life, whereas insecurely attached students were even lonelier than they had been prior to college. Similarly, Zirkel and Cantor (1990) found that students who were particularly anxious about the task of independence saw more daily-life situations as relevant to the task and saw larger concerns as relevant to the task than those without such a focus. For example, while both independence-absorbed and -unabsorbed students listed mundane activities such as doing laundry and balancing the checkbook as relevant to independence, only those with an intense focus on independence listed more substantial concerns such as missing high school friends and being away from their parents. Thus, individuals may show considerable continuity in goal focus across diverse tasks during a particular age-graded life period.

Individuals may not only pursue different tasks simultaneously with the same goal, but also may show a continuity in goal focus across different tasks over time. In their analysis of data from the Terman study, Harlow and Cantor (1996) found a functional continuity in people's goals across time, namely that individuals with a strong focus on interpersonal relationships during one life period were quite likely to maintain this focus across life transitions. Specifically, retired persons who reported considerable enjoyment of their interaction with colleagues during middle adulthood were more likely to report engaging in various social activities (e.g., visiting with friends and neighbors, communicating with relatives, entertaining) in later adulthood. Although the broad task they were working on changed with age-graded life transitions (e.g., career achievement to coping with retirement), the specific meaning that individuals brought to the tasks did not. Similarly, an individual with a strong focus on independence may bring this focus to bear on a variety of tasks throughout life in which independence is a relevant goal (e.g., college graduation, death of a spouse, becoming a parent) (Zirkel & Cantor, 1990; Zirkel, 1992). For example, an individual with a strong focus on independence may find a network of sorority friends during college in order to separate from her parents, but she may focus on her career as a means of maintaining independence during adulthood. In fact, students in Zirkel's (1992) study whose anxiety about independence during the transition to college focused on academic pressures turned into a focus on social pressures during the transition to after college. This research, then, shows coherence in individuals' desire for and commitment to involvement in particular types of goals even across life periods.

Moreover, those with strong goals in a given domain are likely to enter particular daily life contexts that afford, and even strengthen, the pursuit of these goals (Buss, 1987; Emmons et al., 1986). Individuals have considerable choice in terms of the situations, people, and activities in which they spend time and hence are likely to seek out situations that are compatible with their own needs and goals (Snyder & Ickes, 1985). For example, in a series of studies with college students, Sanderson and Cantor (1995) demonstrated that students vary in the extent to which they are intently focused on creating communion with a dating partner (e.g., engaging in self-disclosure and mutual dependence). Accordingly, those with strong intimacy goals are more likely to be in steady dating relationships than those without such goals, presumably because the broad context of a close relationship facilitates engaging in self-disclosure and interdependence. Moreover, even among those who are in steady dating relationships, those with strong intimacy goals structure their daily lives in particular ways that are likely to strength their interpersonal focus, including spending considerable time alone with their dating partner and giving and receiving social support to their partner (Cantor & Sanderson, 1998). This research therefore indicates that those with particular goals are likely to structure and shape their daily lives in ways that reinforce these goals (Emmons et al., 1986; Snyder & Ickes, 1985).

Individuals with strong personal goals in a given domain may also be particularly adept at finding ways of reinforcing those goals, even when they are not able to be in specific goal-relevant daily life situations. In fact, Sanderson and Cantor (1997) examined the role of both personal factors (i.e., intimacy goal pursuit) and situational factors (i.e., spending time alone with one's dating partner, receiving social support from one's dating partner, having an intimacy-focused partner) in predicting dating satisfaction and relationship longevity in 57 college-student dating couples. Findings indicated that although both a personal focus on intimacy and the presence of situational factors that facilitated intimacy were associated with greater relationship satisfaction, individuals with a strong focus on intimacy experienced satisfaction regardless of the presence of intimacy-conductive affordances in daily life. On the other hand, those without intimacy goals in dating were particularly dependent on the presence of concrete intimacy-relevant affordances (e.g., spending considerable time alone with a dating partner, having an intimacy-focused partner) to experience satisfaction. Moreover, a discriminant analysis revealed that the only significant predictors of relationship maintenance at the 5-month follow-up were individuals' own intimacy goals and their partner's intimacy goals. Thus, individuals who are intently focused on fulfilling particular goals may be able to flexibly fulfill these goals regardless of the presence of concrete affordances for goal pursuit in their daily lives.

Even when individuals view life transitions as welcome opportunities to experience substantial personality change (e.g., many high school students see the transition to college as a chance to have a "fresh start"), such change may be hard both to initiate and maintain. In fact, as individuals enter new life periods and face new challenges, they may be particularly likely to cling to familiar patterns and habits in an effort to regain control and predictability over the novel situation (Caspi, 1987; Caspi & Moffitt, 1993). For example, a college freshman may want very much to approach the relatively novel task of social dating with a focus on interpersonal communion and self-disclosure. He or she may, however, feel awkward about engaging in such intimate and unfamiliar behavior, and thereby soon slip back into prior patterns of social interaction (i.e., with a focus on self-reliance and self-protection). In fact, high school students often decide to take on new identities and goals as they start college with a "clean slate," but experience "sophomore-year blues" when they find themselves reverting back to their prior selves (Langston & Cantor, 1989). Ironically, individuals' need for establishing predictability and control may be particularly strong precisely in those situations that are most uncertain and therefore provide the greatest opportunities for change (Caspi & Moffitt, 1993). For example, the transition from college is relatively unstructured, in that people pursue a number of different paths ranging from school to full-time work, and hence this transition may be especially likely to encourage a reliance on familiar goals and strategies.

Such novel and stressful situations, which lead people to engage in their most well-learned (and hence largely automatic) behaviors, may also elicit familiar responses from others and thereby further reinforce their prior goals (Caspi & Moffitt, 1993). The newly intimacy-focused college student described previously, for example, may feel more comfortable receiving familiar (and reciprocated) self-protective reactions from potential dating partners than unfamiliar self-disclosing reactions. Individuals' behavior may therefore evoke familiar reactions from others and hence initiate a goal-reinforcing feedback process. Relatedly, in an analysis of data from the longitudinal Berkeley Guidance Study, men with a history of temper tantrums in childhood are more likely to have difficulty in their marriages as adults: Almost half of those with childhood tantrums had divorced by age 40 compared to only 22% of those without such a history (Caspi, 1987). Therefore although life transitions provide opportunities to take on different goals, and some individuals may be able to take on new age-graded tasks in different ways and thereby experience personality change, there is probably considerable stability in how people typically approach their valued tasks.

The Role of Life Transitions in Driving Change in Strategies

As described previously, as individuals enter new life periods, they are likely to experience pressure to take on their new socially valued tasks with new goals, and therefore the strategies they use to pursue these goals will obviously need to change, as shown in Path B of Figure 11.1. Specifically, the strategies that work very effectively for a particular type of goal pursuit during one life period are likely to be entirely ineffective when individuals approach new tasks with different goals following periods of life transition. For example, those who have pursued friendships with work colleagues with instrumental goals (e.g., making business contacts, acquiring useful information) may have relied on particular strategies of goal pursuit (e.g., having monthly lunches, exchanging e-mail) that will be ineffective when they are pursuing the task of "being a good parent" with a focus on expressive goals. Similarly, a college student who approaches the task of making friends with considerable anxiety may use relatively ineffective strategies for social interaction, such as social humility and social constraint (Langston & Cantor, 1989). However, if following graduation, they take on the task of social dating with a focus on communion, they may rely on more effective strategies for managing such relationships, such as expressing intimate thoughts and feelings and engaging in mutual dependence. In sum, as individuals take on new tasks with new goals, they then need to find appropriate strategies to use to work on goal fulfillment.

On the other hand, even when individuals maintain the same goal focus across time, they will need to change the strategies they use to work on these goals because different life periods set forth different challenges and constraints (see Path C in Figure 11.1). For example, the strategies for working on intimacy in dating as a high school student (e.g., "going steady," attending the prom) are obviously quite different from those used as a divorced or widowed adult (e.g., integrating one's own children with a new dating partner). Similarly, older adults may need to change their strategies of goal pursuit related to health to take into account their increasing physical limitations (e.g., although the strategy may change from running to walking, both involve the goal of exercise). Thus, the distinct strategies that individuals use for goal pursuit will change across life transitions, even if the particular goals of such pursuit do not.

Moreover, specific daily life contexts also differ in the extent to which they encourage the use of particular types of strategies, and thus individuals may need to rely on the use of different strategies in different situations. For example, Sanderson and Cantor (1995) found that college students with strong intimacy goals who were in steady dating relationships had the lowest levels of risky sexual behavior, whereas those with strong intimacy goals who were in casual dating relationships had the highest levels of risky behavior. This patterning makes sense because these different dating contexts differ in the extent to which they encourage the use of particular strategies for regulating behavior. Specifically, the serious relationship is a dating context that encourages the use of intimacy-relevant strategies for regulating safer sex (e.g., engaging in open self-disclosure, interdependence, etc.), and hence those with strong intimacy goals are able to rely on the use of such goal-relevant strategies for behavior regulation. On the other hand, those with strong intimacy goals who are in a casual dating context may avoid discussion of sensitive topics such as condom use (that might thereby potentially disrupt the interaction) because this context does not afford the use of interpersonally focused strategies. (Unfortunately, although the desired outcome of increasing intimacy is likely to be achieved in both of these cases, albeit through the use of different strategies, the use of condoms is much more likely to occur via the first strategy than via the latter.) Therefore, even when individuals maintain the same goal pursuit across the life course, the distinct strategies they use to pursue these goals may change over time as a function of the opportunities and constraints of their life period and daily life situation.

The Role of Outcomes in Driving Change in Goals and Strategies

Although life transitions in general break the structuring and selecting of daily interactions and thereby allow for change in type of goal and / or strategies of pursuit, the timing of such life events influences the outcome of goal pursuit, which has implications for personality coherence (see Path D of Figure 11.1). As described by Helson and colleagues (Helson et al., 1984), individuals are differentially affected by major life events depending on when they experience such events (e.g., doing the "right" thing at the "right" time and in the "right" context is important for well-being). Specifically, life events that occur at normative or "socially sanctioned" times tend to be less stressful than those that occur at nonnormative times, in part because events that occur at predicted ages allow for anticipation and preparation on the part of the individual as well as that person's social environment (Caspi & Moffitt, 1993; Neugarten, 1968, 1979). For example, research on the behavioral responses of adolescent girls who experienced the onset of menarche at a typical or "on time" versus atypical or "off-time" period revealed various behavioral problems, including lower academic success and conduct problems in school (Caspi & Moffitt, 1991; Simmons & Blyth, 1987; Stattin & Magnusson, 1990). Goal pursuit is therefore associated with more positive outcomes when it is pursued at normative times as opposed to less culturally sanctioned times (Helson et al., 1984; Neugarten, 1968, 1979).

In addition to taking on certain tasks at certain times, individuals also need to take on these tasks with appropriate (i.e., realistic) goals and strategies to experience positive outcomes. The pursuit of socioculturally prescribed tasks is particularly important for life satisfaction because these tasks are typically those that individuals have considerable opportunities to pursue in daily life (e.g., cultures provide opportunities for individuals to pursue such tasks). For example, retired individuals who continue to focus on goals related to career achievement may experience considerable feelings of loss, given that their daily life context does not facilitate the fulfillment of such goals. In fact, in the Terman longitudinal study, the link between social life participation and life satisfaction was particularly strong for those who were retired and hence can no longer derive the social rewards of interacting with work colleagues (Harlow & Cantor, 1996). In contrast, retired individuals who do not find ways to engage in social interaction may experience considerable feelings of loss, which should in turn motivate a change in how they approach the retirement task. Relatedly, this study also revealed that individuals may find new ways of experiencing positive outcomes across the life course by pursuing different goals during different life periods. Specifically, men who had previously pursued self-focused goals in their friendships were able to approach this task with interpersonally focused goals during retirement, perhaps due to the relaxation of sex-role expectations during older adulthood, which in turn led to greater enjoyment of this task. In sum, individuals who do not take on the culturally valued tasks, or who pursue these tasks with nonnormative goals, are likely to experience negative outcomes, which may motivate changes in tasks, goals, and/or strategies.

Furthermore, those who do not engage in the valued tasks of their culture are likely to experience considerable negative outcomes, such as feelings of personal and social inadequacy. For example, a longitudinal study of women who were seniors at Mills College in the late 1950s, and who again completed questionnaires in the early 1980s, when they were between 42 and 45 years of age, revealed two different types of normative patterning, namely an initial focus on marriage and children ("the feminine social clock") versus a focus on career achievement ("the masculine social clock"), as well as a subset of the women who were not pursuing either family or career goals by age 28 (Helson et al., 1984). Those women who were not pursuing either normative task tended to have lower self-images, feel incompetent, and yearn for social support and approval from others. Furthermore, their findings indicate that at least a subset of these women had not pursued normative tasks and goals for some time; as one "nonclock" subject wrote, "I never went through what seems now to be the 'normal' teenage period of dating boys, kissing, and partying with the gang. So by the time I got to college I felt backward, inhibited, and quite petrified of boys, and covered up with either sarcastic remarks or noncommittal silence" (Helson et al., 1984, p. 1090). These women also showed decreases over time in tolerance and communality, suggesting alienation (Helson & Moane, 1987). In turn, individuals who are experiencing such negative outcomes are likely to be motivated to change their goals or strategies of pursuit.

Summary

This chapter has described the life task perspective on personality coherence and specifically how such coherence can include both stability and change, albeit in distinct components of personality. In summary, the life task perspective is a contextualized view of personality in that it examines not only individuals' age-graded tasks, but also the meaning they bring to these tasks, their distinct strategies of task pursuit, and the outcome of this pursuit. Given these different levels of personality, stability and change are not seen as opposites, but rather as integrally connected (i.e., individuals may at times change their precise strategy of goal pursuit to remain stable in their overarching goal pursuit or in their desired outcomes; individuals who experience negative outcomes may change their goals or strategies of pursuit to receive positive outcomes). This perspective also sees personality change as small and incremental as opposed to broad and sweeping: Given the push and pull of the units driving change versus those driving stability, personality change will be gradual and small. This approach, then, allows for change and stability on several dimensions, including what the person is supposed to be doing (i.e., the broad sociocultural task), what he or she wants to do (i.e., personal goals), how he or she is trying to do it (i.e., the strategies of goal pursuit), and why he or she is trying to do it (i.e., the outcome of goal pursuit).

LINGERING ISSUES AND IMPLICATIONS

Do Different Subcultures Facilitate versus Discourage Personality Change?

Although this chapter has emphasized the role of broad cultures in encouraging the pursuit of age-graded tasks with socially valued goals, specific subcultures may in fact vary in the extent to which they facilitate the pursuit of these goals. As described previously, many college students approach the age-graded task of identity formation with a focus on self-exploration and personal growth (Stewart, 1982). However, research by Cantor and Prentice (Cantor & Prentice, 1996; Prentice, 1997) on the patterning and experience of activities for over 1,500 college sophomores at three distinct institutions revealed striking differences in the extent to which different campus subcultures emphasize an openness to change versus conserving prior goals. Specifically, this data revealed that certain tight-knit social groups (e.g., fraternities and sororities, varsity athletic teams) may attract individuals with similar goals and strategies of goal pursuit (i.e., norms of behavior). In turn, to the extent that individuals in these groups then spend considerable amounts of time together (e.g., if they are living together or spending considerable time practicing and on road-trips together), these groups may reinforce individuals' prior goals and preclude an openness to change and self-exploration. For example, the patterning and strategies of daily life used by those in the athlete subculture are quite disparate from their nonathletic peers: They spend less time at cultural events, are less likely to pursue new activities and interests, and are less likely to meet people from new and different backgrounds compared to other college students. Although the time pressure that athletes typically experience obviously accounts for part of this lack of exposure, other students with heavy time commitments to nonathletic activities (e.g., extracurricular groups such as singing groups, orchestra, and drama productions) spend considerable amounts of time in these broadening activities. Thus, even during a life period in which the broad cultural task emphasizes personal growth and an openness to change, individuals are likely to gravitate toward particular groups that support and validate their own values and goals.

Are There Individual Differences in Rates and/or Patterning of Change?

Although we have posited that the effects of changing life tasks across the life span exert similar effects on all individuals, individuals may themselves vary in the extent to which their goals are influenced by various situational factors and life events (Campbell, Chew, & Scratchley, 1991; Kernis, 1993; Kernis, Cornell, Sun, Berry, & Harlow, 1993). For example, a daily diary study by Campbell and colleagues (1991) examined the appraisals of positive and negative life events and mood ratings of 67 college students and found that students who were low in self-esteem overall rated daily events as having more impact on mood and as more personally important. In turn, those who are lower in self-esteem may be more influenced by life events and thereby more likely to show changes in goals and/or strategies in response to life transitions or changes in life circumstances. Similarly, research suggests those who are high in self-monitoring, namely those who act in different ways in different situations, may be more influenced in terms of their goal pursuit by situational factors than low self-monitors (Snyder & Gangestad, 1986). Thus, because individuals differ in their responsiveness to situational forces, life events such as periods of transitions may have different effects on personality coherence for different people.

Can Life Transitions Include Changes in Developmental Needs as Well as Changes in Life Tasks?

Although we have focused on the role of changes in broad tasks during life transitions in leading to changes in personal goals, changes in one's developmental needs may also lead to changes in an individual's personal goals (Erikson, 1950; Stewart, 1989; Stewart & Healy, 1985, 1989). In other words, as individuals mature and grow over time, they may feel ready to take on normative tasks with new goals. For example, Erikson's (1950) psychosocial model of development posits that adolescence is a time of focus on issues of independence and identity. However, once individuals have successfully resolved these issues, they may be ready to approach socially valued tasks with new goals, namely communion and interdependence. In fact, Sanderson and Cantor (1995) have shown that adolescents who are low on interpersonal achievement and ideological ego achievement are more likely to approach the age-graded task of social dating with a focus on identity and independence needs than those who more successfully "resolved" their current identity issues (e.g., have formed a more unified identity). Thus, individuals' own maturation and development may also lead to changes in goal focus over time.

Why Does a Particular Person Pursue Particular Goals?

Because our life task perspective sees individuals' goals as the primary force behind personality coherence over time, an obvious question is how do such goals develop? For example, five-factor models of personality suggest that individuals' traits or dispositions lead to the pursuit of particular goals. However, our perspective places considerable weight on the power of individuals to set agendas and make progress working toward them. Thus, abstract trait approaches that imply a level of static and passivity are not particularly relevant to our perspective. Instead, we posit that personal goals emerge from a complex interaction of traits, situations, and cultural contexts. Finally, although we have emphasized the role of goals in leading to personality coherence over time, goals may also change (e.g., in response to feedback and pressure from the sociocultural environment, in response to negative outcomes from goal pursuit, etc.).

Can Goals Also Lead to Cross-Situational Coherence?

Although this chapter has examined how individuals' goals may lead to coherence across time, such a perspective would readily apply to coherence across situations during a given life period. Specifically, individuals with strong personal goals in a given domain would likely bring this focus to their work on diverse life tasks, albeit with different strategies and potentially different outcomes. For example, Zirkel's research has demonstrated that those with a particular concern about the task of independence bring this issue to bear on a variety of daily life situations (Zirkel & Cantor, 1990; Zirkel, 1992). However, the pursuit of independence in the social dating task may involve the strategy of dating several casual partners to avoid dependence on a single person and hence could be associated with positive outcomes such as personal growth for someone who is truly interested in self-reliance. On the other hand, the pursuit of independence in the "getting good grades" task may involve the strategy of avoiding asking others for assistance (e.g., professors and peers), which could obviously be associated with negative outcomes such as poorer grades. In this way, individuals' goals could lead to personality coherence across different daily life situations, although their tasks, strategies, and outcomes could still differ.

CONCLUSIONS

Although we believe that individuals probably remain fairly stable in some components of personality, namely their overarching goal pursuit across time, we also believe that substantial change can and does occur in other aspects of personality, namely how people are actively living their lives (e.g., the tasks they are working on, the strategies they are using to work on these tasks, and the outcome of this task pursuit). Thus, we believe that personality does change, even if it is not "deep" change (Cantor et al., 1993). Therefore even if people are remaining relatively focused on a particular goal pursuit (e.g., the pursuit of intimacy, the pursuit of independence, etc.), their distinct patterns and consequences of task pursuit have substantial implications for how they live their lives (e.g., experiencing satisfaction, engaging in functional behavior). For example, Caspi has shown that while shyness is considered a liability for boys during childhood, shy boys are likely to be caring fathers as adults (e.g., Caspi & Bem, 1990; Caspi et al., 1989). In turn, being a nurturing parent is seen positively, and hence men who were shy as boys are able to approach one of the valued tasks of adulthood (e.g., raising children) in a way that is seen positively. Similarly, Harlow and Cantor (1996) found that people who had not previously found satisfaction in their task pursuits during adulthood were able to do so during retirement to the extent that they were currently participating in activities relevant to their tasks. In other words, even individuals who were not particularly congenial or social during earlier life periods were able to experience satisfaction during retirement, as long as they were now engaging in social participation. Because different subcultures value the pursuit of different goals, adopting a particular goal with particular strategies will therefore have different consequences during different life periods, and hence individuals can find new ways of experiencing positive outcomes throughout the life course.

REFERENCES

Buss, D. (1987). Selection, evocation, and manipulation. *Journal of Personality and Social Psychology, 53,* 1214–1221.

Campbell, J. D., Chew, B., & Scratchley, L. S. (1991). Cognitive and emotional reactions to daily events: The effects of self-esteem and self-complexity. *Journal of Personality, 59,* 473–506.

Cantor, N. (1990). From thought to behavior: "Having" and "doing" in the study of personality and cognition. *American Psychologist, 45,* 735–750.

Cantor, N. (1994). Life task problem-solving: Situational affordances and personal needs. *Personality and Social Psychology Bulletin, 20,* 235–243.

Cantor, N., & Fleeson, W. (1994). Social intelligence and intelligent goal pursuit: A cognitive slice of motivation. In W. D. Spaulding (Ed.), *Nebraska Symposium on Motivation: Vol. 41. Integrative views of motivation, cognition, and emotion* (pp. 125–179). Lincoln: University of Nebraska Press.

Cantor, N., & Kihlstrom, J. F. (1987). *Personality and social intelligence.* Englewood-Cliffs, NJ: Prentice-Hall.

Cantor, N., Norem, J., Langston, C., Zirkel, S., Fleeson, W., & Cook-Flannagan, C. (1991). Life tasks and daily life experiences. *Journal of Personality, 59,* 425–451.

Cantor, N. E., & Prentice, D. A. (1996, March). *The life of the modern-day student-athlete: Opportunities won and lost.* Paper presented at the Princeton Conference on Higher Education, Princeton, NJ.

Cantor, N., & Sanderson, C. A. (1998). Social dating goals and the regulation of adolescent dating relationships and sexual behavior: The interaction of goals, strategies, and situations. J. Heckhausen & C. Dweck (Eds.), *Motivation and self-*

regulation across the life span (pp. 185–215). New York: Cambridge University Press.

Cantor, N., Zirkel, S., & Norem, J. K. (1993). Human personality: Asocial and reflexive? *Psychological Inquiry, 4,* 273–277.

Carstensen, L. L. (1993). Motivation for social contact across the life span: A theory of socioemotional selectivity. In J. E. Jacobs (Ed.), *Nebraska Symposium on Motivation: Vol. 40. Developmental Perspectives on Motivation* (pp. 209–254). Lincoln: University of Nebraska Press.

Caspi, A. (1987). Personality in the life course. *Journal of Personality and Social Psychology, 53,* 1203–1213.

Caspi, A., & Bem, D. J. (1990). Personality continuity and change across the life course. In L. A. Pervin (Ed.), *Handbook of personality: Theory and research* (pp. 549–575). New York: Guilford Press.

Caspi, A., Bem, D. J., & Elder, G. H., Jr. (1989). Continuities and consequences of interactional styles across the life course. *Journal of Personality, 57,* 375–406.

Caspi, A., Elder, G. H., Jr., & Bem, D. J. (1988). Moving away from the world: Life-course patterns of shy children. *Developmental Psychology, 24,* 824–831.

Caspi, A., & Moffitt, T. E. (1991). Individual differences are accentuated during periods of social change: The sample case of girls at puberty. *Journal of Personality and Social Psychology, 61,* 157–168.

Caspi, A., & Moffitt, T. E. (1993). When do individual differences matter? A paradoxical theory of personality coherence. *Psychological Inquiry, 4,* 247–271.

Costa, P. T., & McCrae, R. R. (1980). Still stable after all these years: Personality as a key to some issues in adulthood and old age. In P. B. Baltes & O. G. Brim, Jr. (Eds.), *Life span development and behavior* (Vol. 3, pp. 65–102). New York: Academic Press.

Deutsch, F. M., Ruble, D. N., Fleming, A., Brooks-Gunn, J., & Stangor, C. (1988). Information-seeking and maternal self-definition during the transition to motherhood. *Journal of Personality and Social Psychology, 55,* 420–431.

Elder, G. H., Jr. (1975). Age differentiation and the life course. In G. H. Elder, Jr. (Ed.), *Life course dynamics: Trajectories and transitions, 1968–1980* (pp. 23–49). Ithaca, NY: Cornell University Press.

Emmons, R. A. (1989). The personal striving approach to personality. In L. A. Pervin (Ed.), *Goal concepts in personality psychology* (pp. 87–126). Hillsdale, NJ: Erlbaum.

Emmons, R. A., Diener, E., & Larsen, R. J. (1986). Choice and avoidance of everyday situations and affect congruence: Two models of reciprocal interactionism. *Journal of Personality and Social Psychology, 51,* 815–826.

Erikson, E. H. (1950). *Childhood and society.* New York: Norton.

Gollwitzer, P. (1993). Goal achievement: The role of intentions. In W. Stroebe & M. Hewstone (Eds.), *European review of social psychology* (Vol. 4, pp. 141–185). London: Wiley.

Harlow, R. E., & Cantor, N. (1996). Still participating after all these years: A study of life task participation in later life. *Journal of Personality and Social Psychology, 71,* 1235–1249.

Havighurst, R. J. (1953). *Human development and education.* New York: Longmans, Green.

Havighurst, R. J. (1972). *Developmental tasks and education* (3rd ed.). New York: David McKay.

Hazan, C., & Shaver, P. R. (1987). Romantic love conceptualized as an attachment process. *Journal of Personality and Social Psychology, 52,* 511–524.

Helson, R., Mitchell, V., & Moane, G. (1984). Personality and patterns of adherence and nonadherence to the social clock. *Journal of Personality and Social Psychology, 46,* 1079–1096.

Helson, R., & Moane, G. (1987). Personality change in women from college to midlife. *Journal of Personality and Social Psychology, 53,* 176–186.

Higgins, E. T., & Eccles-Parsons, J. E. (1983). Social cognition and the social life of the child: Stages as subcultures. In E. T. Higgins, D. N. Ruble, & W. W. Hartup (Eds.), *Social cognition and social development: A sociocultural perspective* (pp. 15–62). New York: Cambridge University Press.

Kernis, M. (1993). The role of stability and level of self-esteem in psychological functioning. In R. Baumeister (Ed.), *Self-esteem: The puzzle of low self-regard* (pp. 167–182). New York: Plenum Press.

Kernis, M. H., Cornell, D. P., Sun, C., Berry, A., & Harlow, T. (1993). There's more to self-esteem than whether it is high or low: The importance of stability of self-esteem. *Journal of Personality and Social Psychology, 65,* 1190–1204.

Langston, C. A., & Cantor, N. (1989). Social anxiety and social constraint: When making friends is hard. *Journal of Personality and Social Psychology, 56,* 649–661.

Levinson, D. J. (1978). *The seasons of a man's life.* New York: Ballantine.

Little, B. (1989). Personal projects analysis: Trivial pursuits, magnificent obsessions, and the search for coherence. In D. M. Buss & N. Cantor (Eds.), *Personality psychology: Recent trends and emerging directions* (pp. 15–31). New York: Springer-Verlag.

Livson, N., & Peskin, H. (1967). Prediction of adult psychological health in a longitudinal study. *Journal of Abnormal Psychology, 72,* 509–518.

McCrae, R. R., & John, O. P. (1992). An introduction to the five-factor model and its applications. *Journal of Personality, 60,* 175–215.

Mischel, W., Cantor, N., & Feldman, S. (1996). Principles of self-regulation: The nature of willpower and self-control. In E. T. Higgins & A. W. Kruglanski (Eds.), *Social psychology: Handbook of basic principles* (pp. 329–360). New York: Guilford Press.

Neugarten, B. L. (1968). The awareness of middle age. In B. L. Neugarten (Ed.), *Middle age and aging: A reader in social psychology* (pp. 93–98). Chicago: University of Chicago Press.

Neugarten, B. L. (1979). Time, age, and the life cycle. *American Journal of Psychiatry, 136,* 887–894.

Omoto, A. M., & Snyder, M. (1990). Basic research in action: Volunteerism and society's response to AIDS. *Personality and Social Psychology Bulletin, 16,* 152–165.

Prentice, D. A. (1997, April). *The student–athlete.* Paper presented at Princeton University's 250th Anniversary Symposium, Princton, NJ.

Sanderson, C. A., & Cantor, N. (1995). Social dating goals in late adolescence: Implications for safer sexual activity. *Journal of Personality and Social Psychology, 68,* 1121–1134.

Sanderson, C. A., & Cantor, N. (1997). Creating satisfaction in steady dating relationships: The role of personal goals and situational affordances. *Journal of Personality and Social Psychology, 73,* 1424–1433.

Shaver, P. R., & Hazan, C. (1993). Adult romantic attachment: Theory and evidence. In

D. Perlman & W. H. Jones (Eds.), *Advances in personal relationships* (Vol. 4, pp. 29–70). Philadelphia: Jessica Kingsley.

Simmons, R. G., & Blyth, D. A. (1987). *Moving into adolescence: The impact of pubertal change and school context.* New York: de Gruyter.

Snyder, M. (1981). On the influence of individuals on situations. In N. Cantor & J. Kihlstrom (Eds.), *Personality, cognition, and social interaction* (pp. 309–329). Hillsdale, NJ: Erlbaum.

Snyder, M. (1993). Basic research and practical problems: The promise of a "functional" personality and social psychology. *Personality and Social Psychology Bulletin, 19,* 251–264.

Snyder, M., & Gangestad, S. (1986). On the nature of self-monitoring: Matters of assessment, matters of validity. *Journal of Personality and Social Psychology, 51,* 125–139.

Snyder, M., & Ickes, W. (1985). Personality and social behavior. In G. Lindsey & E. Aronson (Eds.), *Handbook of social psychology* (pp. 883–947). New York: Random House.

Stattin, H., & Magnusson, D. (1990). *Pubertal maturation in female development.* Hillsdale, NJ: Erlbaum.

Stewart, A. J. (1982). The course of individual adaptation to life changes. *Journal of Personality and Social Psychology, 42,* 1100–1113.

Stewart, A. J. (1989). Social intelligence and adaptation to life changes. In R. S. Wyer & T. K. Srull (Eds.), *Advances in social cognition* (Vol. 2, pp. 187–196). Hillsdale, NJ: Erlbaum.

Stewart, A. J., & Healy, J. M., Jr. (1985). Personality and adaptation to change. In R. Hogan & W. Jones (Eds.), *Perspectives on personality: Theory, measurement, and interpersonal dynamics* (pp. 117–144). Greenwich, CT: JAI Press.

Stewart, A. J., & Healy, J. M., Jr. (1989). Linking individual development and social change. *American Psychologist, 44,* 30–42.

Taylor, S. E. (1983). Adjustment to threatening events: A theory of cognitive adaptation. *American Psychologist, 38,* 1161–1173.

Taylor, S. E., & Brown, J. D. (1988). Illusion and well-being: A social psychological perspective on mental health. *Psychological Bulletin, 103,* 193–210.

Veroff, J. (1983). Contextual determinants of personality. *Personality and Social Psychology Bulletin, 9,* 331–344.

Watson, D., & Clark, L. A. (1992). On traits and temperament: General and specific factors of emotional experience and their relation to the five-factor model. *Journal of Personality, 60,* 441–476.

Zirkel, S. (1992). Developing independence in a life transition: Investing the self in the concerns of the day. *Journal of Personality and Social Psychology, 62,* 506–521.

Zirkel, S., & Cantor, N. (1990). Personal construal of life tasks: Those who struggle for independence. *Journal of Personality and Social Psychology, 58,* 172–185.

Indexes

Author Index

Subject Index